BRITISH MUSLIMS, ETHNICITY AND
HEALTH INEQUALITIES

BRITISH MUSLIMS, ETHNICITY AND HEALTH INEQUALITIES

Edited by Sufyan Abid Dogra

EDINBURGH
University Press

Edinburgh University Press is one of the leading university presses in the UK. We publish academic books and journals in our selected subject areas across the humanities and social sciences, combining cutting-edge scholarship with high editorial and production values to produce academic works of lasting importance. For more information visit our website: edinburghuniversitypress.com

Edinburgh University Press Ltd
The Tun – Holyrood Road
12 (2f) Jackson's Entry
Edinburgh EH8 8PJ

Typeset in 11/15 Adobe Garamond by
IDSUK (DataConnection) Ltd, and
printed and bound by CPI Group (UK) Ltd,
Croydon, CR0 4YY

A CIP record for this book is available from the British Library

ISBN 978 1 3995 0265 8 (hardback)
ISBN 978 1 3995 0267 2 (webready PDF)
ISBN 978 1 3995 0268 9 (epub)

CONTENTS

PART 4 BRITISH MUSLIMS PROMOTING HEALTH

FIGURES AND TABLES

Figures

Tables

NOTES ON CONTRIBUTORS

Sufyan Abid Dogra is a Principal Research Fellow at Bradford Institute for Health Research. His research explores ways to encourage healthy dietary habits and increase physical activity among children and young people from ethnic and religious minorities living in deprivation in the UK. He has conducted pioneering research on how mosques and madrassas in the UK can be used for health promotion. He views religion, physical activity, art, culture, poetry, spirituality, health and music as ways to create synergies for active civic life, better mental health and happiness for young people living with structural inequalities.

Anya Ahmed is the Professor of Wellbeing and Communities at Manchester Metropolitan University. As a social scientist and academic, her research has extensively explored the social aspects of ageing, migration, housing and homelessness, focusing on the experiences of Black and minoritised communities. Much of her work has involved the interrogation of the theoretical, conceptual and applied nature of 'community' in national and international contexts. Professor Ahmed's background in social policy has informed her research exploring the social and structural inequalities experienced by marginalised communities across the life-course.

Ishtiaq Ahmed was the general manager of the Khidmat Centre (a local community centre) and strategic policy adviser to the Council of Mosques in Bradford. For forty years he worked on community development, equality and diversity in Bradford. He was the first Black and Minority Ethnic (BME) head of Bradford Metropolitan Council for Voluntary Services and Director of Doncaster and

Bradford Race Equality Council. He has written many reports on British Muslims, including Muslim women in prison, Muslim children's education and community engagement.

Zlakha Ahmed MBE founded and is the current CEO of Apna Haq, a survivor-led organisation that supports BME women and girls in Rotherham, South Yorkshire, who are experiencing any form of violence or abuse. She has over thirty years' experience developing and overseeing at a local level support services concerning violence against women, while influencing strategy, policy and procedure at regional, national and European level.

Parveen Ali is a Professor in the School of Health Sciences at the University of Sheffield. She is the first UK Professor in Nursing of Pakistani origin, a Registered Nurse, Registered Midwife (Pakistan), Registered Nurse Teacher, Senior Fellow of Higher Education Academy and Fellow of the Royal Society of Arts. Professor Ali is an associate editor of *Nursing Open* and an editorial board member of the *Journal of Advanced Nursing* and the *Journal of Interpersonal Violence*. Her research interests include domestic violence and abuse, gender-based violence, the impact of domestic violence and abuse on victims' lives, and the training of healthcare professionals.

Razia Bhatti-Ali is an experienced clinical psychologist who has worked with diverse populations in both the NHS and the private sector. She works closely with local universities and was appointed Chair of the Behavioural Sciences Department in a renowned university in Pakistan, a position she held for two years. She has a BSc (Hons) degree in Behavioural Science, an MSc in Applied Psychology and another in Clinical Psychology, and a PhD in Clinical Psychology. She continues to have strong international academic links and has an active interest in Islamic psychological interventions.

Daniel Bingham is a Senior Research Fellow on the Born in Bradford project at the Bradford Institute for Health Research. He began his work with Born in Bradford in 2012 and has been a PhD student (2012–16), Research Assistant (2013–15), Research Fellow (2015–17) and Senior Research Fellow (2017–present). His primary research interests are the measurement, correlates, determinants, intervention design and intervention evaluation of children and young people's physical activity, sedentary behaviour and obesity. He is currently part of the Born in Bradford research team evaluating the Join Us: Move. Play (JU:MP) programme and is Chair of School Engagement in Bradford's Centre for Applied Education Research.

Aysha Divan is a Professor in the Faculty of Biological Sciences at the University of Leeds with a background in biochemistry, genetics and cancer biology. **Ghazala Mir** is an Associate Professor in the Faculty of Medicine and Health at the University of Leeds. Her research covers disadvantaged ethnic and faith communities, women and people with learning disabilities. **Mehrunisha Suleman** is currently Director of Medical Ethics and Law Education at the University of Oxford and a member of the Nuffield Council on Bioethics. **Arzoo Ahmed** is the ethics lead at Genomics England. **Ataf Sabir** is a practising clinician at Birmingham Women's and Children's NHS Foundation Trust working with patients with genetic disorders.

Yasmin Ghazala Farooq is a social researcher and has worked as a lecturer in Social Work at the University of Sheffield. She completed her PhD at the University of Manchester in 2014 where she subsequently worked as a lecturer in Social Statistics. Her research interests include migration, identity, ethnicity, race and health inequalities. She is particularly interested in exploring the experiences of elite migrants. Her doctoral research focused on the migration and identity experiences of overseas-trained South Asian doctors in the UK.

Melanie Haith-Cooper is a Reader in Maternity and Migrant Health at the University of Bradford, with a clinical background as a nurse and midwife. Her research interests focus on reducing health inequalities in people from ethnic minority backgrounds by co-designing, developing and evaluating interventions to support their interaction with health services and improve their health. This includes the use of digital technology and peer-support interventions. Her most recent project involves an intervention to increase cancer screening uptake in women from a South Asian Muslim background through working with families.

Jennifer Hall is a Senior Research Fellow on the Born in Bradford project at the Bradford Institute for Health Research. She is a qualitative researcher with expertise in intervention development and process evaluation, and is currently evaluating a whole systems approach to increasing physical activity in children and families in Bradford.

Shadim Hussain is CEO of My Foster Family, a community interest company he founded in 2019. He successively launched My Adoption Family, a faith-sensitive and diverse fostering and adoption recruitment and training organisation that supports agencies to find the best placements to meet the needs of children coming into care. He spearheaded the much-acclaimed Muslim Fostering Project, achieving positive change for unaccompanied asylum-seeking children and Muslim children living in care.

Shahid Islam has, for over a decade, been involved in engaging and supporting communities through activities that can increase rates of involvement and participation in a variety of spheres spanning health service research and delivery. His research has focused on reducing health inequalities and inequities especially among under-served communities. In 2015 he was awarded the Community Star Award for his work in Bradford. He is currently employed by the ActEarly City Collaboratory to propagate the research methods that fall under the citizen science and co-production paradigm.

Aqib Khan is currently a final-year medical student at Barts and the London Medical School. He is actively involved in various community initiatives based within the Muslim student sphere, such as the Federation of Student Islamic Societies, and has also volunteered within the Muslim charity sector. He has been actively involved in organising health promotion for student groups including Reconnecting Our Community through Kindness and has participated in health promotion activities with the British Islamic Medical Association.

Asma Khan is a Research Fellow in British Muslim Studies at Cardiff University's Centre for the Study of Islam in the UK. Her research interests include labour market inequalities, migration and the everyday lives of British Muslims. She leads a project team developing an online course entitled Understanding Muslim Mental Health. Generously funded by the Jameel Research Programme, this project aims to facilitate a better understanding of experiences of mental health illness among health professionals and religious pastoral care providers who work within British Muslim communities.

Stephen Abdullah Maynard has a BSc (Hons) in Psychology from the University of Surrey, an MA in Social Policy from Middlesex University and a diploma in Humanistic Counselling. He has worked as a counsellor since 1984. In 1990 he developed the first Transcultural Counselling certificate courses specifically for Black and Asian participants. A revert to Islam, he studied Tasawwuf and in 1995 was given permission, along with his colleague Sabnum Dharamsi, to develop and practise a coherent therapeutic model based on Islamic teachings. In 2010 he founded the Lateef Project, the longest-running Islamic counselling service in the UK, where he continues to work.

Aamnah Rahman is a Research Fellow based at the Bradford Institute for Health Research, working with local communities on engagement and co-production community-based research. She is a graduate of the University of Bradford with a BA (Hons) in Social Studies and an MSc in Advanced Practice (Psychological

Therapies). She has a keen interest in mental health and working with people with mental health issues in therapeutic settings.

Rukhsana Rashid is a research consultant. She worked as a Senior Research Fellow at the Bradford Institute for Health Research, managing a quasi-experimental study exploring the life-course health impact of a city-wide intervention to improve air quality in a Yorkshire city. Her other research interests include weight management, sleep, behavioural change and novel interventions. She has a personal interest in UK race relations, issues of identity and critical race theory.

Mohammed Akhlak Rauf MBE is founder and director of Meri Yaadain, a community interest company working to raise awareness of dementia and access to dementia care among BME communities. Meri Yaadain has been recognised nationally for providing good practice on engaging with and supporting BME communities given the challenges and barriers these communities face. He received an MBE in 2016 in recognition of his services to people living with dementia and to their families.

Alison Scott-Baumann is Professor of Society and Belief and Associate Director of Research (Impact and Engagement) at SOAS, University of London. She and her research team were awarded a three-year Arts and Humanities Research Council grant to analyse representations of Islam and Muslims on campus (2015–18). She speaks on BBC Radio 4, writes for the *Guardian* and several higher education blogs, and applies philosophy to social justice issues. She currently leads a research project called Influencing Corridors of Power, working with academics on one-page briefings of evidence-based findings for every MP and peer. She recently launched an All Party Parliamentary Group on Communities of Inquiry across the generations.

Hina J. Shahid is a GP in London and Chair of the Muslim Doctors Association, a non-profit organisation working to reduce health inequities affecting marginalised and minority communities in the UK. She holds an MSc in Public Health from the London School of Hygiene & Tropical Medicine where her dissertation was part of a UN project analysing the socioeconomic determinants of chronic disease outcomes among refugee populations in Lebanon. She has worked in a number of research, teaching and humanitarian roles in Europe, the Middle East and South Asia. In the UK her work focuses on community engagement, advocacy and policy reform through an intersectional lens to address the multiple structural barriers to health affecting marginalised communities.

Aaliyah Shaikh is a psychotherapist, certified clinical trauma professional and PhD researcher in health psychology. She graduated from St Catharine's College, University of Cambridge with an MEd in Psychotherapeutic Counselling, has an MA in Muslim Community Studies from the University of Loughborough, and completed training in Psychodynamic Skills at the University of Leicester. She is an Aziz Foundation Scholar and has been awarded a scholarship from the Centre for Maternal and Child Health at City University, London for her PhD research, which explores experiences of pregnancy and birth in the British Muslim community.

Mohammad Shoiab is a pain specialist physiotherapist who for several years worked for the NHS in Bradford, which influenced his interest in exploring the differences in expectations of patients presenting with pain in the musculoskeletal outpatient and pain services. He was an invited speaker at the World Physiotherapy Congress in Geneva in 2019 and co-convenor of the Chartered Society of Physiotherapy's BME network 2018–20.

Salman Waqar is a GP in Berkshire and a Research Fellow at the Nuffield Department of Primary Care Health Sciences, University of Oxford. He is the General Secretary of the British Islamic Medical Association, an award-winning voluntary non-profit association of Muslim health professionals that has been proactive in community health promotion for many years.

FOREWORD

There has been a Muslim presence in Britain since the sixteenth century, with Muslims arriving in substantial numbers around 300 years ago into port towns following their recruitment as sailors from South Asia by the East India Company. Yet, despite this long period of interaction, which included the colonisation by the British Empire of many predominantly Muslim countries, Islam and Muslims remain something of an enigma in Britain. This persistent lack of familiarity is disturbing and, more importantly, has consequences in many facets of life, including suboptimal healthcare provision and poor health outcomes among British Muslims.

Two decades ago I, together with my colleague Professor Abdul Rashid Gatrad, co-edited *Caring for Muslim Patients* (Radcliffe Publishing, 2008) in which we attempted to provide an insider's perspective for healthcare professionals of the rich, complex, multifaceted relationship between Islam and health as experienced by British Muslims. Our hope was (and remains) that a deeper appreciation of this worldview would enable emergence of more culturally sensitive, personalised approaches to healthcare delivery and health promotion than had hitherto been the case.

Much has changed over the past twenty years, including the emergence of a large, increasingly diverse and more educated, financially secure and assertive British Muslim community, but as the contributors to *British Muslims, Ethnicity and Health Inequalities* remind us, many challenges persist. Dr Dogra and colleagues highlight in particular the complexities resulting from people of faith trying to navigate an essentially secular healthcare system. Added to this are the adverse health effects, whether direct or indirect, resulting from experiencing racial and religious discrimination, and the lack of voice and agency still often afforded to Muslims in identifying their own health goals and priorities. The contributors to this book lament the many missed opportunities for engaging with religious institutions and structures in intersectional ways to support the delivery of health-care and the development of key health promotional interventions. Helpfully, they also offer some more promising examples of grassroots initiatives such as the emergence of Islamic counselling and pain management services, and detailed case studies of the British Islamic Medical Association's Lifesavers initiative and the work of Bradford's Council of Mosques in responding to the COVID-19 pandemic.

There will, I hope, be something of interest in the eclectic series of essays that comprise this volume to all those interested in understanding how health inequalities operate and are experienced. Whilst the focus is clearly on British Muslims, there are many potentially transferable insights to other marginalised communities. Readers are likely to benefit hearing directly from contributing authors who are deeply embedded in their communities and who as a result have first-hand experience of understanding how the battle for health is experienced. These passionate voices may at times inspire, challenge and provoke, but they should above all be seen as a call to more inclusive dialogue and debate about how we *together* realise the potential and promise of the NHS, namely to deliver humane care for all – irrespective of colour or creed, and whilst respecting deeply held beliefs and values.

Two decades on, I remain convinced that this is a goal worth striving for and to this end I welcome the contribution made by Dr Dogra and colleagues focusing on the needs of an important sub-section of our increasingly religiously, ethnically and culturally diverse British society.

Aziz Sheikh OBE
Chair of Primary Care Research and Development,
Usher Institute,
University of Edinburgh
Edinburgh, July 2022

PART 1

CONTEMPORARY ISSUES AND DEBATES

1

BRITISH MUSLIMS, ETHNICITY AND HEALTH INEQUALITIES: CONTEMPORARY ISSUES AND DEBATES

Sufyan Abid Dogra ⓘ

This book presents social diagnoses on how and why British Muslims live with health inequalities and how they experience difficulties in accessing health services. It explores the scope of British Muslims' involvement in health promotion initiatives and in the delivery of preventive health interventions. We use religion, ethnicity, deprivation and marginalisation as representative sites of embodiment and context in which British Muslim bodies negotiate being fit or unfit when juxtaposed with prevalent health standards. We debate British Muslims' patterns of engagement with healthcare systems in the UK and the subsequent marginalisation they encounter when benefiting from those systems. We discuss the unequal distribution of health benefits to British Muslims that are otherwise universally offered to all citizens through the UK healthcare system. Using reflexive, interpretive, critical and evidence-based, data-driven scenarios from across the country, we identify loopholes in the British healthcare system and what is missing in its policy, delivery and health promotion initiatives for marginalised communities living with disadvantages. We provide contemporary situation analysis on what makes British Muslims live with the worst health outcomes from within all deprived social groups and ethnicities in the country.

The idea of a pioneering edited book on this topic was conceived during a national conference on the health experiences of British Muslims that I organised in 2018 at the University of Bradford in collaboration with the Muslims in Britain

ⓘ https://orcid.org/0000-0001-9896-9503
✉ Sufyan.Dogra@bthft.nhs.uk

Research Network and the Born in Bradford (BiB) study. Participants and speakers shared their learning, observations and findings on how British Muslims experience structural inequalities that result in higher chances of them living with ill-health indicators by virtue of their religious, ethnic, migration and working-class identities and positionalities. The health indicators become worse when children, women and minorities within minority British Muslims are exposed to these multiple layers of systematic inequalities. Targeted health interventions and health promotion initiatives in the UK are generally designed by experts who rely upon data that is collected by making ethnicity and economic class in the UK a unit of analysis. The data collected for health promotion interventions on indicators such as ethnicity and economic class has its advantages in certain areas of health promotion, for example cancer screening, obesity rates and diabetes. In most cases, this data keeps health promotion interventions and initiatives unreflective of the changes in society that have taken place during the last two decades and how those changes shape the experiences of deprivation among British Muslims. The practice of designing and developing health interventions based on indicators such as ethnicity and economic class ignores the role that intersectionality plays in the distribution of deprivation within disadvantaged communities in general, and among British Muslims in particular, and there is a lack of reliable data in this regard (Sheikh 2007).

This book answers the questions that are becoming increasingly relevant for preventive health interventions and health promotion initiatives for high-risk groups in contemporary Britain. Experts may be familiar with questions regarding ill-health experience, but a new insight and a revisiting of current policy and practice is increasingly necessary. The questions include: what frequently goes wrong with targeted health interventions for disadvantaged communities in the UK? Why are these interventions not effective in delivering the outcomes they aspire to achieve at the planning stage? Why is available health data not reflective of the comprehensive and in-depth description of ill health that British Muslims live with? How do applied health research methodologies on collecting data disenfranchise British Muslims? How does data analysis based on these methodologies overlook the constituting factors of ill health for Muslim research participants? Why are health promotion initiatives not co-produced, why do they lack local or place-based adaptations and ownership, and why are they are often unsustainable? Why are available community assets in deprived neighbourhoods and localised resources designed to improve health among British Muslims not part of health planning, policy and delivery? Why do applied health researchers, policy makers and experts shy away from acknowledging the established and evidence-based relationship between racism, Islamophobia and discrimination with ill-health indicators and health inequalities? To answer these questions, it is imperative that we revisit and re-address five key themes, outlined below, in relation to health promotion and targeted health interventions in the UK. This book will attempt to find answers through multidisciplinary interpretations by researchers, academics and practitioners.

Religious identity is a wider determinant of health for British Muslims along with ethnicity, racism, social class and deprivation. This book argues that religion, religious identity and the lived experience of religion for British Muslims should be considered as a wider determinant for their health outcomes. I expand this broader argument of the book by deliberating on the following major issues in relation to health inequalities, ethnicity and British Muslims.

What Has Religion Got to Do with Health (and Health Promotion)?

For the religious, the human body and its composition is more than a physical body. This might sound an odd statement to most British academics, health practitioners, applied health researchers and experts trained in the secular intellectual and medical tradition, mainly because they might imagine this implies re-inventing the very familiar story of medieval Christian European history where the Church always maintained a stake in temporal affairs with a retrogressive worldview towards social progress. It is argued that modern scientific medical practice takes its theoretical inspiration from Cartesian dualism (a belief in the separation of mind and body) that naturally results in the adoption of reductionist and linear approaches towards contemporary health problems (Daykin 2020). Islamic bioethics, on the other hand, can be located at the intersection of tradition, modernity, spirituality and clinical practice (Padela 2021). Hence the understanding of the human body among religious minorities in contemporary Britain cannot be conceptually approached using the prism of the Christian European historical experience. Religious traditions other than Christianity, Islam in particular, had a different attitude towards and experience with the human body and medicine during the era infamously known as the Dark Ages in Europe. These times can be arguably viewed as the 'golden age' in Muslim societies (Edriss et al. 2017). Muslim scientists, medics and physicians during this golden age were eclectic in their approach and well versed in poetry, philosophy and politics, and happened to be Islamic scholars simultaneously (Moosa 2021). They set a historic pattern by laying the foundations of how medicine, the relationship between medical interventions and the human body, and health guidelines would be interpreted and practised among Muslim communities, where 'temporal' has traditionally been inspired by the 'religious'.

Another aspect that goes often unnoticed during the implementation of targeted health interventions for deprived communities is the lived experience of British Muslims and how they use a huge canon of Islamic literature to maintain a healthy body. This Islamic literature and guidelines on the relationship between body and health is available to them in the forms of Qur'anic verses, *Sunnah* (the practices of Prophet Muhammad) and hadith (the sayings of Prophet Muhammad) written in sacred Islamic texts, and the writings of Islamic scholars who excelled in medicine. This Islamic literature and guidelines on health and body are regularly disseminated to what is a captive audience of Muslims through Friday sermons and religious learnings in mosques, during the month of Ramadan, in women's Islamic study circles, and through daily prayers and other religious events in the Islamic calendar. Recent evidence shows that the Islamic narrative on health is used within Islamic religious settings in the UK to form an active part of British Muslims' health practices and health promotion initiatives (Rai et al. 2019; Dogra et al. 2021). Furthermore, the Islamic narrative is culturally adapted in different ways for various health outcomes among diverse communities of British Muslims and operates as a supplementary medical system or set of instructions in combination with the mainstream British medical guidelines issued by the National Health Service (NHS) and Public Health England. The ways in which Islamic literature and guidelines on health and body are used, received and culturally adapted among diverse British Muslims depend upon the gender, age, ethnic origins, migration histories and social class of the users. Preventive health interventions and guidelines for targeted communities in the UK can capitalise on Islamic narratives on health and can use them as a community asset when implementing health promotion programmes.

Double Deprivation and the Triple Whammy of Inequalities for British Muslims

The majority of British Muslims are from migrant ethnic minority backgrounds, are working class and live in deprived neighbourhoods. In the changed political climate after the 9/11 attacks in the USA in 2001 and the 7/7 bombings in the UK in 2005, discrimination based on religious profiling and scrutiny on the basis of Muslim identity has only doubled the deprivation that Muslims already experienced by virtue of their disadvantaged background (Jones 2020). In addition, there is a triple whammy of structural inequalities (Mir and Sheikh 2010), physiological inequalities such as high adiposity (Nightingale et al. 2011) and cultural or societal inequalities such as acculturation (Smith et al. 2012). These factors play a key role for British Muslims living with chronic health conditions and experiencing health disadvantages. Constituting factors for ill health, such as low levels of physical activity, unhealthy dietary practices, gendered notions of fitness and taboos around certain physical activities, together with deprivation, racism and inequality, require open and informed discussions between academic researchers, clinicians, policy makers and those active within British Muslim communities in order to approach and understand the causes of ill health. However, these issues and questions are often drowned out in the public sphere and policy debates by the overarching political narratives about British Muslims. One major consequence of the changing political landscape in the past two decades has been the disappearance of debate, discussion, policies and initiatives aimed at health promotion among British Muslims and ethnic minorities; instead, securitisation has taken precedence at institutional and structural levels (Jones 2020) over indicators such as health, wellbeing and education.

The Marmot Review (2010) identified the disproportionate health risks to different social groups and ethnic minorities and advocated responding to the wider determinants of health to tackle health inequalities. Recent reports and research on the disproportionate impact of COVID-19 on Black and Minority Ethnic (BME) populations offered new evidence on how marginalised groups in Britain from disadvantaged backgrounds are far more vulnerable to COVID-19 either because of underlying health conditions or by virtue of living with ill-health indicators (Hu 2020; Qureshi et al. 2020; Shahid and Scott-Baumann 2020). These reports emphasise that structural, systemic and environmental factors including living in poor and congested housing, long working hours, poor working conditions and being employed as a key worker play a more significant role in making BME populations more vulnerable to pandemics such as COVID-19 than factors relating to biological and genetic disposition. At the same time, there are more nuanced reports on the disproportionate long-term impact of COVID-19 on British Muslims within BME communities (CMPR 2020; MCB 2020). These reports point out that Islamophobia plays a role in harming the health of British Muslims.

The Impact of Racism and Islamophobia on the Health of British Muslims

In the wake of COVID-19, evidence has emerged on how racism and Islamophobia have a direct impact on British Muslims' ill health and significantly enhances the chances of their contracting COVID-19 or chronic diseases such as diabetes or asthma (Iacobucci 2020). Stigmatisation, fear, discrimination, blame and religious hatred against Muslims in Britain make them vulnerable to ill health or depression during a pandemic (Sarkar 2020; Gopal et al. 2020). Recent media coverage of the spread of COVID-19 in Britain during July and August 2020 has pointed to Muslims living in northern England being responsible for the second wave of the virus (Sarkar 2020). Demonisation, prejudice and hate speech against British Muslims have historically exacerbated their chances of living with chronic diseases and a number of mental health conditions (see Chapters 2, 3, and 10 for details). Racism and Islamophobia take the form of institutional and structural oppression when the NHS or other health promotion and delivery organisations apply protocols such as the PREVENT framework to identify racialised Muslims as suspects (Younis and Jadhav 2019). At the same time, medical history, records and assessments are still generally defined and interpreted from a biomedical perspective. Social epidemiology is not a prominent narrative of diagnosis in medical practice. This curtails new social realities of structural violence like Islamophobia to become part of the holistic diagnosis of people living with ill health or underlying health conditions. There is clear evidence that experiencing any form of structural violence, racism or Islamophobia has a direct impact on and relationship with ill health and makes British Muslims and BME communities more susceptible to pathogens (Bentley 2020; Conching and Thayer 2019).

This book advocates that acknowledging the Islamophobia and racism experienced by British Muslims will only improve environmental conditions and will help reduce ill health indicators and enable those affected to overcome historical trauma (Conching and Thayer 2019). New health policies for vulnerable groups in the UK need to acknowledge how racism and Islamophobia have been instrumental in allowing the consequences of structural health inequalities to trickle down among British Muslims. For future health improvement policy, nuanced and intersectional approaches are inevitable for in-depth social diagnoses of ill-health indicators among high-risk groups like the majority of British Muslims. Public health science in UK needs to improve its evidence base to link social and biological factors with a nuanced approach in granularity with regard to 'groups living with social disadvantages' as the existing evidence is inadequate (Kelly 2021).

Neo-eugenics: Issues with Applied Health Research and Methodologies

Another critical issue concerning mainstream applied health experts such as practitioners, researchers and academics is the prevalence of speculation and assumptions made about British Muslims and ethnic minorities, accommodating the mindset that these groups choose to live an unhealthy lifestyle. These stereotypical assumptions are not substantiated with evidence and are counter-productive in addressing the factors behind British Muslims' ill health. The cognitive constructs of applied health experts are influenced by their sociopolitical context, which reinforces stereotypes and assumptions and becomes instrumental in shaping their epistemologies and ontologies regarding health issues in society. This leads health experts to work with what I call the 'neo-eugenics mindset' while they assess, analyse and interpret ill health among high-risk groups such as British Muslims. This neo-eugenics mindset is inspired by the puritanistic and ambitious desire of applied health experts to see particular health outcomes achieved among ethnic minorities and British Muslims. These experts, when designing any health promotion intervention or initiative, will come up with theories, logic models, and selective and biased data interpretations to create health promotion solutions that aim at rapidly yet insensitively changing dietary habits, bodily discipline, physical movements, sexual, marital and reproductive choices, health practices, family structure, fitness ideals and bodily conduct such as posture or appearance in public among ethnic minorities and British Muslims. Applied health experts do this with a strong belief in the efficacy of biomedical supremacy to shape, discipline and produce 'standardised ideal type bodies' of ethnic minorities and British Muslims at the cost of ignoring the severity of the societal, cognitive and environmental factors that cause vulnerable and ill bodies. This neo-eugenics mindset behind knowledge production only leads to epistemological incommensurability between social and biomedical scientists (Kelly 2021) when they translate scientific knowledge into practice for shaping policy.

In the past three decades, the available literature and data in applied health research and social sciences has interpreted ill health among ethnic minorities and British Muslims through identifying and associating cultural and religious practices as barriers for healthy lifestyles. Ironically, the language of culture or religion as a barrier disappears when these applied health experts interpret similar ill-health indicators among majority British populations. This differential attitude of experts towards interpreting data with a neo-eugenics mindset is manifested more openly in certain areas of applied health research, such as physical activity, dietary habits, genetics and health, smoking and alcohol consumption during pregnancy, marital choices with close relatives and vaccine hesitancy, where the findings of data from bi-ethnic or multi-ethnic samples are interpreted using different language for minority ethnic and majority British populations (Dickerson et al. 2021; Lockyer 2021; Taylor et al. 2021; Collings et al. 2020; Sheridan et al. 2013). The mainstream media takes inspiration from the language used by health researchers who, consciously or unconsciously, interpret and present a commentary driven by a neo-eugenics mindset on ethnic minorities as scientific analysis. Consequently, the mainstream media ends up presenting the neo-eugenics driven health research with racist buttressing about the markers of the cultural and religious identities of ethnic minorities and British Muslims (BBC 2013) while ignoring the same about the majority population when broadcasting research findings on the ill health of that group (Macnamara 2021). Experts in applied health research often strongly advocate introducing, and in some cases enforcing, certain practices as 'scientific solutions' among post-World War Two second-, third- or fourth-generation ethnic minorities and British Muslims in the name of encouraging a good diet, physical activity and other healthy behaviours. The standardisation of ethnic bodies in Britain with the aim of reshaping them into 'healthy bodies' is pursued on similar neo-eugenics inspired thinking patterns that were tested in the early twentieth century by health experts in Australia who believed in eugenics, and were used to standardise, tame and discipline the Aboriginal populations. The research inspired by the neo-eugenics mindset about the lived experience of ethnic minorities with regard to their health is generally published by research teams that do not include any members from ethnic minority backgrounds. Diversity and inclusivity among the health research teams working on programmes involving ethnic minorities can ensure the nuanced multifacetedness of the analyses and reflexivity (Mathijssen et al. 2021) which is part of describing the complexity of health issues among high-risk groups. This diversity and inclusivity of ethnic minorities should be visible at the point when health research teams plan, design and co-produce research, disseminate research findings, prepare clear and simple research summaries and write publications, and in the overall processes of knowledge production about ethnic minorities. This book points out that the consequences of the neo-eugenics mindset in applied health research are the exclusion of researchers from ethnic minority backgrounds from the processes of knowledge production and ethnic minorities themselves being taken for granted and stereotyped when they are in the role of 'research participants'.

Harnessing the Potential of Islamic Settings in the UK for Health Promotion

Islamic settings such as mosques, madrassas (schools for Islamic learning), women's circles for the study of Islam, Muslim charities or sports organisations in the UK are very influential and can be effective settings for encouraging healthy behaviours or delivering health promotion interventions or initiatives for high-risk groups. Islamic narrative, teachings and faith leaders play an important role in mobilising and influencing the life choices of Muslims (Dogra 2019). A recent scoping review and systematic mapping on using Islamic religious settings for health promotion found that people in these settings are already actively engaged in delivering physical activities, encouraging healthy dietary habits, and organising various educational and informative sessions and workshops, whether on their own initiative or in collaboration with mainstream healthcare organisations such as the NHS or other public health authorities (Rai et al. 2019). However, the review also found that these health promotion interventions are mostly delivered voluntarily and are unfunded and unrecorded, and that there is a need to evaluate how effective Islamic religious settings can be for health promotion, particularly for delivering childhood obesity prevention interventions. The BiB study found that 91 per cent of British Muslim children attend a mosque or a madrassa most days after school for Islamic learning and that their parents and Islamic leaders would welcome a tailored health promotion intervention delivered by involving and using these faith settings (Dogra et al. 2021). Such Islamic settings are attended not only by the children themselves, but also by the parents and members of the broader community living in the neighbourhood. This captive audience can be instrumental in delivering health promotion interventions and successfully ensuring community ownership.

Using the COM-B model (capability, opportunity and motivation for behaviour change) as a framework (Michie et al. 2014), this book views Islamic settings as *capability*, British Muslims as the captive audience in those settings as an *opportunity*, the availability of Islamic teachings on healthy living, the Islamic narrative on health promotion and its preferential use among British Muslims for the adopting of healthy behaviours and the delivery of any health promotion intervention as *motivation* for behaviour change. Equally, we note that the application of the COM-B model to develop the theory of change and logic models has its limitations when designing delivery programmes for health promotion among British Muslims. The COM-B model's realism of assessment does not address or take into account the impact of structural inequalities and violence which defines health inequalities among ethnic minorities and British Muslims. Logic models for health promotion programmes driven by the COM-B framework ignore how structural inequalities affect the COM-B framework's constituent elements of capability, opportunity and motivation for behaviour change among British Muslims. This book advocates that the potential of Islamic settings needs to be harnessed for the delivery health promotion interventions and initiatives that target high-risk groups. The 2019 Cochrane Review informs us that the majority of health and obesity prevention interventions in the UK in the past twenty-five years have addressed down-to midstream variables such as biological and individual lifestyle factors. This has not been very effective and so there is a need to address midstream to upstream variables, for example social, community and wider environmental factors, as well as working conditions (Nobles et al. 2021). Involving Islamic settings can ensure that midstream to upstream factors for health promotion are addressed, including family, peer groups, neighbourhoods, political governance at local level and so on. Islamic settings as community assets can adopt place-based approaches and ensure effective involvement and ownership of communities in the government's health promotion initiatives. More work, research and involvement is needed to highlight health promotion in Islamic settings. This will ensure public and funding bodies on health promotion acknowledge the value of religious settings as a stakeholder in addressing health inequalities.

The Scope of this Book

The book offers a fresh insight into the health inequalities and ethnic disadvantages that British Muslims have been living with and continue to live with. It comprises eighteen single- or multi-authored chapters. The authors are academics, researchers, GPs, practitioners and activists in the fields of health research and the promotion and delivery of health programmes, as well as third-sector professionals and community activists. Each chapter discusses a different dimension of the health inequalities that British Muslims live with and offers a sound alternative for improved health around that theme.

The book begins its main argument in the first chapter, written by Dr Sufyan Abid Dogra: that religion is a wider determinant of health for British Muslims. The chapter emphasises that British Muslims are a high-risk group for many ill-health indicators, and hence utilising Islamic literature on health, addressing health inequalities, acknowledging the role of racism and Islamophobia in British Muslims' ill health, avoiding a neo-eugenics inspired mindset and assumptions, and using Islamic settings as place-based localised venues for health promotion can ensure effective outcomes for the delivery of healthcare in the UK. The chapter argues that having a new perspective and a strategy with regard to involving the public in health promotion initiatives in the UK has become essential and that the existing health promotion policy and strategy require revisiting. Due to the disproportionate impact of COVID-19 on British Muslims and ethnic minorities, there is a pressing need for a new perspective and strategy with regard to health promotion initiatives and interventions that target high-risk populations. The conception, design and delivery of such interventions, methodologies and evaluations for high-risk groups requires a careful process of adaptability for the targeted audiences of such interventions.

Chapter 2, led by Dr Sufyan Abid Dogra, highlights the disproportionate impact of COVID-19 on British Muslims and how the pandemic exposed prevalent health inequalities in the UK public sphere. This chapter provides a critique and discussion around faith in relation to COVID-19, highlights victim blaming by experts and authorities, and demonstrates the impact of COVID-19 and how the subsequent socioeconomic consequences of lockdown have further marginalised British Muslims. By focusing on the experiences of British Muslims, this chapter discusses the interplay of ethnicity, religion and deprivation in negotiating the particular challenges of living through COVID-19. The chapter goes on to assess the impact of COVID-19 on British Muslim families, children, chaplains, charitable and voluntary organisations, mental health and wellbeing, and how national Muslim medical organisations in the UK responded to the crisis. It also includes a multidisciplinary perspective of academics and explores lived experiences in relation to the pandemic, lockdown and the socioeconomic implications of COVID-19 in the UK.

Chapter 3, led by Dr Hina J. Shahid, presents gendered reflections on health inequalities among British Muslim women through the intersectionality of religion, culture, racism and marginalisation. The chapter discusses the lived experience of British Muslim women with health inequalities and how it is shaped by ethnicity, migration, health indicators such as gendered structural inequalities, physical inactivity, access to health services, cancer screening, marriage patterns, Islamophobia and racism, domestic abuse, and upward social mobility, or the lack thereof. This chapter reveals how British Muslim women rise to prominence and challenge or shape the discourses, policies and practices around healthcare and women's rights, and goes on to present the services Muslim women provide within the NHS and other healthcare sectors.

Chapter 4, by Aaliyah Sheikh, presents an epistemological critique of the colonisation of knowledge production and how it becomes relevant when various research methodologies are used in health psychology, health research and in other social sciences where British Muslims are participants. The chapter points out the absence of meaningful representative research on the health experiences of British Muslims, in particular in health psychology through a non-oriental lens. Chapter 4 discusses Islamic ontology as a concept, with an emphasis on decolonising research methodologies by acknowledging colonial epistemicide. The chapter advocates the consideration of living with continuous trauma as a feature of conducting research when it comes to studying South Asian British Muslim women's experiences of womb and birth.

Chapter 5, led by Dr Aysha Divan, is a collaborative work that analyses the genetic health of British Muslims and its relationship with consanguinity, therapeutic interventions and sociocultural contexts. The chapter emphasises the need to improve access to genetic testing and subsequent counselling amongst minority ethnic groups in the UK. It identifies the absence of national-level policy aimed at improving birth outcomes for those in consanguineous relationships. The chapter also offers appropriate alternative choices for those in such relationships and discusses the lessons learned from previous interventions before going on to highlight the role of families in decision making.

Chapter 6, by Dr Mehrunisha Suleman, discusses caring for Muslim patients and families at the end of life. This chapter shares an analysis of the data from seventy-six interviews with Muslim patients and families and juxtaposes how different values and moral frameworks require careful negotiation when these patients and their families encounter the healthcare system. The chapter provides examples and suggestions on how policy, training and education can enhance services for Muslim patients and families who receive end-of-life care and also support healthcare professionals in the UK.

Chapter 7, by Mohammed Akhlak Rauf, elaborates on dementia among Muslim communities in the UK. This chapter discusses various factors that impact the lives of Muslims who are either caring for someone with dementia or living with the condition themselves. It introduces some areas of dementia where further training and a greater understanding of how services can provide support to family carers are required. It goes on to introduce the idea of how British Muslims themselves can rise to the challenge of supporting dementia care needs while living in Western societies.

Chapter 8, co-authored by Professor Parveen Ali and Zlakha Ahmed, discusses domestic violence and abuse and how this impacts the health of British Muslims.

The chapter provides details on factors affecting access to healthcare for victims of domestic violence and abuse from British Muslim backgrounds. The chapter argues that Muslim women in Britain experience additional barriers in accessing healthcare and receiving support provided by the healthcare system for victims of domestic violence and abuse.

Chapter 9, by Dr Yasmin Ghazala Farooq, explores reciprocity of expressions of marginalisation in the medical encounters between overseas-trained South Asian doctors and patients from working-class backgrounds in the UK. The chapter discusses the widely debated privileged position of doctors and how relevant it remains in the case of UK doctors who have been trained overseas. It finds that the standard theories concerning the sociocultural dimension of Western medicine do not fully reflect the experiences of overseas-trained South Asian GPs in their interactions with patients.

Chapter 10, by Dr Hina J. Shahid, discusses the health cost of Islamophobia for the NHS. She presents a conceptual framework on how Islamophobia creates pathologies among British Muslims through intersectional systems of oppression, which functions at global, structural, social and individual levels and results in negative health outcomes. The chapter emphasises that an intersectional approach towards various identities must be taken into consideration while planning and implementing health promotion programmes in the UK.

Chapter 11, by Rukhsana Rashid, discusses how second- and third-generation British Muslims experience identity struggles while seeking health information. The chapter analyses the stereotypical assumptions, perceptions and speculations among health practitioners in the UK and how they can be instrumental in discouraging young British Muslims from trying to access the wider benefits of mainstream healthcare services. This chapter elaborates the importance of sensitive narratives and how health practitioners need to remain up to date through regular training on meeting the needs of diverse communities.

Chapter 12, by Stephen Abdullah Maynard, considers the relationship between faith, mental health and mental illness among British Muslims. The focus of the chapter is on mental health problems such as anxiety, depression and post-traumatic stress disorder, and the social contexts of these conditions within Muslim communities. It considers the significance of the Islamic faith to Muslims with regard to its function as a 'cognitive schema' within Muslim communities enabling interpretation of experience and mental wellbeing. The chapter advocates the need to consider research on Muslim mental health as a theme in the mainstream study of psychology.

Chapter 13, by Aamnah Rahman, discusses mental health among British Muslims by taking the case of their lived experience in Bradford, in the north of England. The chapter discusses how British Muslims experience mental health issues while living in a predominantly homogeneous social environment. The majority of Muslims in Bradford have the same migration roots and origins. The chapter expands on the relationship between mental health issues and racism, inequalities, COVID-19 and a general sense of deprivation in northern England. It highlights the intergenerational differences in experiencing mental health issues and offers unique insights into the cultural and Islamic concepts around it.

Chapter 14, co-authored by Dr Razia Bhatti-Ali and Mohammad Shoaib, reiterates the need for culturally adapted healthcare services for approaches to pain management. The chapter states that with the growing awareness of discrimination in healthcare, it is imperative that clinical practice adopt self-management and lifestyle approaches to pain. It discusses how different psychological therapies for pain management can incorporate Islamic concepts such as *sabr* (patience), *shukr* (gratitude) and *muraqba* (mindfulness). The authors discuss how pain management therapies have changed and adapted to cultural contexts in the UK over the years.

Chapter 15, by Shahid Islam, presents how actively engaged fathers have an important influence on their children's social and emotional wellbeing. This chapter explores some of the reasons why we still have very few fathers from British Muslim backgrounds who attend training courses for the health and wellbeing of children. Drawing on the fields of social epidemiology, psychology and sociology, the chapter forms a coherent critical analysis which highlights the gaps in policy and practice and how these continue to maintain health inequalities for British Muslim fathers and children.

Chapter 16, co-authored by Dr Salman Waqar and Aqib Khan, informs us about the role that the British Islamic Medical Association (BIMA), a national Muslim organisation of doctors, is playing in improving the health and wellbeing of British Muslims. The authors state that culturally appropriate interventions are known to be effective and can induce behavioural change but question whether this extends to those that are tailored to faith? Using the case study of BIMA's Lifesavers project, this chapter explores the potential of community health promotion in mosques using Muslim health professionals.

Chapter 17, led by Dr Sufyan Abid Dogra and co-authored with Ishtiaq Ahmed, explores the role that different Islamic settings in Bradford such as mosques, madrassas and Muslim organisations have played in health promotion. The chapter introduces Born in Bradford, a research project that laid the foundation of the Trailblazer Childhood Obesity Prevention Progamme, aimed at harnessing the potential of mosques and madrassas to address the issue of childhood obesity. The chapter provides a case study of a local Muslim organisation, Council of Mosques Bradford, and shows how it has played an active role in health promotion. Chapter 17 goes on to discuss Bradford-based initiatives that advocate using religious settings for health promotion. These case studies delineate how the health needs of first-generation migrants in Bradford in the 1960s and 1970s resulted in the formation of the Council of Mosques and how this organisation continues to fulfil the dual functions of health promotion and religious needs.

Chapter 18, by Dr Sufyan Abid Dogra, concludes this edited volume and presents the way forward in the light of the findings and recommendations revealed in this book. He proposes culturally adaptable and useful recommendations that a new health policy targeting disadvantaged populations, British Muslims and ethnic minorities might wish to consider in their efforts to reduce health inequalities in the UK.

References

BBC (2013). 'Bradford study finds higher birth defect risk in married cousins'. Available at: www.bbc.co.uk/news/uk-england-leeds-23183102 (last accessed 28 April 2022).

Bentley, G. R. (2020). 'Don't blame the BAME: ethnic and structural inequalities in susceptibilities to COVID-19'. *American Journal of Human Biology*, 32(5), e23478.

Centre for Muslim Policy Research (2020). 'Impact of COVID-19 on the Muslim community: assessment of key risk factors'. Available at: https://cmpr.org.uk/wp-content/uploads/2020/11/20201123-COVID19-and-the-Impact-on-the-Muslim-Community_vF-.pdf (last accessed 28 April 2022).

Collings, P. J., Dogra, S. A., Costa, S., Bingham, D. D. and Barber, S. E. (2020). 'Objectively-measured sedentary time and physical activity in a bi-ethnic sample of young children: variation by socio-demographic, temporal and perinatal factors'. *BMC Public Health*, 20(1), 1–15.

Conching, A. K. S. and Thayer, Z. (2019). 'Biological pathways for historical trauma to affect health: a conceptual model focusing on epigenetic modifications'. *Social Science & Medicine*, 230, 74–82.

Council for Muslims in Britain (2020). 'Together in tribulation: British Muslims and the COVID-19 pandemic'. Available at: https://mcb.org.uk/report/covid-and-muslims (last accessed 28 April 2022).

Daykin, N. (2020). *Arts, Health and Well-Being: A Critical Perspective on Research, Policy and Practice*. London: Routledge.

Dickerson, J., Lockyer, B., Moss, R. H., Endacott, C., Kelly, B., Bridges, S., Crossley, K. L., Bryant, M., Sheldon, T. A., Wright, J., Pickett, K. E., McEachan, R. R. C., Bradford Institute for Health Research COVID-19 Scientific Advisory Group (2021). 'COVID-19 vaccine hesitancy in an ethnically diverse community: descriptive findings from the Born in Bradford study'. *Wellcome Open Research*, 6, 23.

Dogra, S. A. (2019). 'Living a piety-led life beyond Muharram: becoming or being a South Asian Shia Muslim in the UK'. *Contemporary Islam*, 13(3), 307–24.

Dogra, S. A., Rai, K., Barber, S., McEachan, R. R., Adab, P. and Sheard, L. (2021). 'Delivering a childhood obesity prevention intervention using Islamic religious settings in the UK: what is most important to the stakeholders?'. *Preventive Medicine Reports*, 22, 101387.

Edriss, H., Rosales, B. N., Nugent, C., Conrad, C. and Nugent, K. (2017). 'Islamic medicine in the Middle Ages'. *The American Journal of the Medical Sciences*, 354(3), 223–9.

Gopal, D. P., Waqar, S., Silverwood, V., Mulla, E. and Dada, O. (2020). 'Race and racism: are we too comfortable with comfort?'. *BJGP Open*, 4(5). https://doi.org/10.3399/BJGPO.2020.0143

Hu, Y. (2020). 'Intersecting ethnic and native–migrant inequalities in the economic impact of the COVID-19 pandemic in the UK'. *Research in Social Stratification and Mobility*, 68, 100528.

Iacobucci, G. (2020). 'Covid-19: PHE review has failed ethnic minorities, leaders tell BMJ'. *BMJ*, 369, m2264.

Jones, S. H. (2020). *Islam and the Liberal State: National Identity and the Future of Muslim Britain*. London: Bloomsbury Publishing.

Kelly, M. P. (2021). 'The relation between the social and the biological and COVID-19'. *Public Health*, 196, 18–23.

Lockyer, B., Islam, S., Rahman, A., Dickerson, J., Pickett, K., Sheldon, T., Wright, J., McEachan, R. and Sheard, L. (2021). 'Understanding COVID-19 misinformation and vaccine hesitancy in context: findings from a qualitative study involving citizens in Bradford, UK'. *Health Expectations*, 24(4), 1158–67.

Macnamara, F. (2021). 'Bradford researchers contribute to major report on smoking in pregnancy'. *Telegraph & Argus*, 27 May, www.thetelegraphandargus.co.uk/news/19334000.bradford-researchers-contribute-major-report-smoking-pregnancy/?ref=twtrec (last accessed 28 April 2022).

Majeed, A. (2005). 'How Islam changed medicine'. *BMJ*, 331, 1486–7.

Marmot, M. (2010). 'Fairer society, healthy lives: the Marmot Review'. Available at: www.parliament.uk/globalassets/documents/fair-society-healthy-lives-full-report.pdf (last accessed 8 July 2022).

Mathijssen, B., McNally, D., Dogra, S., Maddrell, A., Beebeejaun, Y. and McClymont, K. (2021). 'Diverse teams researching diversity: negotiating identity, place and embodiment in qualitative research'. *Qualitative Research*. https://doi.org/10.1177%2F14687941211006004

Michie, S., Atkins, L. and West, R. (2014). *The Behaviour Change Wheel. A Guide to Designing Interventions*. Sutton: Silverback Publishing, pp. 1003–10.

Mir, G. and Sheikh, A. (2010). '"Fasting and prayer don't concern the doctors . . . they don't even know what it is": communication, decision-making and perceived social relations of Pakistani Muslim patients with long-term illnesses'. *Ethnicity & Health*, 15(4), 327–42.

Moosa, E. (2021). *Medicine and Shariah: A Dialogue in Islamic Bioethics*. Notre Dame, IN: University of Notre Dame Press.

Nobles, J., Summerbell, C., Brown, T., Jago, R. and Moore, T. (2021). 'A secondary analysis of the childhood obesity prevention Cochrane Review through a wider determinants of health lens: implications for research funders, researchers, policymakers and practitioners'. *International Journal of Behavioral Nutrition and Physical Activity*, 18(1), 22.

Padela, A. (2021). *Medicine and Shariah: A Dialogue in Islamic Bio-ethics*. Notre Dame, IN: Notre Dame Press.

Qureshi, K., Meer, N. and Hill, S. (2020). 'Different but similar? BAME groups and the impacts of Covid-19 in Scotland', in N. Meer, S. Akhtar and N. Davidson (eds), *Taking Stock*. London: Runnymede, pp. 22–4.

Rai, K. K., Dogra, S. A., Barber, S., Adab, P., Summerbell, C., on behalf of the Childhood Obesity Prevention in Islamic Religious Settings' Programme Management Group (2019). 'A scoping review and systematic mapping of health promotion interventions associated with obesity in Islamic religious settings in the UK'. *Obesity Reviews*, 20(9), 1231–61.

Sarkar, S. (2020). 'Religious discrimination is hindering the covid-19 response'. *BMJ*, 369, m2280.

Shahid, H. and Scott-Baumann, A. (2020). 'An intersectional approach during Covid-19: disaggregating data to protect BAME communities'. SOAS COP Policy Briefings. Available at: https://blogs.soas.ac.uk/cop/wp-content/uploads/2020/04/An-Intersectional-Approach-during-Covid-19-Disaggregating-data-to-protect-BAME.pdf (last accessed 28 April 2022).

Sheikh, A. (2007). 'Should Muslims have faith based health services?' *BMJ*, 334(7584), 74.

Sheridan, E., Wright, J., Small, N., Corry, P. C., Oddie, S., Whibley, C., Petherick, E. S., Malik, T., Pawson, N., McKinney, P. A. and Parslow, R. C. (2013). 'Risk factors for congenital anomaly in a multiethnic birth cohort: an analysis of the Born in Bradford study'. *The Lancet*, 382(9901), 1350–9.

Smith, N. R., Kelly, Y. J. and Nazroo, J. Y. (2012). 'The effects of acculturation on obesity rates in ethnic minorities in England: evidence from the Health Survey for England'. *The European Journal of Public Health*, 22(4), 508–13.

Taylor, K., Elhakeem, A., Thorbjørnsrud Nader, J. L., Yang, T. C., Isaevska, E., Richiardi, L., Vrijkotte, T., Pinot de Moira, A., Murray, D. M., Finn, D., Mason, D., Wright, J., Oddie, S., Roeleveld, N., Harris, J. R., Nybo Andersen, A.-M., Caputo, M. and Lawlor, D. A. (2021). 'Effect of maternal prepregnancy/early-pregnancy body mass index and pregnancy smoking and alcohol on congenital heart diseases: a parental negative control study'. *Journal of the American Heart Association*, 10, e020051.

Younis, T. and Jadhav, S. (2019). 'Islamophobia in the National Health Service: an ethnography of institutional racism in PREVENT's counter-radicalisation policy'. *Sociology of Health & Illness*, 42(3), 610–26.

2

COVID-19, HEALTH INEQUALITIES AND THE LIVED EXPERIENCE OF BRITISH MUSLIMS

Sufyan Abid Dogra, ⓘD *Hina J. Shahid, Salman Waqar, Daniel Bingham, Aamnah Rahman, Stephen Abdullah Maynard, Shadim Hussain and Alison Scott-Baumann*

COVID-19, Health Inequalities and British Muslims

Black and Minority Ethnic (BME) communities have been disproportionately affected by COVID-19: death rates are higher and survival rates are lower, with statistics varying in different BME communities (Public Health England 2020b). BME communities are at risk of higher infection rates and mortality rates due to certain pre-disposed health conditions and living in poorer, overcrowded housing (Meer et al. 2020). These higher infection and mortality rates together with the fear of spreading the virus or catching it from others have caused further distress. Ethnic minorities in Britain have experienced a disproportional impact of COVID-19, as for these groups the pandemic was translated as a syndemic pandemic (Bambra et al. 2020) because of pre-pandemic inequalities on all social determinants of health such as unhealthy dietary practices, poor housing and working conditions, unemployment, poor access to healthcare, high levels of inactivity and discrimination that ethnic minorities and the majority of British Muslims live with.

ⓘD https://orcid.org/0000-0001-9896-9503

✉ Sufyan.Dogra@bthft.nhs.uk

This chapter highlights the disproportionate impact of COVID-19 on British Muslims and how the pandemic exposed prevalent health inequalities in the UK. We critically analyse the discussions around faith in relation to COVID-19, victim blaming, its impacts and the socioeconomic consequences of COVID-19 lockdowns on marginalised British Muslims. We evaluate the vulnerabilities of British Muslims working in the NHS and healthcare and the responses by professional Muslim organisations providing healthcare awareness. We explore the interplay of ethnicity, religion and deprivation in negotiating the particular challenges of living through COVID-19. We critically evaluate and problematise the notions around 'vaccine hesitancy', and question the emphasis on national religious organisations of British Muslims for responses to COVID-19 instead of professional medical organisations or small-scale community-based organisations. We assess the impact of COVID-19 on British Muslim families, children, charity and voluntary organisations, physical activity, mental health and wellbeing, and how British Muslims living in deprived neighbourhoods responded to the pandemic through engaging with community groups. We highlight the work of neighbourhood and community-based organisations and services for healthcare awareness by professional Muslim groups. This chapter also includes multidisciplinary perspectives of academics and practitioners on the pandemic, lockdown, vaccination and subsequent socioeconomic implications of COVID-19 with regard to British Muslims' lived experience.

The Impact of COVID-19 on British Muslims

Unequal and low levels of physical activity in children from British Muslim families and ethnic minorities during COVID-19

'Physical activity' is a simple term that encompasses one of the most complex of human behaviours, which is how and why we move our physical bodies. The most commonly known definition of physical activity – 'any bodily movement produced by skeletal muscles that results in energy expenditure' (Caspersen et al. 1985) – along with its more specifically defined cousin, exercise – 'planned, structured, repetitive, and purposively for improvement of health well-being' (ibid.) – have been the main reference points for the study of human movement in relation to medical and public health research. However, such definitions can be limiting when comprehending what it means to move our bodies throughout our lives, from the cultural importance of dance and celebration, taking part in games and sports, travelling to see friends, being able to get to work or being an asset of our work (in jobs involving manual labour). Experience of physical activity for a child begins during pregnancy and continues from birth, with family, culture and environment shaping the lived experience around it. A newer and broader representative definition of physical activity is 'people moving, acting and performing within culturally specific spaces and contexts, and influenced by a unique array of interests, emotions, ideas, instructions and relationships' (Piggin 2020). Our co-author Dr Daniel Bingham, who has more than a decade of experience in this field, views being physically active as a foundation of basic human dignity. He maintains that the inequalities of physical activity between ethnicities goes beyond standard calculations of minutes of daily physical activity and is related to mental health outcomes (WHO 2018). The inequalities in activity have been exacerbated by the COVID-19 pandemic on the lines of ethnicity and religion in Britain.

Low levels of physical activity of people from ethnic minorities were well documented even before the COVID-19 pandemic. National and international population data reports that up to 80 per cent of children and young people are not sufficiently physically active to ensure good health and wellbeing (i.e. 60 minutes of moderate to vigorous physical activity per day) (Steene-Johannessen et al. 2020; Guthold et al. 2020). There was already an increased concern that levels of inactivity were higher in children from ethnic minority groups, especially those with South Asian and Pakistani heritage (Love et al. 2019; Eyre and Duncan 2013). Such low levels of physical activity place children at risk of poor physical and mental wellbeing and school performance (Bailey et al. 2013; Janssen and Leblanc 2010; Ekelund et al. 2012; Wu et al. 2017; WHO 2018). Such risks are higher and more impactful among children from these ethnic minority backgrounds who already have increased risk and rates of obesity and type 2 diabetes compared to White majority ethnic groups (Nightingale et al. 2009). Although this inequality in physical activity and associated health problems was prevalent before the outbreak of COVID-19, what is concerning is that COVID-19 has hit ethnic minority groups even harder and they are more likely to suffer more than any other group as society recovers over the next decade (Sallis et al. 2020; Van Lancker and Parolin 2020; Douglas et al. 2020).

The Born in Bradford (BiB) study is one of the world's largest research programmes and has tracked and monitored the determinants of health of over 30,000 Bradford residents (parents and children) since 2007 (Wright et al. 2012). BiB had amassed a wealth of knowledge of children from ethnic minority backgrounds before the pandemic began, has been able to track their health and wellbeing during the pandemic and will continue to evaluate the impact of the pandemic on the health and wellbeing trajectories of the children and their families (McEachan et al. 2020). Using BiB data collected before the pandemic and during the first lockdown, Dr Daniel Bingham and colleagues (Bingham et al. 2021) found from a sample of 643 children that the 60 minutes or more a day of moderate to vigorous physical activity recommended by health guidelines reduced for all children by nearly 50 per cent to 69.4 per cent during the first UK-wide lockdown. This is not entirely unsurprising due to the necessary restrictions to everyday life implemented in order to curtail the spread of the virus. However, what was especially concerning was a clear ethnic difference, with White British children reportedly meeting physical activity guidelines more than their peers of Pakistani heritage (34 per cent vs 23 per cent) during the first lockdown, a statistic explained through a large minority of children of Pakistani heritage (40 per cent) reporting that they had not left the house at all in the last week, while a drastically lower percentage of White British children (18 per cent) reported the same. This study did not ask children directly to explain why they had not left the house, but previous studies indicate that the children who took part in this study mostly live in areas of high deprivation, with their mothers reporting numerous difficulties during the spring 2020 lockdown, including a number of insecurities (financial, employment, housing, clinical symptoms of anxiety and depression) and high levels of anxiety about becoming ill or dying from COVID-19 (Dickerson et al. 2020). Anxiety and fear of ill health and death is probably greater within people from of Pakistani heritage, which leads to their not wanting to leave the home environment (Dickerson et al. 2020). It should also be mentioned that negative media reporting on ethnic minorities, particularly those of Muslim faith, who were accused of violating lockdown protocols and government guidelines and spreading the virus (Swerling 2020; Rahim 2020), with no evidence for such claims, could logically lead to a fear of being labelled when outside the home.

COVID-19 and the mental health of British Muslims: findings of the Lateef Project

Sixty-three per cent of healthcare workers who died from COVID-19 were from ethnic minorities (British Medical Association 2021). There is growing evidence of specific mental health consequences from significant COVID-19 infection, with increased rates of not only PTSD, anxiety and depression, but also specific neuropsychiatric symptoms. Given the higher risks of mental illnesses and complex care needs among ethnic minorities and also in deprived inner-city areas, COVID-19 seems to deliver a double blow. Physical and mental health vulnerabilities are inextricably linked, especially as a significant proportion of healthcare workers (including those employed in mental health services) in the UK are from BME groups (King et al. 2021). It is unlikely that ethnicity in itself is the cause of differences in the impact of the pandemic on mental health and wellbeing. Instead, ethnicity may be correlated with other factors that bring about these differences. It remains difficult to draw conclusions about ethnicity, interactions with gender and mental health during the pandemic (Public Health England 2020b). People of the Muslim faith experience poorer recovery rates in improving access to psychological therapies services than any other faith group, as reported in NHS advancing mental health equalities strategy in 2020 (Rethink

2007). It is important to note that only 33 per cent of Muslims would discuss any concerns they had regarding mental health with mental health professionals (Rethink 2007).

Pre-existing racial and socioeconomic inequalities, resulting in disparities in co-morbidities between ethnic groups, have been amplified by the pandemic and significant differences have been revealed in people's ability to cope physically, mentally or economically, to protect themselves or their families and to shield from COVID-19. According to a Runnymede Trust Survey (Haque et al. 2020):

- Black and minority ethnic (BME) people face greater barriers in shielding from coronavirus as a result of the types of employment they hold (BME men and women are over-represented among key worker roles); having to use public transport more; living in overcrowded and multigenerational households more; and not being given appropriate PPE (personal protective equipment) at work.
- One in twenty BME people (5%) have been hospitalised with the virus, compared with one in a hundred white people (1%).
- 15% of black people say they personally knew someone who had died with the virus, with this figure rising to 19% for people of African Caribbean backgrounds.
- BME people are also more likely than white people to live with someone (including children) who may be vulnerable to coronavirus due to a disability or health condition (38% of BME groups vs 31% of white groups).
- Greater proportions of BME key workers (32%) reported that they were not given adequate PPE compared with their white counterparts (20%). Among those in this position, 50% of Bangladeshi, 42% of Pakistani and 41% of Black African respondents reported that they had not been given adequate Personal Protective Equipment (PPE).
- People of Bangladeshi and Black African origin (34% and 33%, respectively), followed closely by people of Pakistani origin (29%), were the most likely to report that they had experienced all of the three forms of racism – racially motivated attack, being treated unfairly because of their ethnicity or an increase in racism/racial abuse since the start of COVID-19.

The Lateef Project provides religiously appropriate mental health services to British Muslims. From August 2020, with minimal advertising the service expanded its service through time-limited funding to work across England with a team of ten part-time Islamic counsellors in recognition of the heightened need. It worked with adults with common mental health problems. The service was offered to those who were COVID-19 bereaved, those whose ongoing mental health problems had been exacerbated by the impact of the pandemic and those with new mental health problems.

For some clients of the Lateef Project, the various lockdowns resulted in continued confinement in an ongoing abusive relationship and with this a worsening of previous mental health conditions, sometimes specifically exacerbating their experiences of PTSD. Such experiences have not been exclusive to female clients, nor have they been exclusively within the traditional model of a singular relationship with an abuser. Violent abusive relationships have been central to the presentations of anxiety in some male clients in lockdown. In some multigenerational households abusive relationships have been further complicated by the client's need to negotiate a number of relationships with abusers simultaneously. Often in these circumstances there have been additional issues regarding the safety or welfare of children. The re-traumatisation of people with previous experiences of PTSD has also been present in a number of clients, specifically issues related to childhood abuse where lockdown has led to the client being confined within the home in which they experienced this abuse.

Income instability has been a concern for a number of professionals leading specifically to pandemic-related issues of anxiety, particularly in relation to locum doctors, teaching staff and pharmacists. There have been job losses among Muslim clients across different income brackets, reflecting the job insecurity that has resulted for the community during the pandemic. In many respects Muslim key workers, irrespective of any underlying previous histories, have often had to address competing needs regarding the risk personally experienced through COVID-19 exposure and isolation as well as attempt to safeguard their families. Where such individuals have been long-term carers there have been experiences of fear or guilt exacerbating anxiety specifically when they have been exposed to COVID-19.

Within multigenerational households there have also been issues of anxiety and anger management in relation to the inconsistent behaviour of family members, leading to multigenerational risks. An additional complication has been the exhaustion, lack of motivation and related depression experienced within the community by individuals who have experienced COVID-19 or long COVID but whose economic need has meant they are unable to isolate or recuperate. Often in concert with depression or anxiety there have been immense feelings of guilt and concern as individuals make decisions that are known to potentially have serious impact, such as going back to work when ill.

COVID-19 and the experiences of British Muslims living in deprivation

COVID-19 lockdowns impacted double-marginalised Muslim communities living in already marginalised Northern England due to a variety of factors such as self-isolation, loss of life, loss of income due to being furloughed or out of work, and not being able to socialise with family and friends who are usually their biggest social support network. Muslims in Northern England are generally from ethnic minority groups and tend to be self-employed and/or own small businesses. Loss of income has been a bigger issue for these communities compared to others as British Muslims were already on the lower end of the economic spectrum (Northern Data Hub 2018). The fact that their social life was curtailed in many respects, such as not being able to participate in the five-times daily congregational prayers at local mosques, Taraweeh (additional voluntary evening prayer during Ramadan), visiting the sick (especially those at end of life) in hospital, saying funeral prayers and taking part in funeral rites or paying condolences for the deceased, was instrumental in creating mental distress for many.

During lockdown, food poverty and the inability to pay for basic essential sanitary products were an issue for those already living in poverty and deprivation. The social stigma associated with receiving food from the food banks operating in the city has enhanced food poverty among South Asian Muslims in particular. In addition, the food banks did not always stock items needed for staple ethnic diets and there was a language barrier in the referral process, both of which contributed to Muslims' further deprivation (Islam et al. 2020). The recent research on COVID-19 carried out by the BiB birth cohort study reveals that 40 per cent of respondents had depression or anxiety (Dickerson et al. 2020). BME communities are at risk of higher infection and mortality rates due to certain predisposed health conditions and living in poorer, overcrowded housing (Meer et al. 2020). On a positive note, whilst West Yorkshire has been identified as one of the hotspots for COVID-19 infection, initial statistics from Bradford Teaching Hospitals NHS Foundation Trust state that BME communities are not disproportionately affected by COVID-19 in Bradford as compared to other cities (Quantrill 2020). This may be attributed to the early closure of mosques and schools, and the stringent self-isolation measures taken before the first national lockdown began in the UK. However, BME hospital admissions state that people from these groups are more unwell and for a longer period of time and this has been attributed to underlying health conditions, poor living conditions and population density in deprived neighbourhoods (Dickerson et al. 2021).

According to a national survey conducted by Muslim Women's Council in the UK (Think Tank Programme 2020), 42 per cent of women reported that COVID-19 had had a detrimental impact on their interpersonal relationships during the first lockdown period. Furthermore, 61 per cent of women reported experiencing stress, anxiety and loneliness during the pandemic. There were other negative impacts on physical health, such as weight gain, lack of exercise, restrictions on movement and difficulty in accessing healthcare.

In addition, 17 per cent of women reported that they had lost their jobs, had their salary reduced or had been furloughed, which impacted negatively on their household financial management, as costs were already higher with children being at home. The biggest challenges for British Muslim women were home-schooling children and being unable to exercise (Dickerson et al. 2021), which led to effects on mental health such as depression, a feeling of being unable to cope with having to adapt to a virtual working environment, and anxieties around social distancing and returning to work. The same survey indicated however that for 86 per cent of British Muslim women, spending more time with family and having time to focus on spirituality was a positive experience of COVID-19, with many respondents stating that during lockdown they had learned how to appreciate life more, experienced an increase in spirituality, had become more patient and had learned new skills. Some women made personal commitments and resolutions, such as being less materialistic, living more modestly, becoming more involved in community affairs and challenging their fears in the future.

BiB research found that COVID-19 and the associated lockdowns affected BME communities significantly due to existing health inequalities and other wider social determinants of health (McEachan et al. 2020). The trust of the public in the NHS and health professionals is paramount to successful vaccination programmes; however, in the case of COVID-19 it has been termed as the 'crisis of trust' (Khurshid 2020).

While the impact of COVID-19 has been disproportionate for ethnic minorities and British Muslims, their response to the pandemic has been phenomenal. In the next sections, we describe the work of small-scale grassroots and local community groups and how they helped individuals, families and communities at the neighbourhood level. We go on to describe the nationwide response by national organisations of Muslim medical professionals and how these organisations were instrumental in providing religious and culture-specific guidelines for British Muslims, shaping their response to COVID-19.

Responses of British Muslims to COVID-19

We present the responses to COVID-19 by two small-scale, local community organisations of British Muslims (the KML Project and the Bradford Foundation Trust) and two national organisations of Muslim health professionals (the Muslim Doctors Association and the British Islamic Medical Association) to capture how the Muslim community and professional associations were, locally and nationally, at the forefront of the COVID-19 response and give an insight into the challenges they faced.

COVID-19 and small-scale neighbourhood and community-based organisations

Small charity and community organisations were impacted profoundly by the COVID-19 pandemic. The crisis itself has reshaped the work that small charities normally undertake. We present two case studies of small- to medium-sized community-based organisations from Bradford and how they adapted their response to COVID-19.

The KML Project

KML is a voluntary organisation set up in 2019 and named after a deceased family member of some Bradford residents (Alam 2019). It provides essential hygiene products such as soap, hand sanitiser and toothbrushes to vulnerable adults including refugees, asylum seekers, women affected by domestic violence and trafficked women and children. This small-scale organisation is 100 per cent reliant on donations for its services and products and is dependent on the goodwill of volunteers to provide services to people in need.

KML had been working in collaboration with fifteen other organisations, but this number started to reduce during the pandemic. This was largely because of the extent of crossover between organisations as the crisis forced other small charities to adapt their services and take on new activities due to increased demand. KML worked with faith centres and food banks to provide services to poor and needy families who were significantly impacted because of lockdown and faith centres being closed. It responded to referrals made by the NHS and local council when they identified a resident or family in need through their own work in tackling hygiene problems.

KML services its users by setting up a table at local food banks once a month, and has found this to be the best way to make donations last longer. The organisation has connections with local supermarkets, such as Morrisons, and receives supplies of personal hygiene products and toiletries. COVID-19 affected the finances of the project, mainly because the number of packs of products distributed tripled due to the city's worsening economic conditions. In addition, panic buying during the first wave of the pandemic had negatively impacted supply, thus raising costs. KML also helped young volunteers to update their CVs to include the voluntary work they did during the pandemic.

The Bradford Foundation Trust

The Bradford Foundation Trust (BFT) helps asylum seekers and refugees who have no recourse to public funds, as well as single parents in the community.

Their *zakat* (compulsory giving for Muslims) distribution programme means that they also have the ability to help any Muslims in distress. Their service users face problems around integration as they are new arrivals in the country, so there are issues with fitting into the community, as well as the main issues of housing and welfare. Poor English-language proficiency means that service users lack confidence and struggle to tackle these issues themselves.

There was a concern as to whether families would be able to understand COVID-19 guidelines and safety information because of language barriers. BFT responded to this by translating NHS advice independently. They also started a befriending telephone service to tackle mental health problems. There was a need to adapt the way funds were raised, so the group launched an internet crowdfunding campaign to raise £10,000 for asylum seekers. They also organised a 'fasting Friday' event where non-Muslims would fast to improve integration among the community during COVID-19 and ran a forum for asylum-seeker organisations with the aim of keeping members informed about the COVID-19 situation.

BFT helps clients to find suitable housing by contacting the local authority on their behalf. In situations where a private landlord is involved the organisation will often try to negotiate for them. In emergencies they will also deliver food parcels. In order to boost the confidence of service users, pre-pandemic the organisation would host social gatherings, for example a 'monthly mingle' so that issues of isolation and loneliness could be tackled. Importantly, it also acts as a signpost to other similar facilities across the city, such as social service organisations.

BFT is funded by private donors, council funds and through the National Lottery. The organisation has maximised all funding access points and crowdfunding sources. During COVID-19, it was challenging to complete the detailed funding applications required, as the language used was difficult for small charity organisations to understand and respond to. They received information on available COVID-19 funds after the deadlines expired. They believe that COVID-19 funds were being allocated based on track record and relationships with authorities to the established organisations working regionally or nationally.

COVID-19 and national organisations of British Muslim health professionals

The Muslim Doctors Association: research, advocacy and community empowerment

The Muslim Doctors Association & Allied Health Professionals CIC (MDA) is a non-profit organisation established in 2004 as a voluntary organisation serving the health needs of the local community in Luton. It has grown into a national organisation with three main areas of work: (1) empowering Muslim, minority and marginalised communities to optimise health outcomes through outreach campaigns; (2) research and advocacy on health issues affecting these communities to inform policy reform; and (3) improving diversity and inclusion in the NHS to support compassionate workplaces with a specific focus on eliminating Islamophobia. Drawing on over fifteen years of outreach work nationally with the British Muslim community, MDA has used a multilevel framework driven by community wisdom during the pandemic to mitigate the risks and impact of the pandemic on the community, predicting early on the disproportionate impact that the pandemic would have on the community. The following are the four key areas on which MDA focused their COVID-19 response to inform and shape policy towards COVID-19 in relation to British Muslims.

Community wisdom

The rich community insights drawn from lived experiences have been vital in shaping MDA's policy, advocacy and community empowerment response. At a time when most of the discourse was centred on biological explanations for disparities, MDA was among the first to explain the multilevel disadvantages and discrimination embodied by Muslim communities in contributing to unequal impact from COVID-19 in the UK, integrating structural, social, cultural and biological explanations, as shown in Figure 2.1. Further synthesising literature on pre-exist-

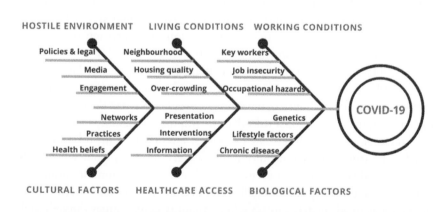

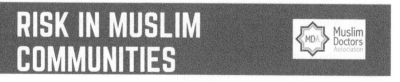

Figure 2.1 Multilevel framework for excess COVID-19 risk in Muslim communities.

ing health inequalities in the British Muslim community with community wisdom, MDA published its first report on health disparities from COVID-19 in the British Muslim community in May 2020 (MDA 2020a). This was followed by a second report, published by the Centre for Muslim Policy and Research, to which MDA contributed, highlighting specific risk factors and policy recommendations (CMPR 2020).

Evidence-based advocacy and engagement

Using a multilevel framework as an advocacy tool, MDA worked with a range of partners including academia, government, NHS and Public Health England, and third-sector organisations to encourage whole system transformation focused on community-led, culturally and contextually sensitive solutions. Through policy briefings in a project with SOAS University of London linking academia with Westminster, MDA highlighted the need for an intersectional rights-based approach and disaggregating data on ethnicity and faith (Shahid and Scott-Baumann 2020b), the role of religion-based discrimination in contributing to unequal outcomes from COVID-19, and proposed a syndemic model necessary to understand and respond to the multiple and overlapping health needs of the British Muslim community during the pandemic and beyond (Shahid and Scott-Baumann 2020a).

In addition to written submissions MDA engaged with government, policy and system leaders to provide oral evidence to advocate for policy reform and ethical and sustainable community-based approaches, emphasising the role of Islamophobia as a form of structural discrimination and oppression and as a fundamental cause of health disparities among British Muslims. MDA contributed to the Public Health England report on PHE disparities (Public Health England 2020b) in which many recommendations aligned with MDA's policy recommendations, the Labour-commissioned Lawrence Review (Lawrence 2020) highlighting the intersectional risks that the Muslim community faces embodying structural, social and healthcare inequities, and presented the role of religion as a determinant of health outcomes at the Conservative Party Conference 2020. MDA formed advocacy coalition groups with other ethnic minority healthcare organisations to hold to account policy and decision makers and government in their failings to adequately protect ethnic minority communities through multiple letters and roundtable events.

Early in the pandemic, members from the Muslim community reported the difficulties they experienced in self isolating due to a lack of income protection and highlighted the 'lives versus livelihood' dilemma they faced. MDA advocated for income protection which helped influence the policy of £500 being offered to people from low-income households who were isolating. Additionally,

MDA supported and won a legal challenge against the government to provide health and safety protection to gig economy workers, a large proportion of whom are from ethnic minority backgrounds. Furthermore, as a significant proportion of people from the Muslim community are born overseas (ONS 2020), MDA highlighted the disproportionate impact that the current hostile policy environment towards migrants would have on these communities accessing healthcare, which contributed to public health communications emphasising that COVID-19 related care is free at the point of care.

Death and discrimination on the frontline

Muslim healthcare workers have been disproportionately impacted during the pandemic. During the first wave, MDA collated data based on media reports and crowdsourced community knowledge on the Muslim doctors who had died from COVID-19, creating a digital gallery to commemorate and honour their sacrifice and legacy (MDA 2020a). Preliminary analysis reveals that up to 60 per cent of doctors who died on the frontline were Muslim, despite making up only 10 per cent of the medical workforce (NHS Digital 2016). MDA contributed to a large ITV survey (Morgan 2020) in which over 50 per cent of over 2,000 respondents were Muslim which, together with insights from the frontline, demonstrated the role of bullying, harassment, discrimination, unfair deployment to high-risk areas, lack of access to culturally appropriate PPE and risk assessments, and lack of access to testing in contributing to excess deaths among Muslim doctors. MDA also highlighted the stress and burnout faced by Muslim doctors and the lack of culturally sensitive psychological support available.

In a series of roundtables with stakeholders in the NHS, MDA raised concerns around the need for culturally sensitive PPE and risk assessments, which were taken on board and implemented. Additionally, MDA provided safe spaces for colleagues to discuss their experiences through virtual mental health cafés and created a toolkit for mental health support for Muslim healthcare workers. MDA also contributed to prayer guidance for Muslim NHS staff (NHS Muslim Network 2021) to support employers to better understand and accommodate prayer requests as an important part of psychospiritual wellbeing. MDA highlighted the need to include discrimination and bullying support for GPs as part of the annual NHS GP Appraisal in response to a consultation on how to provide more inclusive appraisals for staff from ethnic minority backgrounds. MDA also campaigned for vaccine priority for ethnic minority healthcare staff and a reduction in the 12-week schedule.

Shifting discourse

MDA's advocacy centring the role of religion as a neglected protected characteristic and important determinant of health has contributed to shifting the narrative on racial disparities to a more intersectional approach that includes culture and religion and has also challenged epistemic racism inherent in evidence-based medicine and healthcare evaluation that delegitimises lived experiences (Shahid and Waqar 2020). MDA has written and contributed to articles (Shahid 2020b) and blogs, and has delivered webinars to health and social care professionals on recognising and understanding the role of Islamophobia, structural discrimination and racism in contributing to health disparities among the Muslim community and how to eliminate these through combining interpersonal actions based on cultural humility and recognising privilege and bias with system change.

MDA has highlighted the negative media reporting on the Muslim community as a structural driver of health disparities, outlining the ways in which divisive scapegoating narratives create stigma, impede access to healthcare, contribute to community transmission and undermine public health efforts, worsening health disparities (Mahase 2020). MDA has used its research and policy analyses to challenge and provide an evidence-based counter-narrative to the cultural stereotyping of the Muslim community and has been involved with advising journalists across mainstream channels on the need for positive and destigmatised media reporting. During Eid al-Adha 2020, MDA ran a national campaign to commemorate all the NHS Heroes (MDA 2020b) who had died on the frontline across mosques by reading prayers for the deceased, as a mark of respect and appreciation which was covered by the national media, and united with other faith groups on the 70th anniversary of the founding of the NHS to celebrate the work of faith-based organisations during the pandemic.

Hidden work and future directions of MDA

MDA's current focus areas are: building a digital platform for social prescribing and community resources as a one-stop portal to access faith, cultural and linguistically sensitive information for the Muslim community on health and its wider determinants; and promoting sustainable whole-system transformation centred on community empowerment, ethical resourcing and cultural humility, especially as ethnic disparities in mental health and chronic disease are predicted to worsen post-pandemic. While doing this MDA continues to hold decision makers to account through advocacy that is driven by community wisdom and principles of public health and human rights, centring the voices of marginalised and stigmatised Muslim communities whose health needs have been neglected for too long. It continues to campaign for faith and disaggregated data to be routinely collected and published for all health outcomes across the healthcare system.

Advocacy work is however invisibilised in grant-making processes and funding models which focus predominantly on immediate tangible outcomes rather than long-term structural changes. Authentic advocacy requires complex, difficult and nuanced negotiations and dialogue that take place out of the public view and continuous sustained efforts which are difficult to quantify; direct cause and effect can be difficult to demonstrate in multi-component interventions. However, a multi-system response which addresses upstream drivers of health outcomes is essential to meaningfully address disparities. This has been highlighted by MDA's work during the pandemic where a notable change in policy and discourse has been observed with widespread societal benefit. However, the work of community-based organisations cannot continue to rely on goodwill exploitation and cultural taxation of minoritised groups who are desperate to change the unjust and unequal systems that govern their lives. This hidden work needs to be recognised and adequately resourced and supported to truly amplify voices, empower the health and wellbeing of Muslim communities, and hold to account those whose decisions shape the lives of millions.

British Islamic Medical Association and COVID-19 response

The British Islamic Medical Association (BIMA) is a non-profit, volunteer-led and -delivered, national democratic membership body of Muslim healthcare professionals in Britain. For many years BIMA has been conducting health promotion activities with its members in mosques and with Muslim faith leaders, as well as advocating for the needs of Muslim communities in public policy. BIMA's approach has been to bring a health agenda delivered by known and trusted local health professionals into their own community spaces. BIMA is also an affiliate of the Muslim Council of Britain (MCB) and the Federation of Islamic Medical Associations (FIMA) and enjoys close links with many of the main Muslim charities, activist groups and scholarly bodies. These relationships with grassroots Muslim leaders, mosques and community voices proved to be pivotal during the COVID-19 response both at home and abroad.

Prior to COVID-19, the literature made clear that British Muslims were more likely to report poor health, have higher rates of metabolic disease, live in multigenerational housing and have frequent extended social contacts – all of which were to put them at an increased risk of adverse events during a pandemic. As BIMA saw the devastating toll of COVID-19 on Italy in mid-March 2020, it became clear to healthcare practitioners and public health experts that Britain was a few days behind and would be following the same trajectory. The British Muslim community would be hit harder and had to act quickly if lives were to be saved.

BIMA first wrote guidance for the Muslim community on 6 March 2020, highlighting these risk factors and the possibility of suspending communal activities. This guidance also encouraged mosques to take proactive steps to establish lines of communication with local public health experts, combat fake news and develop contingency plans. A further guidance document was issued six days later with the MCB, stating explicitly that congregational activity was likely to be suspended, recommending the establishment of support systems for vulnerable members of the congregation, and reinforcing hand hygiene and social distancing advice.

On 16 March 2020, one week before the UK Government announced lockdown, BIMA wrote an open letter to the Muslim community urging 'that it is unsafe and harmful to continue business as usual, or even with significant adjustments'. The same day the MCB wrote to affiliates quoting BIMA's position and took the unprecedented step of asking for the suspension of congregational activity in mosques, which was quickly heeded by mosques across the UK. Leading up to this statement, BIMA was engaged in an intense nationwide community engagement with scholarly bodies, representatives of mosques and local leaders to help them understand the scientific and public health aspects of the pandemic. These conversations were mostly outside the public eye and allowed for robust and critical conversations to take place.

The COVID-19 pandemic put BIMA in a leading role for the Muslim community. Under the MCB, several COVID-19 Response Groups (CRGs) were created which focused on various elements that were of importance to British Muslims, with BIMA leading the Medical CRG and having a strong steer on other areas. During the first lockdown, in spring 2020, the MCB hosted weekly briefings where BIMA appraised the latest evidence and contextualised the public health messaging to our communities. The Mental Health CRG also brought together various Muslim mental health organisations and delivered regular webinars.

As COVID-19 raged on, one of the concerns from Muslim communities was around the religio-cultural customs in sickness and death, due to the difficulties in managing the surge of admissions and care bring rationalised. These included worries around hospital visitation, burials and funerary rites, and end-of-life care. BIMA produced flyers to help patients and communities navigate the stressful experience of not being able to contact relatives who were admitted with COVID-19, dying at home or being refused intensive care – recognising that health experiences were already poor in these communities – as well as producing videos to explain palliative care, why care is rationed and how end-of-life care can be arranged in the community. These resources were novel and welcomed by the palliative care community and hospices, and were also translated into Arabic.

Ramadan started one month into the first lockdown in the UK and was a nervous time for the Muslim community. For the first time there would be no congregational night prayers or sharing of iftar meals, and questions were also being asked about the safety of fasting during a pandemic. BIMA quickly organised a rapid evidence review and published a pioneering Ramadan Rapid Review that provided guidance for clinicians in managing chronic diseases and acute illness in Ramadan; many of these sections are published in high-quality peer-reviewed journals and endorsed by specialist medical societies. For the public, a series of Health Ramadan videos were also created to help with common queries, and videos on mental health in lockdown were also produced in response to demand from the community. With Ramadan and Eid being highly social events, there was a strong community-led response to #StayAtHomeThisEid with BIMA producing several social media assets and providing credible Muslim health professional voices. Later research found that there was no increase in COVID-19 mortality amongst British Muslims during Ramadan 2020.

As the UK emerged from its first lockdown in the summer of 2020, BIMA worked closely with the MCB to produce a nine-step guidance document on re-opening mosques safely. Many other policy documents were issued later, covering a range of issues such as roadmaps out of lockdown, dealing with COVID-19 in mosques, burial guidance, new variants, and celebrating Eid and Ramadan safely.

As winter came, attention turned towards COVID-19 vaccination. In September 2020, BIMA had already launched a campaign called Operation Vaccination, in partnership with the MCB, the NHS Muslim Network and the British Board of Scholars and Imams. This was aiming to increase the uptake of influenza vaccination among adults and children and was especially important as childhood vaccination rates in some Muslim communities were very low. This was in part due to the inequity of not providing a non-porcine derived alternative influenza vaccine in England and Wales, unlike in Northern Ireland and Scotland, and since overturned because of COVID-19 and lobbying by BIMA. The conversations in the community started as the flu season kicked off allowing Muslim populations to be primed for the later conversations around COVID-19 vaccination.

Furthermore, knowing that some elements of the Muslim community would be vulnerable to disinformation and conspiracy from the historic sociopolitical isolation and marginalisation of Muslims in Britain, BIMA sought to quickly produce a public health information campaign to deconstruct the false narratives that were emerging around COVID-19. The highly popular 'Answering the Myth' series was very well received by Muslim communities and helped deconstruct some of the popular anti-vax stories. The series was also heavily promoted by the NHS, local government and public health bodies. It was also translated into fourteen languages and was used in various campaigns abroad to help with COVID-19 and vaccine misinformation.

In January 2021, the UK faced another crisis with a third lockdown looming and congregational activities being suspended once more. BIMA wrote again to the community, in an open letter explaining the situation and highlighting options for mosques to make informed decisions and encouraging them to continue their efforts with supporting the COVID-19 vaccination programme. Towards the end of January, BIMA started encouraging mosques to sign up as COVID-19 vaccination centres – an offer which dozens of centres took up and formed a vital part of increasing confidence and ensuring underserved communities had access to the vaccine.

Ramadan 2021 coincided with the rollout of the UK's COVID-19 vaccination programme. Like before, British Muslims were targeted with misinformation about the ingredients of the COVID-19 vaccines in the UK market and around the permissibility of being vaccinated whilst fasting. For the first time in the pandemic, BIMA received funding from a public body. NHS England supported BIMA to produce a video on vaccination and Ramadan featuring prominent UK Muslim scholars and funded a hotline for Muslim NHS staff who had questions about vaccination. BIMA was also supported by Facebook, who selected the organisation as one of their global partners in supporting equitable access to COVID-19 vaccines.

BIMA also had several high-profile engagements with the UK Chief Medical Officer Prof. Chris Whitty, vaccines minister Nadhim Zahawi MP, Secretary of State for Health and Social Care Matt Hancock MP and HRH Prince Charles during the COVID-19 pandemic. Several UK Government departments, such as the Foreign Commonwealth Office, Department for Digital, Culture, Media and Sport, and the Department of Health and Social Care also collaborated with BIMA on projects, ranging from addressing COVID-19 misinformation to helping pilot lateral flow tests in areas of high Muslim populations. Throughout the COVID-19 vaccine rollout, BIMA organised over 150 webinars with grassroots Muslim organisations, appeared in over fifty news shows, had over 150 media articles mentioning its work and worked with at least ten other countries across the world in creating their own CRGs and disseminating information to Muslim communities abroad.

Critical issues on representation and projection of British Muslims during COVID-19

Representing British Muslims during the COVID-19 response

British academics and health practitioners (Al-Astewani 2021) often overestimate and unnecessarily privilege the MCB or other national religious organisations as authoritative bodies of British Muslims dictating and defining British Muslims' response to COVID-19 or other issues concerning their wellbeing. This tendency to glorify and privilege these organisations often overlooks and ignores the meaningful and tangible response to COVID-19 made by neighbourhood or community-based organisations affiliated with mosques or madrassas, and those working in deprived neighbourhoods among disadvantaged communities across the UK.

Small or medium-sized neighbourhood or community-based organisations of British Muslims work with a religious ethos and enjoying a direct relationship of exchange, reciprocity and active involvement with ordinary British Muslims in matters concerning their everyday lives. However, their contributions are often ignored at the expense of priority given to national religious or political organisations of British Muslims. Equally, the work and impact of national organisations of British Muslim health professionals goes unnoticed when more media attention is given to national religious or political organisations. We look at this pattern critically and emphasise highlighting the role of small-scale and national organisations of British Muslim health professionals more than national religious or political organisations in response to COVID-19.

The unwarranted privileging of national religious organisations and placing authority with them in relation to the response to COVID-19 or other issues concerning the wellbeing of British Muslims has unintended consequences. First, it compromises the spirit of authority in Islam which is vested in the Qur'an and Sunnah and how these translate into the everyday lives of British Muslims as there is no space for papal authority in Islam (something that national religious and political organisations often aspire to imitate). Second, it silences the public promotion and vitality of the good work done by neighbourhood and community-based organisations that live with and are from within British Muslim communities, whose work makes a huge difference in the everyday lives of children and young people, families and derived communities, unlike national religious or political organisations of British Muslims who are mostly busy talking, representing, gatekeeping, and safeguarding certain vested interests directly or indirectly. Third, the unnecessary privileging of the responses of national religious or political organisations takes public attention and focus away from real-life issues such as education, health, mental health, housing, unemployment, youth violence, domestic abuse, political participation, drugs and antisocial behaviour, access to green spaces and so on. Professional or small-scale organisations of British Muslims strive to make a difference in these areas whereas national religious or political organisations will deflect the focus on these issues towards the epiphenomenon of Islam or politicisation of deprivation. Fourth, national religious organisations through their apologetic responses limit the scope of public debates on issues such as the COVID-19 response within liberal and/or neo-liberal political debates in the mainstream media and the public sphere by deflecting the narratives towards extremism and securitisation in relation to British Muslims instead of locating the disproportionate impact of COVID-19 on British Muslims and ethnic minorities within the scope of inequalities they experience in their in daily lives. Finally, national religious organisations sometimes express partisan views favouring any particular political party in Britain which compromises the interests of British Muslims.

We believe that national organisations such as the MDA and BIMA are well placed and better equipped to respond to COVID-19, policy debates around the pandemic and other issues concerning the health and wellbeing of British Muslims. It is for that reason that we chose to focus on the experience and response to COVID-19 by professional Muslim groups of medics and neighbourhood or community-based organisations of British Muslims, how they were impacted by the pandemic and what difference they made in the responses to COVID-19 for ordinary British Muslims living in deprivation.

The problematic use of the term 'vaccine hesitancy' and victim blaming by academics and researchers

The internalisation of racist stereotypes and promotion of dismissive attitudes towards ethnic minorities during the pandemic among applied health researchers, academics and health promotion managers led to the causes of ill health to be attributed to and associated with markers of identity such as the ethnicity and religion of people living with disadvantages. Recent research on low or delayed uptake of the COVID-19 vaccine among ethnic minorities was called 'vaccine hesitancy' by academics and applied health researchers (Lockyer et al. 2021), with the term used by a number of people in counterproductive ways, resulting in the fuelling of racist narratives in the popular media. The ways in which ethnic minorities made an informed choice on getting vaccinated were framed, conceptualised and projected as them being 'vaccine hesitant'. This epistemicidal take from academics and applied health researchers buttresses the resurgence of the neo-eugenics mindset of knowledge production (see Chapter 1) during the pandemic. This mindset in applied health research conveniently blames ethnic minorities living with disadvantages for being 'hesitant' in saving the lives of their loved ones, viewing members of these groups as victims of conspiracy theories when they expressed their doubts and concerns on the way government and major pharmaceutical companies were handling COVID-19. In recent studies (Lockyer et al. 2021; Dickerson et al. 2021), applied health researchers interpreted the responses of community members living in deprivation by taking an epistemicidal academic and analytical position. Equally, the academic analysis on COVID-19 vaccine hesitancy happened to be politically buttressing racist narratives on vaccine uptake among ethnic minorities during the pandemic.

Equally, this neo-eugenics mindset, reflected in the works of some academics and applied health researchers, ignores how the doubts and concerns of ethnic minorities and British Muslims have deep roots in the structural inequalities and historical experiences of discrimination and racism. It is unfair to locate these doubts and concerns of communities living in deprivation in their individual choices, lifestyles, social capital or worldviews.

Ironically, researchers in applied health would generally use the term 'low uptake' or 'fidelity' instead of 'hesitancy' for other health interventions aimed at the majority British population when these interventions receive less approval or acceptance among the targeted audience. The implications of neo-eugenics inspired knowledge production processes during the pandemic reinforce the regimes of bodily control by policy makers and practitioners who view ethnic minorities and disadvantaged populations as passive recipients of interventions and would prefer to dub their concerns as 'irrational' and having no place in the modern world, believing they should be criminalised or penalised. Generally, research on the problematic use of the jargon 'vaccine hesitancy' in relation to ethnic minorities is conducted by teams with no representation or involvement of researchers or academics from an ethnic minority background. Some publications on vaccine hesitancy involved researchers from ethnic minority backgrounds who happened to be co-authors but were not leading the research projects. We argue that diversity among research teams who are publishing on ethnic minorities can help avoid interpretations of findings that reinforce 'victim blaming' by academia in the name of scientific knowledge production. We believe diverse research teams contribute to a better understanding of complex social phenomena (Mathijssen et al. 2021), such as ethnic minorities' and British Muslims' experience of the pandemic.

A Way Forward

Analysis reveals that equality, diversity and inclusion in the workplace are clearly still predicated upon White male presumptions of selfhood and are thus perforce blind to disadvantages imposed by racism and other discriminatory mechanisms (Scott-Baumann et al. 2019a). This phenomenon can be clearly seen on university campuses: the biggest data sets yet collected demonstrate the ways in which people of colour are considered to have views less worthy of attention than the views of their White contemporaries, leading to a form of epistemic injustice, of not being heard (Scott-Baumann et al. 2020). In addition, as this book shows, COVID-19 exaggerates these existing systemic disadvantages and thereby clearly reveals the racial and ethnic injustices that create cracks and fault lines through our country (Atewologun et al. 2019). Having shown the epistemic injustices that play out on campus, we are in a better position to recognise and explain them when people of colour or of a recognisable faith, mainly Muslims, are denied the PPE they request or have their concerns about risk dismissed (Shahid and Scott-Baumann 2020b).

This pandemic is set to continue for some years yet and a simple four-point plan is urgently needed to transform the situation for Muslims and other minority groups (Scott-Baumann 2010):

1. Test, track and trace systems must be made efficient and a system of compensation should be in place to ensure that those who are infected with COVID-19 do actually stay off work
2. All training programmes for teachers and health workers must include clear education in anti-discrimination, unconscious bias, conflict resolution and assertiveness training.
3. Reciprocal mentoring (already used to an extent by the NHS) must be introduced to cut through hierarchies by pairing senior and junior staff, especially those of colour. Reciprocal mentoring breaks down the barriers of privilege by facilitating conversations in which entrenched personal views can be challenged and replaced with a more balanced, negotiated understanding of career development.
4. Development is needed of relatively new and further career pathways such as chaplaincy in health services to improve dialogue and understanding between those of faith and those of none in workplaces and places of study.

References

Alam, Y. (2019). 'Project aims to tackle hygiene poverty "crisis"'. *Telegraph & Argus*, 30 December, www.thetelegraphandargus.co.uk/news/18125190.project-aims-tackle-hygiene-poverty-crisis (last accessed 28 April 2022).

Al-Astewani, A. (2021). 'To open or close? Covid-19, mosques and the role of religious authority within the British Muslim community: a socio-legal analysis'. *Religions*, 12(1), 11.

Atewologun, D., Kline, R. and Ochieng, M. (2019). 'Reducing disproportionality in fitness to practise concerns reported to the GMC'. Available at: www.gmc-uk.org/-/media/documents/fair-to-refer-report_pdf-79011677.pdf (last accessed 8 July 2022).

Bailey, R., Hillman, C., Arent, S. and Petitpas, A. (2013). 'Physical activity: an underestimated investment in human capital?' *Journal of Physical Activity and Health*, 10(3), 289–308.

Bambra, C., Riordan, R., Ford, J. and Matthews, F. (2020). 'The COVID-19 pandemic and health inequalities'. *Journal of Epidemiology and Community Health*, 74(11), 964–8.

Bingham, D. D., Daly-Smith, A., Hall, J., Seims, A., Dogra, S. A., Fairclough, S. A., Ajebon, M., Kelly, B., Hou, B., Shire, K. A., Crossley, K. L., Mon-Williams, M., Wright, J., Pickett, K., McEachan, R., Dickerson, J. and Barber, S. E. (2021). 'Covid-19 lockdown: ethnic differences in children's self-reported physical activity and the importance of leaving the home environment. A longitudinal and cross-sectional study from the Born in Bradford birth cohort study'. medRxiv. https://doi.org/10.1101/2021.02.26.21252543

British Medical Association (2021). 'COVID-19: the risk to BAME doctors'. Available at: www.bma.org.uk/advice-and-support/COVID-19/your-health/COVID-19-the-risk-to-bame-doctors (last accessed 29 April 2022).

Caspersen, C. J., Powell, K. E. and Christenson, G. M. (1985). 'Physical activity, exercise, and physical fitness: definitions and distinctions for health-related research'. *Public Health Reports*, 100(2), 126–31.

Centre for Muslim Policy and Research (2020). 'Impact of COVID-19 on the Muslim community: analysis of key risk factors'. Available at: https://cmpr.org.uk/wp-content/uploads/2020/11/20201123-COVID19-and-the-Impact-on-the-Muslim-Community_vF-.pdf (last accessed 29 April 2022).

Dickerson, J., Kelly, B., Lockyer, B., Bridges, S., Cartwright, C., Willan, K., Shire, K., Crossley, K., Bryant, M., Sheldon, T. A., Lawlor, D. A., Wright, J., McEachan, R. R. C. and Pickett, K. E., on behalf of the Bradford Institute for Health Research Covid- 9 Scientific Advisory Group (2020). 'Experiences of lockdown during the COVID-19 pandemic: descriptive findings from a survey of families in the Born in Bradford study, version 1'. *Wellcome Open Research*, 5, 228. Available at: https://doi.org/10.12688/wellcomeopenres.16317.1 (last accessed 29 April 2022).

Dickerson, J., Lockyer, B., Moss, R. H., Endacott, C., Kelly, B., Bridges, S., Crossley, K. L., Bryant, M., Sheldon, T. A., Wright, J., Pickett, K. E., McEachan, R. R. C., Bradford Institute for Health Research COVID-19 Scientific Advisory Group (2021). 'COVID-19 vaccine hesitancy in an ethnically diverse community: descriptive findings from the Born in Bradford study'. *Wellcome Open Research*, 6, 23. Available at: https://wellcomeopenresearch.org/articles/6-23/v2 (last accessed 29 April 2022).

Douglas, M., Katikireddi, S. V., Taulbut, M., McKee, M. and McCartney, G. (2020). 'Mitigating the wider health effects of covid-19 pandemic response'. *BMJ*, 369, m1557.

Ekelund, U., Luan J., Sherar, L. B., Esliger, D. W., Griew, P. and Cooper, A. (2012). 'Moderate to vigorous physical activity and sedentary time and cardiometabolic risk factors in children and adolescents'. *JAMA*, 307(7), 704–12.

Eyre, E. L. J. and Duncan, M. J. (2013). 'The impact of ethnicity on objectively measured physical activity in children'. *ISRN Obesity*, 4, 757431.

Guthold, R., Stevens, G. A., Riley, L. M. and Bull, F. C. (2020). Global trends in insufficient physical activity among adolescents: a pooled analysis of 298 population-based surveys with 1.6 million participants'. *The Lancet Child & Adolescent Health*, 4(1), 23–35.

Haque, Z., Bécares, L. and Treloar, N. (2020). 'Over-exposed and under-protected – the devastating impact of COVID-19 on Black and minority ethnic communities in Great Britain'. A Runnymede Trust and ICM Survey. Available at: https://assets-global.website-files.com/61488f992b58e687f1108c7c/61c31c9d268b932bd064524c_Runnymede%20Covid19%20Survey%20report%20v3.pdf (last accessed 29 April 2022).

Islam, S., Albert, A., Haklay, M. and McEachan, R. (2020). 'Nothing about us without us'. Available at: https://actearly.org.uk/wp-content/uploads/2022/03/Co-production-Strategy-May-2022-V3.pdf (last accessed 7 July 2022).

Janssen, I. and Leblanc, A. G. (2010). 'Systematic review of the health benefits of physical activity and fitness in school-aged children and youth'. *International Journal of Behavioral Nutrition and Physical Activity*, 7, 40.

Khurshid, A. (2020). 'Applying blockchain technology to address the crisis of trust during the COVID-19 pandemic'. *JMIR Medical Informatics*, 8(9), e20477.

King, C., Bennett, M., Fulford, K. W. M., Clarke, S., Gillard, S., Bergqvist, A. and Richardson, J. (2021). 'From preproduction to coproduction: COVID-19, whiteness, and making black mental health matter'. *The Lancet Psychiatry*, 8, 2, 93–5.

Lawrence, D. (2020). 'An avoidable crisis. The disproportionate impact of Covid-19 on Black, Asian and minority ethnic communities'. Available at: www.lawrencereview.co.uk (last accessed 29 April 2022).

Lockyer, B., Islam, S., Rahman, A., Dickerson, J., Pickett, K., Sheldon, T., Wright, J., McEachan, R. and Sheard, L. (2021). 'Understanding COVID-19 misinformation and vaccine hesitancy in context: findings from a qualitative study involving citizens in Bradford, UK'. *Health Expectations*, 24(4), 1158–67.

Love, R., Adams, J., Atkin, A. and van Sluijs, E. (2019). 'Socioeconomic and ethnic differences in children's vigorous intensity physical activity: a cross-sectional analysis of the UK Millennium Cohort Study'. *BMJ Open*, 9(5): e027627.

Mahase, E. (2020). 'COVID-19: Tighter restrictions imposed in the north of England as cases spike'. *BMJ*, 370, m3066.

Mathijssen, B., McNally, D., Dogra, S., Maddrell, A., Beebeejaun, Y. and McClymont, K. (2021). 'Diverse teams researching diversity: Negotiating identity, place and embodiment in qualitative research'. *Qualitative Research*, 14687941211006004. https://doi.org/10.1177/14687941211006004

McEachan, R. R. C., Dickerson, J., Bridges, S., Bryant, M., Cartwright, C., Islam, S., Lockyer, B., Rahman, A., Sheard, L., West, J., Lawlor, D. A., Sheldon, T. A., Wright, J. and Pickett, K. E., on behalf of the Bradford Institute for Health Research COVID-19 Scientific Advisory Group (2020). 'The Born in Bradford COVID-19 research study: protocol for an adaptive mixed methods research study to gather actionable intelligence on the impact of COVID-19 on health inequalities amongst families living in Bradford'. *Wellcome Open Research*, 5, 191.

Meer, N., Qureshi, K., Kasstan, B. and Hill, S. (2020). 'The UK COVID-19 response ignores impact of social inequalities'. Blogs.ED. University of Edinburgh. Available at: https://blogs.ed.ac.uk/COVID-19perspectives/2020/05/01/the-social-determinants-of-COVID-19-and-blame-disproportionality-by-nasar-meer-kaveri-qureshi-ben-kasstan-and-sarah-hill (last accessed 29 April 2022).

Moore, L. (2021). 'We must do more to protect Muslim women in the UK'. Available at: https://publicpolicyprojects.com/newsdit-article/340abd2655757863edc1260eb5c66b65/we-must-do-more-to-protect-muslim-women-in-the-uk (last accessed 29 April 2022).

Morgan, E. (2020). '"Discrimination" on frontline of coronavirus outbreak may be factor in disproportionate BAME deaths among NHS staff'. ITV News, 13 May. Available at: www.itv.com/news/2020-05-13/discrimination-front-line-coronavirus-covid19-black-minority-ethnic-bame-deaths-nhs-racism (last accessed 29 April 2022).

Muslim Council of Britain (2015). 'British Muslims in numbers: a demographic, socio-economic and health profile of Muslims in Britain drawing on the 2011 census'. Available at: https://www.mcb.org.uk/wp-content/uploads/2015/02/MCBCensusReport_2015.pdf (last accessed 29 April 2022).

Muslim Doctors Association (2020a). 'Rapid review of excess burden on Muslim communities from COVID-19'. Available at: https://muslimdoctors.org/wp-content/uploads/2021/02/Impact-of-COVID-19-on-the-Muslim-Community.pdf (last accessed 29 April 2022).

Muslim Doctors Association (2020b). 'Muslims commemorate NHS workers on Eid al Adha'. Available at: https://muslimdoctors.org/muslim-nhs-heroes (last accessed 29 April 2022).

Nazroo, J. and Bécares, L. (2021). 'Ethnic inequalities in COVID-19 mortality: a consequence of persistent racism'. Runnymede/CoDE briefing. Available at: www.runnymedetrust.org/publications/ethnic-inequalities-in-covid-19-mortality-a-consequence-of-persistent-racism (last accessed 29 April 2022).

NHS (2020). 'Advancing mental health equalities strategy'. Available at: www.england.nhs.uk/publication/advancing-mental-health-equalities-strategy (last accessed 29 April 2022).

NHS Digital (2016). 'Hospital and Community Health Services (HCHS) workforce statistics: equality and diversity in NHS Trusts and CCGs in England'. Available at: https://digital.nhs.uk/data-and-information/publications/statistical/independent-healthcare-provider-workforce-statistics (last accessed 8 July 2022).

NHS Muslim Network (2021). 'Islamic prayers: guidance for NHS staff and managers'. Available at: https://nhsmuslimnetwork.co.uk/prayer-time-guidance (last accessed 29 April 2022).

Nightingale, C. M., Rudnicka, A. R., Owen, C. G., Cook, D. G. and Whincup, P. H. (2009). 'Patterns of adiposity and obesity among South Asian and white

European children: Child Heart and Health Study in England'. *Journal of Epidemiology and Community Health*, 63, Suppl. 2, 60.

Northern Data Hub (2018). 'Bradford population – City of Bradford Metropolitan District Council'. Available at: https://datahub.bradford.gov.uk/ebase/datahubext.eb?search=Bradford+population&ebd=0&ebp=10&ebz=1_1572347600121 (last accessed 29 April 2022).

Office for National Statistics (2020). 'Coronavirus (COVID-19) related deaths by religious group, England and Wales: 2 March to 15 May 2020'. Available at: www.ons.gov.uk/peoplepopulationandcommunity/birthsdeathsandmarriages/deaths/articles/coronaviruscovid19relateddeathsbyreligiousgroupenglandandwales/2marchto15may2020 (last accessed 29 April 2022).

Piggin, J. (2020). 'What is physical activity? A holistic definition for teachers, researchers and policy makers'. *Frontiers in Sports and Active Living*, 2, 72.

Public Health England (2020a). 'Research and analysis ethnicity spotlight'. Available at: www.gov.uk/government/publications/covid-19-mental-health-and-wellbeing-surveillance-spotlights/ethnicity-covid-19-mental-health-and-wellbeing-surveillance-report (last accessed 29 April 2022).

Public Health England (2020b). 'COVID-19: understanding the impact on BAME communities'. Available at: www.gov.uk/government/publications/covid-19-understanding-the-impact-on-bame-communities (last accessed 29 April 2022).

Quantrill, T. (2020). 'Bradford Heroes: Going above and beyond for communities'. *Telegraph & Argus*, 15 May, www.thetelegraphandargus.co.uk/news/18446002.bradford-heroes-going-beyond-communities (last accessed 29 April 2022).

Rahim, Z. (2020). 'In the latest sign of Covid-19-related racism, Muslims are being blamed for England's coronavirus outbreaks'. CNN, 6 August. Available at: https://edition.cnn.com/2020/08/06/europe/muslims-coronavirus-england-islamophobia-gbr-intl/index.html (last accessed 29 April 2022).

Rethink (2007). 'Our voice: the Pakistani community's view of mental health and mental health services in Birmingham report from the Aap Ki Awaaz project'. Available at: https://lemosandcrane.co.uk/resources/Rethink%20-%20Our%20Voice.pdf (last accessed 29 April 2022).

Sallis, J. F., Adlakha, D., Oyeyemi A. and Salvo, D. (2020). 'An international physical activity and public health research agenda to inform coronavirus disease-19 policies and practices'. *Journal of Sport and Health Science*, 9(4), 328–44.

Scott-Baumann, A. (2010). 'A community of inquiry: talking to Muslims', in M. Farrar (ed.), *The Study of Islam within Social Science Curricula in UK Universities: Case Studies 1*, pp. 78–84. Available at: www.heacademy.ac.uk/system/files/max_farrar_case_studies.pdf (last accessed 29 April 2022).

Scott-Baumann, A., Gibbs, P., Elwick, A. and Maguire, K. (2019a). 'What do we know about the implementations of equality, diversity and inclusion in the workplace?', in M. F. Özbilgin, F. Bartels-Ellis and P. Gibbs (eds), *Global Diversity Management*. Cham: Springer, pp. 11–23.

Scott-Baumann, A., Ebbiary, A., Ad Duha Mohammad, S., Dhorat, S., Begum, S., Pandor, H. and Stolyar, J. (2019b). 'Towards contextualised Islamic leadership: paraguiding and the Universities and Muslim Seminaries Project'. *Religions*, 10(12), 662.

Scott-Baumann, A., Guest, M., Naguib, S., Cheruvallil-Contractor, S. and Phoenix, A. (2020). *Islam on Campus: Contested Identities and the Cultures of Higher Education in Britain* Oxford: Oxford University Press.

Shahid, H. J. (2020a). 'The pandemic of Islamophobia'. *Journal of the British Islamic Medical Association*, 6(2). Available at: https://jbima.com/wp-content/uploads/2020/12/4_Advocacy_1_The-Pandemic-of-Islamophobia-_-Hinna-Shahid-Z.pdf (last accessed 29 April 2022).

Shahid, H. J. (2020b). 'Coronavirus: Creating a syndemic'. SOAS COP Policy Briefings. Available at: https://blogs.soas.ac.uk/cop/wp-content/uploads/2020/10/Coronavirus-creating-a-syndemic.pdf (last accessed 29 April 2022).

Shahid, H. J. and Scott-Baumann, A. (2020a). 'An intersectional approach during COVID-19: disaggregating data to protect BAME communities'. SOAS COP Policy Briefings. Available at: https://blogs.soas.ac.uk/cop/wp-content/uploads/2020/04/An-Intersectional-Approach-during-Covid-19-Disaggregating-data-to-protect-BAME.pdf (last accessed 29 April 2022).

Shahid, H. J. and Scott-Baumann, A. (2020b). 'Keeping faith during COVID-19: protecting religious minorities experiencing disproportionate impact'. SOAS COP Policy Briefings. Available at: https://blogs.soas.ac.uk/cop/wp-content/uploads/2020/05/Keeping-faith-during-Covid-19.pdf (last accessed 29 April 2022).

Shahid, J. and Waqar, S. (2020). 'Covid-19 and ethnic minority communities – we need better data to protect marginalised groups'. *The BMJ Opinion*. Available at: https://blogs.bmj.com/bmj/2020/07/07/covid-19-and-ethnic-minority-communities-we-need-better-data-to-protect-marginalised-groups (last accessed 29 April 2022).

Smith, K., Bhui, K. and Cipriani, A. (2020). 'COVID-19, mental health and ethnic minorities'. *Evidence Based Mental Health*, 23(3), 89–90.

Steene-Johannessen, J., Hansen, B. H., Dalene, K. E., Kolle, E., Northstone, K., Møller, N. C., Grøntved, A., Wedderkopp, N., Kriemler, S., Page, A. S., Puder, J. J., Reilly, J. J. et al. (2020). 'Variations in accelerometry measured physical activity and sedentary time across Europe – harmonized analyses of 47,497 children and adolescents'. *International Journal of Behavioral Nutrition and Physical Activity*, 17(1), 38.

Swerling, G. (2020). 'Far-right posing as journalists to spread fake news about Muslims, government Islamophobia adviser warns'. *The Telegraph*, 10 May, www.telegraph.co.uk/news/2020/05/10/far-right-posing-journalists-spread-fake-news-muslims-government (last accessed 29 April 2022).

Think Tank Programme (2020a). 'Muslim women's views and experiences on mental health'. Muslim Women's Council. Available at: www.muslimwomenscouncil.org.uk/sites/default/files/documents/Beyond%20Stigma%20Muslim%20women%e2%80%99s%20views%20and%20experiences%20on%20mental%20health.pdf (last accessed 8 July 2022).

Think Tank Programme (2020b). 'The impact of the COVID-19 lockdown on Muslim Women in the UK Ethnic background'. Muslim Women's Council. Available at: https://amhp.org.uk/resources/publications/ (last accessed 8 July 2022).

Van Lancker, W. and Parolin, Z. (2020). 'COVID-19, school closures, and child poverty: a social crisis in the making'. *The Lancet Public Health*, 5(5), e243–e244.

World Health Organization (2018). 'Global action plan on physical activity 2018–2030: more active people for a healthier world'. Available at: https://apps.who.int/iris/bitstream/handle/10665/272722/9789241514187-eng.pdf (last accessed 29 April 2022).

Wright, J., Small, N., Raynor, P., Tuffnell, D., Bhopal, R., Cameron, N., Fairley, L., Lawlor, D. A., Parslow, R., Petherick, E. S., Pickett, K. E., Waiblinger, D. and West, J. (2012). 'Cohort Profile: the Born in Bradford multi-ethnic family cohort study'. *International Journal of Epidemiology*, 42(4), 978–91.

Wu, X. Y., Han, L. H., Zhang, J. H., Luo, S., Hu , J. W. and Sun, K. (2017). 'The influence of physical activity, sedentary behavior on health-related quality of life among the general population of children and adolescents: a systematic review'. *PLoS ONE*, 12(11), e0187668.

3

GENDERED HEALTH INEQUALITIES AND BRITISH MUSLIM WOMEN: AN INTERSECTIONAL APPROACH AND ANALYSIS

*Hina J. Shahid, Asma Khan, Jennifer Hall, Melanie Haith-Cooper, Anya Ahmed and Sufyan Abid Dogra**iD

Narratives of Pathologising Bodies and Mobilities of British Muslim Women

Narratives of pathologising British Muslim women's bodies and mobilities were mostly written between 1980 and 2010 in social sciences, in works by academics such as Haleh Afshar (1989, 2002), Afshar and Barrientos (1999), Afshar and Maynard (1994), Afshar et al. (2005), Pnina Werbner (1990, 2004, 2007) and Robina Mohammad (1999, 2005, 2013). British Muslim women have been portrayed as victims, oppressed and abused because of their families, culture, ethnicity and religion. Biased academics and scholars projected British Muslim women through their imaginations as disadvantaged Muslim women from the countries of origin or with their stereotypical and pathological views about first-generation Muslim women in Britain. These scholars internalised speculation on British Muslim

* This book chapter is funded for open access by Bradford Institute for Health Research. The views expressed are those of the author and not necessarily those of the Bradford Institute for Health Research or the Bradford Teaching Hospitals NHS Foundation Trust.

iD https://orcid.org/0000-0001-9896-9503

✉ Sufyan.Dogra@bthft.nhs.uk

women through orientalist depictions, colonial ethnographies and from the popular or mainstream media. The narratives of pathologies about first-generation British Muslim women are conveniently generalised over the second generation or to some extent the third generation by these scholars without acknowledging the qualitative differences in the lived experiences and struggles of different generations (see Chapter 11). These narratives took a condescending view on the 'culture, values, norms, ethnicity or religion of British Muslim women and projected these as barriers to their emancipation on one hand, and as causes and context of their ill-health experiences on the other. These narratives of pathologising British Muslim women often ignore the impact of structural inequities, discrimination, racism, Islamophobia and deprivation that defines the lived experience of ill health for British Muslim women. Advancing the narratives of pathologising British Muslim women's bodies and mobilities by depicting their vulnerabilities, victimhood and helplessness because of the 'moral economy of kin' (Afshar 1989) functioning through their family, culture, ethnicity and religion is the reproduction of the racist, neo-eugenics and neo-colonial mindset that latently aspires to discipline Muslim women's bodies and mobilities on a standardised secular, liberal expression of living a public life in Britain. Such narratives of pathologies depicting third-generation British Muslim women as 'Pakistani women' and 'no different to their grandmothers' (Afshar 1989), not only undermine the upward mobility of British Muslim women but also shore up the racist and Islamophobic environment in the UK with the potential to do further harm to public mobilities, visibilities and diverse expressions.

At the same time, these narratives of pathologising British Muslim women that originate in social sciences indirectly inform the perceptions of researchers and practitioners in the domains of health studies and applied health research. When applied health researchers review the literature while formulating research questions on the diet, physical activity or other health practices of British Muslim women, they end up reproducing narratives of pathologising by ignoring the disconnect of these narratives with lived experience of, in particular, third-generation Muslim women, and as a consequence cite family, culture, ethnicity and religion as barriers to their healthy lives. It was interesting to observe in 2020 a group of applied health researchers, health practitioners and members of the public working on a Born in Bradford (BiB) programme to prevent obesity. The groups were searching for published literature on the food habits and healthy diet of South Asian families and found that most of the available literature was redundant, not reflective of the food habits of third-generation British Muslim women and had been written about the food habits of first-generation migrants and generalised over the second and third generation. We emphasise the need for a renewed approach to studying health inequalities by understanding how structural inequalities, deprivation, marginalisation, racism and Islamophobia create conditions of ill health for British Muslim women. We advocate critically examining the narratives of pathologising that deflect the focus of debate on health inequalities by viewing and labelling Muslim women's family, culture, ethnicity and religion as barriers for ill health experiences.

Structural Inequalities, Discrimination and Gendered Health of British Muslim Women

Muslims form one-third of the Black and Minority Ethnic (BME) population in the UK and are an ethnically diverse group (68 per cent being South Asian and 32 per cent non-Asian) (MCB 2015). Muslim women are also socially, culturally, linguistically, historically and geographically diverse, both native-born and migrant, and as such are a part of a heterogeneous 'community of communities' but where shared religious values and beliefs form a central role (Hassan et al. 2020). Studies on maternity care in particular highlight how religious values are embedded within most aspects of the care experience for Muslim women and the dual role they play not only in maintaining wellbeing and resilience but also as a source of anxiety and contention when Muslim women feel misunderstood and stigmatised for their beliefs (Hassan et al. 2019).

Health disparities among minoritised communities are influenced by structural (state-sanctioned or social), institutional and interpersonal aspects of a society and the healthcare system (Ahmad 1993; Kushnick 1998; Adebowale and Rao 2020). For the Muslim community in the UK, Islamophobia, defined by the All Party Parliamentary Group on British Muslims as 'a form of racism that targets expressions of Muslimness' (APPG 2018) is a key contributor to health disparities through functioning as a fundamental cause of health determinants. Additionally, anti-Muslim prejudice and Islamophobia affect individuals differently, with intersectionality describing how multiple aspects of a person's identity may be shaped with overlapping effects; being Muslim, from an ethnic minority, female, overseas-born, a non-UK national, disabled, and other protected characteristics.

Fifty per cent of Muslim households live in poverty (MCB 2015), which is known to be a strong predictor of health disparities (ONS 2011) and healthy life expectancy, and 50 per cent of Muslims in the UK are born overseas (MCB 2015) which impacts access to healthcare information and services. Muslim women are also more likely to report poorer quality of life and disability, and are more likely to have mental health problems, with young Asian women more likely to report attempted suicide (Mental Health Foundation 2020) and older women more likely to experience chronic mental health disorders. In addition, Muslim women are most likely to be affected by hate crimes (Tell MAMA 2018) as an extreme manifestation of violent Islamophobia.

National priorities to eliminate health disparities, in particular for women, must have a holistic, intersectional and multi-level approach. They must seek to understand and address the layers of disadvantage and discrimination that population subgroups face, such as Islamophobia embodied by Muslim women, with compounding effects across the life course.

Below is our overall assessment and recommendations for understanding, approaching and eliminating existing health inequalities that British Muslim women live with. Afterwards the structural analysis, we deliberate on intersectionality and how it translates in the lived experiences to exacerbate health inequalities among British Muslim women.

Agency and cultural humility

There is a plethora of evidence which highlights the stigma and exclusion that Muslim women face in healthcare. Muslim women, especially older Bangladeshi and Pakistani women, experience derogatory stereotypes based on combined racial and religious bias. Anecdotal evidence points towards the widespread use of terms originating from South Asian surnames such as 'Bibi Syndrome', 'Begumitis' or 'bibi-itis', or 'all over body syndrome' for Muslim female patients presenting with non-specific symptoms of complaints perceived to be exaggerated (Sherif 2021). Other common biases in medicine include perceptions that being an observant Muslim poses health risks, Islamic tradition conflicts with Western medicine, Muslims should become more modern and females wearing headscarves and requesting a consultation with a healthcare provider of the same gender or being accompanied to a healthcare consultation by a male relative are oppressed, abused and/or hold 'traditional' views about morality, sexuality and gender roles (Laird et al. 2007).

Such stereotyping impacts on clinical decision making (Puddifoot 2019) and affects patient safety and quality of care through under- or missed diagnoses and breakdown in trust and rapport, and is likely to contribute to the high levels of dissatisfaction persistently reported in Muslim patients in both social care and healthcare, creating a 'dissatisfaction gap' (King's Fund 2006, 2019). These findings highlight the lack of awareness of culturally diverse clinical presentations, for example recognising that expressing emotional distress in somatic terms is common among Muslims from South Asia and North Africa, in part due to the stigma associated with mental illness in these communities (Williams and Hunt 1997). This can result in Muslim patients receiving worse mental healthcare, if any at all (Thornton 2020). Furthermore, these attitudes demonstrate the persistent implicit biases in the healthcare system which erects barriers for Muslim women accessing care, marginalising and excluding their voices and experiences as they feel they are not listened to and do not have their concerns taken seriously.

Improving the quality and accessibility of information and education on women's health

It is well known that cultural background and beliefs, including religion, influence understandings of health and illness, access to and interactions with healthcare services and healthcare professionals (HCPs), acceptance of and adherence to treatment, and perceptions of 'taboo' topics on women's health, such as sexual and reproductive health and mental health. A study in North West England highlighted the intersecting impact of religious, cultural and social beliefs and identities on perceptions of obesity and associated risks which did not correspond to existing educational and behaviour change models, underscoring the need for health education interventions that incorporate these multiple dimensions to facilitate empowered decision making and healthy life choices (Ludwig et al. 2011).

Targeted information and programmes for Muslim women should consider factors such as preferred language and whether it is oral or written, cultural norms, values and knowledge systems, collective history, position in society, living conditions, and environmental and psychological motivations so that cultural adaptations consider 'language, culture and context in a way that is comparable with cultural patterns, meanings and values' (Mosdøl et al. 2017). Interventions should also analyse patterns of media usage, recognising the popularity of ethnic and faith-based media channels and social media platforms such as WhatsApp for mass health communications. In addition to mass media, outreach programmes co-created and delivered in person with community organisations, influencers and leaders can create opportunities for communication, building trust, and deepening understanding and motivation. It is imperative that any targeted approach considers ethical aspects carefully to avoid stereotyping and stigmatising which can be counterproductive (Thornton 2020). Notable examples include campaigns on female genital mutilation (FGM) and sex education where Muslims have been exceptionalised as problematic when in fact FGM has no theological basis in Islam and there has been insufficient consultation and partnership working with faith and community-based organisations which are important sources of knowledge for health promotion campaigns on sex education. This includes the human papilloma virus (HPV) immunisation programme with Muslim girls less likely to accept the HPV vaccine due to concerns about low levels of trust in HCPs, perceived lack of autonomy and low knowledge of HPV, but who have expressed an interest in learning more (Pratt et al. 2019). Studies on Somali American women, who have low rates of breast and cervical cancer screening, identified specific barriers including cultural differences about gender and sexuality, the gender and competence of HCPs and past traumatic experiences, with religiously tailored messages highlighted as an important community asset (Pratt 2020).

Life course approaches for responsive healthcare systems

Research on other health conditions across the life course is limited due to an absence of data on health outcomes by religion. Low uptake of healthcare-seeking behaviours among Muslims can exacerbate health disparities. These are multi-factorial, including a lack of understanding of and familiarity with the health-care system, especially for recent immigrants, a lack of trust in HCP, perceived discrimination, the lack of same-gender HCPs, divergent cultural value systems and the stigma around seeking help (Saritoprak and Exline 2020). Other cultural barriers identified include modesty and privacy among Muslim women, family involvement and presence in care, maintaining religious practices during illness (such as prayer and fasting), fatalism and predestination, low health literacy and language proficiency, preference for traditional remedies and limited healthcare access (Tackett et al. 2018). Due to the diversity of the Muslim population, it is important for healthcare systems and HCPs to deliver tailored care that is not based on assumptions and prejudices but considers individual differences within groups (Tackett et al. 2018; Puthussery 2016).

Spiritual health beliefs such as concepts of endurance and pain as tests of faith as well as prayer and recitation of the Qur'an can be important coping methods in labour for Muslim women, but these beliefs are not consistent. Variability is also noted in narratives around Muslim women's agency and role of male rela-tives (Walton et al. 2014). Additionally, HCPs have gaps in knowledge (Hassan 2020) and may need to have familiarity with the customs and values of their Muslim female patients including Islamic ethical positions on termination of pregnancy, prenatal screening, disability, vaccinations and medications, end-of-life care and organ donation (Laird et al. 2007) and impact of rituals such as Ramadan on health and pilgrimages such as *Hajj* and *Umrah* where women may request medication to delay their menstruation.

Table 3.1 highlights how Muslim women's health outcomes are impacted across the life course and the mechanisms contributing to these.

Table 3.1 Health disparities in Muslim women across the life course.

Impact	Mechanism
Increased perinatal and infant mortality	Pre-existing health inequalities, deprivation, cultural practice of consanguinity, prenatal racism altering uterine environment and epigenetic activity (Pollock 2005; Ajaz et al. 2015; Firdous et al. 2020)
Increased genetic disorders and disability	Limited understanding of genetic risk, oppositions to evidence, taboo, lack of culturally sensitive health services (NHS England 2016; Birmingham City Council 2021)

Impact	Mechanism
Childhood experiences	Islamophobia and adverse childhood experiences (Harrell et al. 2011)
Mental health burden – common and serious mental health disorders	Lack of culturally sensitive and language appropriate services, stigma, taboo, Islamophobia (hate crimes and anticipatory) (Kalmakis and Chandler 2015; Karlsen and Nazroo 2002)
Chronic disease outcomes	Non-attention, reduced medication compliance, reliance on spiritual practices, HCP attitudes and lack of communication skills, interpreters and lack of interest in patient narratives (Elahi and Khan 2017; Ypinazar and Margolis 2006)
Dementia care	Low level of information, stigma, isolation, lack of culturally sensitive services, carer stress (Fagerli et al. 2007)

Building the correct evidence base

In order to eliminate health disparities for Muslim women, data must be strengthened by building the appropriate evidence base. This requires improvements in data collection and monitoring of health outcomes and experiences by disaggregating ethnicities and including data by religion across all health outcomes, experiences and access metrics to better understand where gaps are that need to be addressed. Most research findings tend to use ethnicity as proxy markers or link outcomes to census survey data which can affect accuracy and completeness of the data. Religion is a protected characteristic according to the 2010 Equality Act and in order to reduce health disparities, it is vital that data on health outcomes by religion is collected (Padilla 1994).

Sociocultural approaches through participatory and narrative research that draw on lived experiences are likely to be most effective in obtaining rich and relevant data that explores what information and service priorities are, health beliefs, perceptions, experiences, barriers and facilitators. It is essential that research is not only co-designed but community led to create agency, ownership and empowerment, with appropriate funding and resources. Too often community organisations and individuals are consulted by research bodies without any reimbursement of their time and expertise, thus exacerbating inequities and creating a system of cultural taxation (Knight et al. 2019) which goes against the principles of social justice, the foundations on which health disparities work is based.

We believe that an intersectional analysis is central to understand health inequalities that British Muslim women live with, as discussed above.

Intersectionality, British Muslim Women and Health Inequalities

Intersectionality is described as a theory (Davis 2008), or a heuristic device for understanding social relations (Anthias 2012). Originally coined by Kimberle Crenshaw in the 1980s, it has gained currency in contemporary feminist theories and across other academic disciplines (Davis 2008; Anthias 2012). Intersectionality addresses the differences between women and aims to include those previously marginalised. Interactions between gender, race and class in individual lives are central as structures that create differences between women and the multiple positioning that constitute their everyday lives (Davis 2008). More recently, other social categories of difference, including faith, have been included. The focus is to examine power imbalances, to deconstruct binary oppositions and universalism, and to move away from static conceptualisations of identity. A person may be in a position of dominance and subordination simultaneously, or at different times and in different places (Anthias 2012). For example, whilst a visibly Muslim woman may be subject to both racial and religious discrimination in wider British society, her piety and practice of Islam can be a source of empowerment, status and fulfilment for herself, other Muslim women and British Muslims as a whole.

The concepts of intersectionality and translocation positionality are useful to examine the experiences of British Muslim women because they remind us to consider the multiple social positions and identities occupied and enacted by British Muslim women; few other groups in British society have been subject to such homogenised and static representations. Below are some of the constituting elements for any intersectional analysis of British Muslim women and how this may be helpful in understanding the complexities of the health inequalities that they live with.

Ethnicity

The Muslim population in Britain is increasingly ethnically diverse (MCB 2015). Whilst some ethnic groups, such as Pakistanis and Bangladeshis, are almost exclusively Muslim, there is greater religious diversity among other ethnic groups, for example around a third of Indian and African people in Britain are Muslim. A wide body of literature, based mostly on qualitative and ethnographic studies, shows that their religious identity is more central to the identities of British Muslim women than their ethnic identities (Shaw 2000). British Pakistanis and Bangladeshis are religiously homogeneous, with research on Pakistani and Bangladeshi women often generalised to all British Muslim women; these ethnic groups comprise

53 per cent of the British Muslim population (MCB 2015). The experiences of South Asian Muslim women in the UK may be different from more recent arrivals, and smaller, ethnic groups of Muslims such as those from the Middle East or Africa. The relationship between ethnicity and religion is a complex one; it is difficult to separate the effects of ethnic culture from religious affiliation – not least because of the interplay of ethnicity and religion in the interpretation of religious texts and the transmission of Islamic practices and beliefs (Scourfield et al. 2013; Cheruvallil-Contractor 2012; Gilliat-Ray 2010)

Religious discrimination, racism and Islamophobia

Religion is central to contemporary articulations of racism in Britain, impacting most markedly on Muslims (Shankley and Rhodes 2020). The current societal context of Britain is one where Islamophobic discourse is prevalent in public spheres (Khattab and Modood 2018; Shankley and Rhodes 2020). Muslims in Britain are markedly different from the White majority because of their socioeconomic disadvantage and their distinctive sociocultural identities (Khattab 2012). Most Muslims are visibly different in terms of their ethnic group and they are sometimes an obvious religious group, many Muslim women being publicly visible in their observance of religious symbols, for example through wearing hijab (Velayati 2018). In policy terms, traditional, patriarchal, ethnoreligious cultural norms and values are thought to contribute to the socioeconomic disadvantage of Muslim households and communities, with far less attention paid to structural factors such as racial or religious discrimination (Casey 2016). British Muslim women and men are subject to distinct gendered and racialised stereotypes (Britton 2019). Muslim women are subject to racialised stereotypes, enshrined in policy, that focus on their perceived vulnerability, notably through immigration policies which seek to restrict spousal immigration to 'protect' vulnerable ethnic minority women (Charsley and Liversage 2015). Widely held stereotypes of Muslim women focus on their perceived subservience and powerlessness and Islam is viewed as a constraint to the agency of Muslim women (Cheruvallil-Contractor 2012; Khattab and Modood 2018). Young British women attract public interest and scrutiny and are often reduced to their religious affiliation (Cheruvallil-Contractor 2012). Muslim women are more likely to experience anti-Muslim hatred or Islamophobia than Muslim men: in 2017, 57 per cent of reports came from Muslim women, while 53 per cent of reports were from 'visibly' Muslim women (Tell MAMA 2018).

Social class

Most British Muslim women may be classified as disadvantaged by virtue of their being of lower socioeconomic status (or working class). Although there is socioeconomic diversity among British Muslims with 'pockets of prosperity', they are disproportionately represented in the 'never worked' and 'long term unemployed' categories (MCB 2015). Whilst Muslim women are more likely to be economically inactive, Muslim men are more likely to be unemployed, unaccounted workers and to occupy marginal positions in the labour market (Cabinet Office 2017). Muslim households are more likely to be in poverty than those of other religious affiliations; Heath and Li (2015) found that households of Jewish affiliation are least likely to be found in poverty (13 per cent), in contrast to those from the Muslim community (50 per cent). Muslim households are disproportionately concentrated in areas with high levels of multiple deprivation in already disadvantaged urban areas, affecting their access to diverse social networks that enable social mobility and occupational attainment (Khattab et al. 2010), and their general health (MCB 2015). Just under half (46 per cent) of the Muslim population lives in the 10 per cent most deprived local authority districts in England, based on the Index of Multiple Deprivation measure (MCB 2015). The residential segregation of Muslim families is a matter of social exclusion and discrimination as well as choice (Modood 2004).

Muslim communities and families

Caste- or kinship-based social networks (*biraderi*) framed social relations in the earliest British Pakistani communities and families. A *biraderi* is a flexible social network, essential to understand the socioeconomic position and impetus for the 'chain migration' of British Pakistani families and communities (Anwar 1979; Shaw 1988). These social networks provided essential social and economic support in the face of widespread structural and interpersonal racial discrimination and disadvantages in employment, housing and social interactions (Kalra 2000). Selective and localised migration from parts of Pakistan to certain towns created the conditions for continuity and persistence in social structure and attitudes from place of origin, including those relating to gender norms (Anwar 1979; Shaw 1988; Kalra 2000). Islamic beliefs play an important role in the everyday lives of Muslim women and a central role in the transmission and continuity of religious beliefs, values and practices in their families and communities (Scourfield et al. 2013; Akhtar 2014). Whilst first-generation women see religion as a way of preserving traditional cultural heritage and of protecting their children from British society, second-generation South Asian Muslim women see religion as liberating and a means to assert their rights to go to university, to be economically active and to choose their own marriage partner (Akhtar 2014).

There is evidence that the marginalised position that Muslim men occupy within British society can make them retreat into a defensive position of safeguarding the distinctive moral frameworks of their own ethno-religious minority communities (Kalra 2000; Vertovec 2008). Transnational marriage is the predominant pattern among some groups of Muslim women; in their analysis of Labour Force Survey data from 2004 to 2018, Charsley et al. (2020) found that just over half of British Pakistani women and men are married to a migrant who was born in Pakistan. First-generation partners are seen as better able to maintain ethno-religious values and to impart these to their children (Shaw 2000; Charsley 2006, 2007). Enacting gendered norms may constitute a useful resource for Muslim women in terms of spiritual rewards as a result of adhering to religious prescriptions, as well as being a source of authority and status in their social interactions within their families and communities. More nuanced qualitative studies into marriage practices in Muslim, and particularly Pakistani, families indicate that transnational marriages are the result of considered negotiations and discussions between parents and their children, and the transmission of ethnic and religious norms are often a desired outcome of transnational marriage.

Education

Bagguley and Hussain's (2016) analysis of the Young Cohort Survey of England and Wales in the years 1988, 1995 and 2001 demonstrated improvements in GCSE and A Level performance for Pakistani and Bangladeshi young women between 1980 and 2001. However, rather than overall generational improvement, there is polarisation in the educational attainment of second-generation British Muslim women (Modood 1997; Khattab 2009, 2012); 33 per cent of Muslim women have higher education qualifications whilst 40 per cent have no qualifications (Khattab and Modood 2018). Despite evidence for continued disadvantage, the focus on the literature around education for Muslim women has been on understanding the success of women in attaining higher education qualifications rather than the continued disadvantage faced by a large proportion of second-generation Muslim women. Research conducted from the 1990s onwards shows that Muslim parents were supportive of education of boys and girls (Dale et al. 2002; Abbas 2003). Qualitative studies have shown that young Muslim women are able to make use of religious argumentation in negotiations with their parents to secure access to post-compulsory education and work. Bolagnani and Mellor (2012) suggest that the religious versus culture debate is not a theory but a social construction that describes how second-generation Muslim women use the distinction between oppressive ethnic traditions and cultural and universal interpretation of Islam as a source of empowerment, to access their rights within Islam and to implement change. Muslim women in Britain have used this form of negotiation to attain greater spatial freedoms and access to higher education, to delay marriage arrangements and to secure access to paid employment (Mohammad 1999; Cheruvallil-Contractor 2012). The successful use of religious argumentation is largely seen in educated and middle-class Muslim families (Bolagnani and Mellor 2012; Cheruvallil-Contractor 2012).

Muslim women in the labour market

British Muslims have not met the conventional theoretical expectations of large-scale generational improvements in socioeconomic outcomes for migrants; this is most evident amongst Muslim women than men. The migrant generation is expected to have relatively poor socioeconomic outcomes for reasons that include: the emotional, social and economic costs of migration; downward social mobility due to a lack of fluency in English and recognised qualifications; and racism or discrimination (Heath 2014). Second generations are expected to gradually adopt the values, norms and culture of the majority population and gain the knowledge, qualifications and skills that will allow them to achieve better outcomes in the labour market (Muttarak 2014; Waters 2014). Despite participation in the British education system, Muslims, and particularly Muslim women, have not experienced significant generational improvements in socioeconomic outcomes. It is the case, however, that migrant Muslim women have lower levels of employment than their British counterparts (Charsley et al. 2020).

British Muslim women are the only group in Britain more likely to be economically inactive than active; 56 per cent of British Muslim women were inactive as per the Census of 2001[1] and they are more than twice as likely to be economically inactive than women from most other religious groups (ONS 2020). Looking after home and family is the reason stated to explain the economic inactivity of 57 per cent of Muslim women – they are more likely to state this reason than women of other religious groups (ONS 2020). 'Ethnic penalties' in the British labour market have been identified since the 1990s, referring to any unexplained differences in labour market outcomes after controlling for age, qualification and UK birth. Since the early 2000s a distinct 'Muslim penalty' has been identified; Muslims experience greater labour market penalties than other religious groups, even among those of the same ethnic group. For example, White Muslims were more likely to face a penalty than other White groups (Khattab et al. 2010). A recent comprehensive field experiment found that employers discriminate on the basis of ethnicity and religion when making hiring decisions; minorities from countries with a sizeable Muslim population (Pakistan, Bangladesh, the MENA region) face 'enormous' barriers when applying for jobs, even when their covering letters and CVs are identical to those of other candidates (Zwysen et al. 2021).

Limited opportunities in the labour market for Muslims can lead to the reinforcement of traditional ethno-religious norms in practical as well as cultural ways. British Pakistani and Bangladeshi men were, and remain, concentrated in low-paid work that required long working hours: as manual workers, self-employed workers such as taxi drivers and owners of small businesses (Anwar 1979; Kalra 2000; Cabinet Office 2017). These occupations do not allow for flexible working patterns that would easily allow the sharing of domestic or childcare responsibilities. The previous state benefit system of tax credits deterred women in low-income households from working (Modood 1997). The loss of state benefits income may mean that the formal economic activity of women in these families would not bring any additional financial benefit (particularly when low levels of education limit them to low-paid work) whilst concurrently creating a dual burden for women; this is likely to be a deterrent to undertaking formal economic activity. There is strong evidence that they experience structural discrimination in the labour market and that their low levels of labour market participation increase the incidence of poverty in British Muslim households.

We expand our intersectional analysis on understanding health inequalities with two examples of ill-health indicators (cancer screening and inactivity) that British Muslim women live with and show how these can be helpful in understanding that living with disadvantages shapes Muslim women's health over their life course.

British Muslim women and cancer-screening inequalities

We argue that inequalities in cancer screening uptake lead to South Asian women being more likely to present late with advanced cancer and the associated morbidity and mortality which could be avoided with the timely uptake of cancer screening offered to women nationally. Uptake of breast, bowel and cervical cancer screening in UK South Asian women in Bradford is low when compared to the national average (Public Health England 2020). The majority South Asian population in Bradford is Muslim, and Muslim families tend to live in areas of the city with high levels of deprivation (Department for Education 2020; Public Health England 2020; ONS 2011). South Asian women can face barriers to accessing cancer- screening services and it is argued that these barriers can be linked to the intersectional inequalities faced by these women.

A recent systematic review (Anderson de Cuevas et al. 2018) reported on numerous barriers South Asian women face when accessing cancer screening. These include less understanding of cancer, asymptomatic cancer screening and cancer prevention than other populations of women. The recent 'Wise up to Cancer' project (Almas et al. 2019) found that South Asian (mainly Muslim) women in Bradford lacked knowledge not only about cancer screening services but also the signs and symptoms of cancer, with one-third of participants not being able to name one sign or symptom. This lack of knowledge was more prevalent in older women not born in the UK. The question may be asked as to why this is the case. Women born outside the UK may not have gone through the

UK education system and perhaps face language barriers when receiving public health messages about cancer screening. It could be that due to the deprivation they experience, they are unable to engage with screening for practical reasons including the cost of travel to appointments. In addition to this, Anderson de Cuevas et al. (2018) identified the fatalistic belief that cancer cannot be cured, as well as a lack of understanding the concept of preventative health care or the belief (especially around cervical cancer) that screening is not relevant. Research shows that Muslim male family members can be the decision makers within households and that women have to obtain permission from men to engage with cancer screening (ibid.).

There is a wealth of research around interventions designed to increase cancer screening uptake in BME women. These include interventions to address language and cultural barriers in women (Donnelly and Hwang 2015; Hou et al. 2011; Escribà-Agüir et al. 2016; Agide et al. 2018). To address these barriers, peers with the same cultural background and who spoke the same language were recruited to deliver the intervention (Agide et al. 2018; Hou et al. 2011). This was a principle followed in the Wise Up to Cancer project, with trained peers delivering the intervention to increase uptake of cancer screening. However, these studies do not consider the role of men in influencing cancer screening in South Asian women and it is argued that tailored interventions need to be developed that target men, who can then facilitate women to engage with the screening process. It is easy to problematise Muslim women in relation to cancer-screening services when in reality services may not be accessible for the many reasons described above. It is important that public health interventions are developed that increase the timely accessibility of cancer-screening services. It is argued that educational interventions in themselves are not enough and that tailored interventions need to consider the wider religious, cultural and practical barriers (Anderson de Cuevas et al. 2018). Thought needs to be given to how interventions can be embedded in Muslim women (and men's) belief systems and address the practical barriers to screening, including language.

British Muslim women, physical inactivity and structural inequalities

Data on self-reported physical activity is collected from around 175,000 adults across England twice a year as part of the Active Lives survey conducted by the regulatory body Sport England. According to this data, Muslim women are consistently less likely to meet the physical activity guidelines of 150 minutes of moderate-intensity physical activity a week than Muslim men and non-Muslims. For example, in a November 2018 – November 2019 survey, the reported proportion of different groups meeting the physical activity guidelines was 53.5 per cent of Muslim males, 61.5 per cent of all females and 44.1 per cent of Muslim females (Sport England 2019). Both the media and some of the early research have played a significant role in the framing of religion as the 'cause' of inactivity in female Muslims in Britain and beyond (Lenneis and Pfister 2017; Stride 2014), including an emphasis placed on inconsistencies between appropriate Islamic and sporting attire (Ahmad 2011). Conversely, religious teachings, Islamic leaders and practising Muslims recognise Islam as encouraging of women's participation in physical activity (Dogra et al. 2021; Ige-Elegbede et al. 2019; Lenneis and Pfister 2017; Miles and Benn 2016). Physical activity is seen as 'central to the Muslim way of life' and is consistent with the Islamic narrative surrounding the importance of taking care of the body (Babakus and Thompson 2012).

Recent research has recognised a myriad of barriers that British Muslim women and girls are required to negotiate in order to engage in regular physical activity (for example, Ahmad 2011; Koshoedo et al. 2015; Miles and Benn 2016; Stride 2014; Stride and Flintoff 2018). Crucially, social structural factors including ethnicity, gender and deprivation intersect and manifest as layers of oppression for many British Muslim women (Collings et al. 2020; Ige-Elegbede et al. 2019; Williams et al. 2019). For example, a meta-ethnography of qualitative studies identified fear of personal or institutional racial discrimination as a barrier to engaging in physical activity in BME, and particularly South Asian Muslim, communities in the UK (Koshoedo et al. 2015). Recent participatory research explored the physical activity experiences of South Asian Muslim girls from a secondary school in Yorkshire (Stride 2014; Stride et al. 2018). This work revealed that the gendered and racialised nature of activity spaces creates problems for participating in more organised and formal physical activities. There is evidence that this experience resonates among British Muslim females more broadly, with British Muslim university students highlighting that university facilities not being inclusive of religious and cultural requirements by, for example, providing female-only spaces (Miles and Benn 2016) can lead to the exclusion of British Muslim females. Many of the girls included in the research conducted by Stride et al. (2018) reported finding it easier to engage in activities in their homes, and a recent survey of 1,000 British Muslim women reported that the COVID-19 pandemic and associated proliferation of home workout opportunities provided a more sustainable option for physical activity (MudOrange 2021). British Muslim women and girls have also cited cultural expectations around the acceptability of sporting activities and domestic responsibilities, and the lack of availability of fit-for-purpose sports hijabs as restricting participation in physical activity (Ahmad 2011; Stride et al. 2018; MudOrange 2021). Finally, although there are irrefutable challenges that British Muslim females face in engaging in physical activity, another explanation for the lower activity levels reported in this population group could be methodological, as the questionnaires commonly used to measure activity are focused on traditional sporting activities and often do not capture domestic activities – requiring significant exertion and strength – that British Muslim females have been reported to regularly engage in (Pollard and Guell 2012; Stride 2018).

Examples of how British Muslim women and girls have challenged structures and stereotypes to engage in physical activity are increasingly emerging. For example, in football, before the governing body FIFA authorised wearing head covers during matches in 2014, practising Muslims for whom wearing the hijab is central to their identity were instrumental in developing the Women's Islamic Games, where they could play football whilst observing the hijab (Ahmad 2011). Stride and Flintoff (2016) provide examples of Muslim girls questioning rules and negotiating access, for example one research participant asked, 'What's done there for girls?' when restricted by local community centre management from taking part in (male) jujutsu sessions. Whilst Sport England recognises religious and ethnic activity inequalities through the Active Lives survey, the words 'religion', 'Muslim' and 'Islam' are completely absent from the recently published fifty-four-page strategy 'Uniting the movement' that outlines a ten-year vision to transform lives and communities through sport and physical activity (Sport England 2021). There is an urgent need for a shift in interventions, policy structures and media representation to avoid the perpetuation of activity inequality in British Muslim females. It is important to co-produce programmes with, and tailor them for, British Muslim women, whilst recognising that Muslim women and girls are not a homogeneous group, and considering the implications of this for physical activity participation (Lenneis and Pfister 2017).

The Way Forward to Reduce Health Inequalities for British Muslim Women

As this chapter illustrates, inequalities in the UK are not experienced equally, and Muslim women have the worst rates of reported ill health (16 per cent) and disability (24 per cent) compared to other religious groups (Laird et al. 2007). Evidence also demonstrates that Muslim women experience greater levels of poverty and deprivation (Casey 2016) and live in the 10 per cent most deprived areas of England (MCB 2015), with 50 per cent of Muslim families living in poverty (Heath and Li 2015). In the UK it is the most deprived and vulnerable communities that receive the poorest quality of healthcare provision across a spectrum of services (Morris and Scobie 2020). It has also been found that experiencing socioeconomic disadvantage negatively impacts on employment and social mobility opportunities by limiting access to social networks (Khattab et al. 2010). Using the lens of intersectionality this chapter has demonstrated how religion, gender, culture, being born outside the UK and marginalisation overlap to create multiple disadvantages which are compounded by structural inequalities, discrimination, domestic violence and poor access to appropriate health services.

The Marmot Review (2010) highlighted major health disparities in the UK and illustrated how austerity measures and cuts to budgets in the most deprived areas of the UK increased these disparities for the poorest and most vulnerable in society. This has resulted in a decrease in life expectancy for women living in the 10 per cent most deprived areas, whilst in the most affluent areas life expectancy for women has increased. Alongside this, those experiencing poverty and deprivation are living in poor health for longer (Marmot 2020). This is particularly evident for Muslim women aged over 65, where in fifty local authority districts 40 per cent are in poor health, yet this population group remains under-represented in all areas of health service provision (MCB 2015). Indeed, this chapter has referenced major service failings in the fields of obstetrics, oncology, mental health, cardiology, mental health, chronic disease management and preventative health. The fact that Muslim women are not accessing healthcare denies them the possibility of preventative, curative and palliative treatments for all types of health condition and leaves them at increased risk of mortality, poor quality of life and preventable suffering.

Muslim women are being failed by health service provision and discriminated against by health service providers who lack the necessary knowledge and skills to plan and deliver inclusive care (MCB 2015). Addressing this should be a national priority, specifically in light of the poor health outcomes experienced by Muslim women. It is imperative that health and social care policy encompasses an intersectional and multi-level approach to combat the stigma and exclusion that is currently being experienced. Public health strategies need to be aligned to cultural and contextual characteristics in order to raise receptivity and salience of health information and access to services, through attention to the content, sources and channels of information dissemination. Such targeted interventions should consider language, format, culture and context as well as the mode of delivery across ethnic and faith-based media channels and social media platforms. It is no longer feasible, sustainable or economically viable to consider an 'opt-out' system of service delivery, which does not tailor healthcare to individual groups in society (MCB 2015).

Under-representation of Muslim women in healthcare services exacerbates poor health outcomes. These issues are well evidenced in the UK body of literature and include difficulties in navigating health services, and knowledge of available services (Markham et al. 2014), language and literacy (Taylor et al. 2013), lack of translation (Dixon et al. 2015), having no recourse to public funds and therefore no access to services (Kang et al. 2019), lack of same-gender providers, as well as divergent cultural value systems. Furthermore, negative stereotyping and false perceptions by HCPs about culture and belief systems are creating a situation where the health concerns of Muslim women are being minimised or ignored. This is problematic as there are impacts on patient safety and this culminates in a lack of trust and dissatisfaction with services. For Muslim women, there are specific cultural barriers around modesty, family involvement in care and the importance of maintaining religious practices. These are often not addressed in healthcare environments or clinical practice. There is therefore a need for healthcare providers to provide tailored care which is culturally appropriate and person-centred and which does not rely on stereotypes and assumptions. Removing this implicit bias evident in the healthcare system will help to build trust and allow Muslim women to feel valued and respected, knowing that their concerns are taken seriously – as is their right under the Equality Act (2010).

Public health policy in the UK is designed to protect and improve the nation's health and wellbeing, through health awareness, screening programmes, research and strategic policy design. However, research highlighted in this chapter shows that there are complex failures across all these remits, which negatively impact Muslim women. In particular, cancer-screening programmes and information surrounding risk, symptoms and treatments have identified specific challenges for Muslim women (Anderson de Cuevas et al. 2018). These barriers to accessing services are most apparent in older women, who were born outside the UK and have not accessed UK education systems, and therefore are not able to access public health information on disease prevention, and may experience language difficulties, challenges in travelling to health appointments caused through poverty (Almas et al. 2019), cultural and religious barriers, as well as paternalistic barriers, whereby male family members may not permit women to engage in cancer screening, as these are not in line with their own religious or cultural beliefs (Anderson de Cuevas et al. 2018).

In the UK, public health strategies are generally centralised around the need for healthy lifestyle choices, pushing the responsibility for health onto individuals. This makes it easy for the state to problematise groups or communities, as opposed to policy and decision makers. This can be seen in the case for increasing the nation's activity, which has been the national goal for Sport England, whose report indicated that 41 per cent of Muslim women were less likely to meet the physical activity guidelines (Sport England 2019). However, Muslim women have to negotiate a barrage of challenges to participate in physical activity (Stride and Flintoff 2018), such as personal and institutional racial discrimination (Koshoedo et al. 2015), cultural expectations, lack of female-only spaces for activities and access to sports hijabs, as well as managing their domestic responsibilities (Stride et al. 2018). Importantly, when looking at lifestyle choices, it must be remembered that these 'choices' are massively impacted by poverty and deprivation. Those who live in overcrowded, multi-generational, poor-quality housing in areas where there are high levels of crime have less agency, freedom and access to gyms, equipment and green spaces, which help the affluent members of society to stay healthy and exercise.

Moving forward, it is essential that national data collection methods are strengthened by disaggregating ethnicity, religion and gender, in order to develop a more nuanced (and intersectional) perspective of health outcomes as well as identifying gaps and disparities which need to be highlighted and addressed. Such data can be further enhanced by qualitative research around Muslim women's lived experiences, which often serves to 'humanise' statistical representations, facilitating greater understanding of the everyday struggles and challenges experienced. Tailored service provision is crucial to meet the needs of Muslim women, who have been under-served in research, education and health services, which means that their voices are absent from service design.

References

Abbas, T. (2003). 'The impact of religio-cultural norms and values on the education of young South Asian women'. *British Journal of Sociology of Education*, 24(4), 411–28.

Adebowale, V. and Rao, M. (2020). 'Racism in medicine: why equality matters to everyone'. *BMJ*, 368, m530.

Afshar, H. (1989). 'Gender roles and the "moral economy of kin" among Pakistani women in West Yorkshire'. *Journal of Ethnic and Migration Studies*, 15(2), 211–25.

Afshar, H. (2002). 'Strategies of resistance among the Muslim minority in West Yorkshire: impact on women', in N. Charles and H. Hintjens (eds), *Gender, Ethnicity and Political Ideologies*. London: Routledge, pp. 119–38.

Afshar, H., Aitken, R. and Franks, M. (2005). 'Feminisms, Islamophobia and identities'. *Political Studies*, 53(2), 262–83.

Afshar, H. and Barrientos, S. (1999). 'Introduction: Women, globalization and fragmentation', in H. Afshar and S. Barrientos (eds), *Women, Globalization and Fragmentation in the Developing World*. London: Palgrave Macmillan, pp. 1–17.

Afshar, H. and Maynard, M. (eds) (1994). *The Dynamics of 'Race' and Gender: Some Feminist Interventions*. London: Taylor & Francis.

Agide, F. D., Sadeghi, R., Garmaroudi, G. and Tigabu, B. M. (2018). 'A systematic review of health promotion interventions to increase breast cancer screening uptake: from the last 12 years'. *European Journal of Public Health*, 28(6), 1149–55.

Ahmad, A. (2011). 'British football: Where are the Muslim female footballers? Exploring the connections between gender, ethnicity and Islam'. *Soccer & Society*, 12(3), 443–56.

Ahmad, W. (1993). *Race and Health in Contemporary Britain*. Oxford: Oxford University Press.

Ajaz, M., Ali, N. and Randhawa, G. (2015). 'UK Pakistani views on the adverse health risks associated with consanguineous marriages'. *Journal of Community Genetics*, 6(4), 331–42.

Akhtar, P. (2014). '"We were Muslims but we didn't know Islam": migration, Pakistani Muslim women and changing religious practices in the UK'. *Women's Studies International Forum*, 47(B), 232–8.

All Party Parliamentary Group on British Muslims (2018). 'Islamophobia defined: the inquiry into a working definition of Islamophobia'. Available at: https://static1.squarespace.com/static/599c3d2febbd1a90cffdd8a9/t/5bfd1ea3352f531a6170ceee/1543315109493/Islamophobia+Defined.pdf (last accessed 2 May 2022).

Almas, N., Haith-Cooper, M., Nejadhamzeeigilani, Z, Payne, D. and Rattray, M. (2019). 'Wise Up to Cancer Bradford: improving cancer prevention and earlier diagnosis for South Asian women in Bradford'. Available at: https://bradscholars.brad.ac.uk/bitstream/handle/10454/17320/UoBWUTCFinalReportSept162019.pdf?sequence=2&isAllowed=y (last accessed 2 May 2022).

Anderson de Cuevas, R., Saini, P., Roberts, D., Beaver, K., Chandrashekar, M., Jain, A., Kotas, E., Tahir, N., Ahmed, S. and Brown, S. (2018). 'A systematic review of barriers and enablers to South Asian women's attendance for asymptomatic screening of breast and cervical cancers in emigrant countries'. *BMJ Open*, 8, e020892.

Anthias, F. (2012). 'Transnational mobilities, migration research and intersectionality'. *Nordic Journal of Migration Research*, 2(2), 102–10.

Anwar, M. (1979). *The Myth of Return: Pakistanis in Britain*. London: Heinemann Educational Books.

Babakus, W. S. and Thompson, J. L. (2012). 'Physical activity among South Asian women: a systematic, mixed-methods review'. *International Journal of Behavioral Nutrition and Physical Activity*, 9(1), 1–18.

Bagguley, P. and Hussain, Y. (2016). 'Negotiating mobility: South Asian women and higher education'. *Sociology*, 50(1), 43–59.

Birmingham City Council (2021). Scrutiny Inquiry: Infant Mortality. Available at: https://birmingham.cmis.uk.com/birmingham/Document.ashx?czJKcaeAi5tUFL1DTL2UE4zNRBcoShgo=fJWPz8KUikSi80Zy6tJEoxjbHzeTNenzrEUllHOdYylkevu8vGFgKg%3D%3D&rUzwRPf%2BZ3zd4E7Ikn8Lyw%3D%3D=pwRE6AGJFLDNlh225F5QMaQWCtPHwdhUfCZ%2FLUQzgA2uL5jNRG4jdQ%3D%3D&mCTIbCubSFfX (last accessed 2 May 2022).

Bolagnani, M. and Mellor, J. (2012). 'British Pakistani women's use of the "religion versus culture" contrast: a critical analysis'. *Culture and Religion*, 13(2), 211–26.

Britton, J. (2019). 'Muslim men, racialised masculinities and personal life'. *Sociology*, 53(1), 36–51.

Cabinet Office (2017). 'Race disparity audit: summary findings from the Ethnicity Facts and Figures website'. Available at: www.ethnicity-facts-figures.service.gov.uk/static/race-disparity-audit-summary-findings.pdf (last accessed 2 May 2022).

Casey, L. (2016). 'The Casey Review: a review into opportunity and integration'. Available at: https://assets.publishing.service.gov.uk/government/uploads/system/uploads/attachment_data/file/575973/The_Casey_Review_Report.pdf (last accessed 2 May 2022).

Charsley, K. (2006). 'Risk and ritual: the protection of British Pakistani women in transnational marriage'. *Journal of Ethnic and Migration Studies*, 32(7), 1169–87.

Charsley, K. (2007). 'Risk, trust, gender and transnational cousin marriage among British Pakistanis'. *Ethnic and Racial Studies*, 30(6), 1117–31.

Charsley, K., Bolognani, M., Ersanilli, E. and Spencer, S. (2020). *Marriage Migration and Integration*. London: Palgrave Macmillan.

Charsley, K. and Liversage, A. (2015). 'Silenced husbands: Muslim marriage migration and masculinity'. *Men and Masculinities*, 18(4), 489–508.

Cheruvallil-Contractor, S. (2012). *Muslim Women in Britain: De-mystifying the Muslimah*. London: Routledge.

Collings, P. J., Farrar, D., Gibson, J., West, J., Barber, S. E. and Wright, J. (2020). 'Associations of pregnancy physical activity with maternal cardiometabolic health, neonatal delivery outcomes and body composition in a biethnic cohort of 7305 mother–child pairs: The Born in Bradford study'. *Sports Medicine*, 50(3), 615–28.

Dale, A., Shaheen, N., Kalra, V. and Fieldhouse, E. (2002). 'Routes into education and employment for young Pakistani and Bangladeshi women in the UK'. *Ethnic and Racial Studies*, 25(6), 942–68.

Davis, K. (2008). 'Intersectionality as buzzword: A sociology of science perspective on what makes a feminist theory successful'. *Feminist Theory*, 9(1), 67–85.

Department for Education (2020). 'National statistics: Schools, pupils and their characteristics: January 2020'. Available at: www.gov.uk/government/statistics/schools-pupils-and-their-characteristics-january-2020 (last accessed 2 May 2022).

Dixon, J., King, D., Matosevic, T., Clark, M. and Knapp, M. (2015). 'Equity in the provision of palliative care in the UK: review of evidence'. Available at: www.mariecurie.org.uk/globalassets/media/documents/policy/campaigns/equity-palliative-care-uk-report-full-lse.pdf (last accessed 2 May 2022).

Dogra, S. A., Rai, K., Barber, S., McEachan, R. R., Adab, P. and Sheard, L. (2021). 'Delivering a childhood obesity prevention intervention using Islamic religious settings in the UK: What is most important to the stakeholders?' *Preventive Medicine Reports*, 22, 101387.

Donnelly, T. T. and Hwang, J. (2015). 'Breast cancer screening interventions for Arabic women: a literature review'. *Journal of Immigrant and Minority Health*, 17(3), 925–39.

Elahi, F. and Khan, O. (2017). 'Islamophobia: still a challenge for us all. A 20th-anniversary report'. The Runnymede Trust. Available at: www.runnymedetrust. org/publications/islamophobia-still-a-challenge-for-us-all (last accessed 2 May 2022).

Escribà-Agüir, V., Rodriguez-Gomez, M. and Ruiz-Perez, I. (2016). 'Effectiveness of patient-targeted interventions to promote cancer screening among ethnic minorities: A systematic review'. *Cancer Epidemiology*, 44, 22–39.

Fagerli, R. A., Lien, M. and Wandel, M. (2007). 'Health care style and trustworthiness as perceived by Pakistani-born persons with type 2 diabetes in Oslo, Norway'. *Health*, 11(1), 109–29.

Firdous, T., Darwin, Z. and Hassan, S. M. (2020). 'Muslim women's experiences of maternity services in the UK: qualitative systematic review and thematic synthesis'. *BMC Pregnancy and Childbirth*, 20, 115.

Gilliat-Ray, S. (2010). *Muslims in Britain: An Introduction*. Cambridge: Cambridge University Press.

Harrell, C. J. P., Burford, T. I., Cage, B. N., Nelson, T. M., Shearon, S., Thompson, A. and Green, S. (2011). 'Multiple pathways linking racism to health outcomes'. *Du Bois Review: Social Science Research on Race*, 8(1), 143.

Hassan, S. M., Leavey, C. and Rooney, J. S. (2019). 'Exploring English speaking Muslim women's first-time maternity experiences: a qualitative longitudinal interview study'. *BMC Pregnancy and Childbirth*, 19, 156.

Hassan, S. M., Leavey, C., Rooney, J. S. and Puthussery, S. (2020). 'A qualitative study of healthcare professionals' experiences of providing maternity care for Muslim women in the UK'. *BMC Pregnancy and Childbirth*, 20, 400.

Heath, A. (2014). 'Introduction: Patterns of generational change: convergent, reactive or emergent?'. *Ethnic and Racial Studies*, 37, 1, 1–9.

Heath, A. and Li, Y. (2015). 'Review of the relationship between religion and poverty; an analysis for the Joseph Rowntree Foundation. CSI Working paper 2015-01'. Available at: http://csi.nuff.ox.ac.uk/wp-content/uploads/2015/03/religion-and-poverty-working-paper.pdf I (last accessed 2 May 2022).

Hou, S. I., Sealy, D. A. and Kabiru, C. W. (2011). 'Closing the disparity gap: cancer screening interventions among Asians—a systematic literature review'. *Asian Pacific Journal of Cancer Prevention*, 12(11), 3133–9.

Ige-Elegbede, J., Pilkington, P., Gray, S. and Powell, J. (2019). 'Barriers and facilitators of physical activity among adults and older adults from Black and Minority Ethnic groups in the UK: A systematic review of qualitative studies'. *Preventive Medicine Reports*, 15, 100952.

Kalra, V. (2000). *From Textile Mills to Taxi Ranks: Experiences of Migration, Labour and Social Change*. Aldershot: Ashgate.

Kalmakis, K. A. and Chandler, G. E. (2015). 'Health consequences of adverse childhood experiences: A systematic review'. *Journal of the American Association of Nurse Practitioners*, 27(8), 457–65.

Kang, C., Tomkow, L. and Farrington, R. (2019). 'Access to primary health care for asylum seekers and refugees: a qualitative study of service user experiences in the UK'. *British Journal of General Practice*, 69(685), e537–e545.

Karlsen, S. and Nazroo, J. Y. (2002). 'Relation between racial discrimination, social class, and health among ethnic minority groups'. *American Journal of Public Health*, 92(4), 624–31.

Khattab, N. (2009). 'Occupational attainment in Britain and ethno-religious background as a determinant of educational and occupational attainment in Britain'. *Sociology*, 43(2), 304–22.

Khattab, N. (2012). '"Winners" and "losers": the impact of education, ethnicity and gender on Muslims in the British labour market'. *Work, Employment & Society*, 26(4), 556–73.

Khattab, N., Johnston, R., Sirkeci, I. and Modood, T. (2010). 'The impact of spatial segregation on the employment outcomes amongst Bangladeshi men and women in England and Wales'. *Sociological Research Online*, 15(1), 1–15.

Khattab, N. and Modood, T. (2018). 'Accounting for British Muslim's educational attainment: gender differences and the impact of expectations'. *British Journal of Sociology of Education*, 39(2), 242–59.

King's Fund (2006). 'Access to healthcare and minority ethnic groups'. Available at: www.kingsfund.org.uk/sites/default/files/field/field_publication_file/access-to-health-care-minority-ethnic-groups-briefing-kings-fund-february-2006.pdf (last accessed 2 May 2022).

King's Fund (2019). 'Public satisfaction with the NHS and social care in 2019: Results from the British Social Attitudes survey'. Available at: www.kingsfund.org.uk/publications/public-satisfaction-nhs-social-care-2019 (last accessed 2 May 2022).

Knight, M., Bunch, K., Tuffnell, D., Shakespeare, J., Kotnis, R., Kenyon, S. and Kurinczuk, J. J. (2019). 'Saving lives, improving mothers' care: lessons learned to inform maternity care from the UK and Ireland confidential enquiries into maternal deaths and morbidity 2015–17'. MBRRACE-UK. Available at: www.npeu.ox.ac.uk/downloads/files/mbrrace-uk/reports/MBRRACE-UK%20Maternal%20Report%202019%20-%20WEB%20VERSION.pdf (last accessed 2 May 2022).

Koshoedo, S. A., Paul-Ebhohimhen, V. A., Jepson, R. G. and Watson, M. C. (2015). 'Understanding the complex interplay of barriers to physical activity amongst black and minority ethnic groups in the United Kingdom: a qualitative synthesis using meta-ethnography'. *BMC Public Health*, 15(1), 1–16.

Kushnick, L. (1988). 'Racism, the National Health Service, and the health of black people'. *International Journal of Health Services*, 18(3), 457–70.

Laird, L. D., Amer, M. M., Barnett, E. D. and Barnes, L. L. (2007). 'Muslim patients and health disparities in the UK and the US'. *Archives of Disease in Childhood*, 92(10), 922–6.

Lenneis, V. and Pfister, G. (2017). 'When girls have no opportunities and women have neither time nor energy: the participation of Muslim female cleaners in recreational physical activity'. *Sport in Society*, 20(9), 1203–22.

Ludwig, A. F., Cox, P. and Ellahi, B. (2011). 'Social and cultural construction of obesity among Pakistani Muslim women in North West England'. *Public Health Nutrition*, 14(10), 1842–50.

Markham, S., Islam, Z. and Faull, C. (2014). 'I never knew that! Why do people from Black and Asian Minority Ethnic groups in Leicester access hospice services less than other groups? A discussion with community groups'. *Diversity and Equality in Health and Care*, 11(3), 237–45.

Marmot, M. (2020). 'Health equity in England: the Marmot Review 10 years on'. *BMJ*, 368, m693.

Mental Health Foundation (2020). 'Black Asian and Minority Ethnic (BAME) communities'. Available at: www.mentalhealth.org.uk/a-to-z/b/black-asian-and-minority-ethnic-bame-communities (last accessed 2 May 2022).

Miles, C. and Benn, T. (2016). 'A case study on the experiences of university-based Muslim women in physical activity during their studies at one UK higher education institution'. *Sport, Education and Society*, 21(5), 723–40.

Modood, T. (1997). 'Employment', in T. Modood, R. Berthoud, J. Lakey, J. Nazroo, P. Smith, S. Virdee and S. Beishon (eds), *Ethnic Minorities in Britain: Diversity and Disadvantage*. London: Policy Studies Institute, pp. 83–149.

Modood, T. (2004). 'Capitals, ethnic identity and educational qualifications'. *Cultural Trends*, 13(2), 87–105.

Mohammad, R. (1999). 'Marginalisation, Islamism and the production of the "other's other"'. *Gender, Place and Culture*, 6(3), 221–40.

Mohammad, R. (2005). 'British Pakistani Muslim women: marking the body, marking the nation', in L. Nelson and J. Seager (eds), *A Companion to Feminist Geography*. London: Blackwell Publishing Ltd, pp. 379–97.

Mohammad, R. (2013). 'Making gender ma(r)king place: Youthful British Pakistani Muslim women's narratives of urban space'. *Environment and Planning A: Economy and Space*, 45(8), 1802–22.

Morris, J. and Scobie, S. (2020). 'Quality and inequality in the NHS'. *British Journal of Healthcare Management*, 26(7), 189–91.

Mosdøl, A., Lidal, I. B., Straumann, G. H. and Vist, G. E. (2017). 'Targeted mass media interventions promoting healthy behaviours to reduce risk of non-communicable diseases in adult, ethnic minorities'. *Cochrane Database of Systematic Reviews*, 2(2), CD011683.

Mud Orange (2021). 'British Muslims' attitudes and behaviours towards exercising, activewear, vitamins and fitness supplements'. Available at: www.mudorange. com/m-economy/health-and-fitness (last accessed 2 May 2022).

Muslim Council of Britain (2015). 'British Muslims in numbers: a demographic socioeconomic and health profile of Muslims in Britain drawing on the 2011 Census'. MCB. Available at: www.mcb.org.uk/wp-content/uploads/2015/02/ MCBCensusReport_2015.pdf (last accessed 2 May 2022).

Muttarak, R. (2014). 'Generation, ethnic and religious diversity in friendship choice: exploring interethnic close ties in Britain'. *Ethnic and Racial Studies*, 37(1), 71–98.

NHS England (2016). 'National maternity review'. Available at: www.england.nhs.uk/ wp-content/uploads/2016/02/national-maternity-review-report.pdf (last accessed 2 May 2022).

Office for National Statistics (2011). 'Ethnicity and national identity in England and Wales: 2011'. Available at: www.ons.gov.uk/peoplepopulationandcommunity/ culturalidentity/ethnicity/articles/ethnicityandnationalidentityinenglandan- dwales/2012-12-11 (last accessed 2 May 2022).

Office for National Statistics (2020). 'Religion, education and work in England and Wales: February 2020'. Available at: www.ons.gov.uk/peoplepopulationand- community/culturalidentity/religion/articles/religioneducationandworkineng- landandwales/february2020 (last accessed 2 May 2022).

Padilla, A.M. (1994). 'Ethnic minority scholars, research, and mentoring: current and future issues'. *Educational Researcher*, 23(4), 24–7.

Pollard, T. M. and Guell, C. (2012). 'Assessing physical activity in Muslim women of South Asian origin'. *Journal of Physical Activity and Health*, 9(7), 970–6.

Pollock, L. (2005). 'Experiences of maternity services: Muslim women's perspec- tives'. Available at: www.maternityaction.org.uk/wp-content/uploads/2013/09/ muslimwomensexperiencesofmaternityservices.pdf (last accessed 2 May 2022).

Pratt, R., Mohamed, S., Dirie, W., Ahmed, N., Lee, S., VanKeulen, M. and Carlson, S. (2020). 'Testing a religiously tailored intervention with Somali American Muslim women and Somali American imams to increase participation in breast and cervi- cal cancer screening'. *Journal of Immigrant and Minority Health*, 22(1), 87–95.

Pratt, R., Njau, S. W., Ndagire, C., Chaisson, N., Toor, S., Ahmed, N., Mohamed, S. and Dirks, J. (2019). '"We are Muslims and these diseases don't happen to us": A qualitative study of the views of young Somali men and women concerning HPV immunization'. *Vaccine*, 37(15), 2043–50.

Public Health England (2020). 'National General Practice Profiles'. Available at: https://fingertips.phe.org.uk/profile/general-practice (last accessed 2 May 2022).

Puddifoot, K. (2019). 'Stereotyping patients'. *Journal of Social Philosophy*, 50(1), 69–90.

Puthussery, S. (2016). 'Perinatal outcomes among migrant mothers in the United Kingdom: is it a matter of biology, behaviour, policy, social determinants or access to health care?'. *Best Practice & Research Clinical Obstetrics & Gynaecology*, 32, 39–49.

Saritoprak, S. N. and Exline, J. J. (2020). 'Religious coping among Muslims with mental and medical health concerns', in A. Bagasra and M. Mackinem (eds), *Working with Muslim Clients in the Helping Professions*. Hershey, PA: IGI Global, pp. 201–20.

Scourfield, J., Gilliat-Ray, S., Khan, A. and Otri, S. (2013). *Muslim Childhood: Religious Nurture in a European Context*. Oxford: Oxford University Press.

Shankley, W. and Rhodes, J. (2020). 'Racisms in contemporary Britain', in W. Shankley, B. Byrne, C. Alexander, O. Khan and J. Nazro (eds), *Ethnicity and Race in the UK: State of the Nation*. Bristol: Bristol University Press, pp. 203–28.

Shaw, A. (1988). *A Pakistani Community in Britain*. New York: Basil Blackwell Inc.

Shaw, A. (2000). *Kinship and Continuity: Pakistani Families in Britain*. Reading: Harwood Academic Publishers.

Sherif, J. (2021). 'The impact of unconscious bias on Muslim women's experiences of healthcare'. BJGP Life. Available at: https://bjgplife.com/2021/05/14/the-impact-of-unconscious-bias-on-muslim-womens-experiences-of-healthcare (last accessed 2 May 2022).

Sport England (2019). 'Active Lives adult data', November 2018/19. Available at: https://activelives.sportengland.org/Home/AdultData (last accessed 2 May 2022).

Sport England (2021). 'Uniting the movement: our 10-year vision to transform lives and communities through sport and physical activity'. Available at: www.sport-england.org/why-were-here/uniting-the-movement#readourstrategy-13743 (last accessed 2 May 2022).

Stride, A. (2014). 'Centralising space: the physical education and physical activity experiences of South Asian, Muslim girls'. *Sport, Education and Society*, 21(5), 677–97.

Stride, A. and Flintoff, A. (2018). '"I don't want my parents' respect going down the drain": South Asian, Muslim young women negotiating family and physical activity'. *Asia-Pacific Journal of Health, Sport and Physical Education*, 8(1), 3–17.

Stride, A., Flintoff, A. and Scraton, S. (2018). '"Homing in": South Asian, Muslim young women and their physical activity in and around the home'. *Curriculum Studies in Health and Physical Education*, 9(3), 253–69.

Tackett, S., Young, J. H., Putman, S., Wiener, C., Deruggiero, K. and Bayram, J. D. (2018). 'Barriers to healthcare among Muslim women: A narrative review of the literature'. *Women's Studies International Forum*, 69, 190–4.

Taylor, S. P., Nicolle, C. and Maguire, M. (2013). 'Cross-cultural communication barriers in health care'. *Nursing Standard*, 27(31), 35–43.

Tell MAMA (2018). 'Beyond the incident: outcomes for victims of anti-Muslim prejudice'. Executive summary. Available at: https://tellmamauk.org/wp-content/uploads/2018/07/EXECUTIVE-SUMMARY.pdf (last accessed 2 May 2022).

Thornton, J. (2020). 'Ethnic minority patients receive worse mental healthcare than white patients, review finds'. *BMJ*, 368, m1058.

Velayati, M. (2018). 'Formation of "religious" identity among British Muslim women', in E. Ruspini, G. T. Bonifacio and C. Corradi (eds), *Women and Religion: Contemporary and Future Challenges in the Global Era*. Bristol: Policy Press, pp. 95–116.

Vertovec, S. (2008). 'Religion and diaspora', in P. Antes, A. W. Geertz and R. R. Warne (eds), *New Approaches to the Study of Religion. Volume 2: Textual, Comparative, Sociological, and Cognitive Approaches*. Berlin: Walter de Gruyter, pp. 275–304.

Walton, L. M., Akram, F. and Hossain, F. (2014). 'Health beliefs of Muslim women and implications for health care providers: Exploratory study on the health beliefs of Muslim women'. *Online Journal of Health Ethics*, 10(2), 5.

Waters, M. C. (2014). 'Defining difference: the role of immigrant generation and race in American and British immigration studies'. *Ethnic and Racial Studies*, 37(1), 10–26.

Werbner, P. (1990). 'Economic rationality and hierarchical gift economies: value and ranking among British Pakistanis'. *Man*, 25(2), 266–85.

Werbner, P. (2004). 'Theorising complex diasporas: purity and hybridity in the South Asian public sphere in Britain'. *Journal of Ethnic and Migration Studies*, 30(5), 895–911.

Werbner, P. (2007). 'Veiled interventions in pure space: honour, shame and embodied struggles among Muslims in Britain and France'. *Theory, Culture & Society*, 24(2), 161–86.

Williams, D. R., Priest, N. and Anderson, N. (2019). 'Understanding associations between race, socioeconomic status, and health: patterns and prospects', in J. Oberlander, M. Buchbinder, L. R. Churchill, S. E. Estroff, N. M. P. King, B. F. Saunders, R. P. Strauss, R. L. Walker (eds), *The Social Medicine Reader*, vol. II, 3rd edn. Durham, NC: Duke University Press, pp. 258–67.

Williams, R. and Hunt, K. (1997). 'Psychological distress among British South Asians: the contribution of stressful situations and subcultural differences in the West of Scotland Twenty-07 Study'. *Psychological Medicine*, 27(5), 1173–81.

Ypinazar, V. A. and Margolis, S. A. (2006). 'Delivering culturally sensitive care: the perceptions of older Arabian Gulf Arabs concerning religion, health, and disease'. *Qualitative Health Research*, 16(6), 773–8.

Zwysen, W., Di Stasi, V. and Heath, A. (2021). 'Ethnic minorities are less likely to find good work than their white British counterparts, even when born and educated in the UK'. British Politics and Policy at LSE, blog post, 19 January. |Available at: https://blogs.lse.ac.uk/politicsandpolicy/ethnic-penalties-and-hiring-discrimination (last accessed 2 May 2022).

4

RELEVANCE OF RESEARCH METHODOLOGIES USED IN HEALTH PSYCHOLOGY FOR BRITISH MUSLIMS: AN EPISTEMOLOGICAL CRITIQUE ON THE COLONISATION OF KNOWLEDGE PRODUCTION

Aaliyah Shaikh

Introduction

It has been argued that in order to study Muslims, it is crucial to do so within an Islamic ontological framework (Azram 2011; Elmessiri 2013; Malik 2019; Grosfoguel 2013). There is a distinct lack of meaningful representative research on British Muslims' experiences of health, and in particular health psychology, through a non-orientalised lens. From the outset of my academic journey, I have been concerned about how British Muslims in general and Muslim women specifically are researched and how Western literature reproduces certain dynamics of regressiveness and orientalisation, and the lack of meaningful growth and development in research with Muslim populations. Stonebanks (2008) highlights that there has been a failing in research when it comes to representing Muslims, asserting that 'Muslim communities continue to be dehumanized'. This chapter draws upon my PhD research experience exploring the most appropriate fit of methodology and underlying philosophical inquiries when considering research with British Muslims. I share a broad overview of the considerations, challenges, dilemmas and topics I investigated and/or came across in the context of looking at Muslims' experiences in healthcare of pregnancy and birth and the impact on mental health and intergenerational trauma, with a consideration of intersectional factors, which I did so under the umbrella of decolonising approaches.

Epistemicide

Understanding the role of epistemicide – the destruction of knowledge and knowledge systems, also referred to as intellectual genocide – is crucial. As Savransky (2017) states: 'there is no social and cognitive justice without existential justice, no politics of knowledge without a politics of reality'. Throughout colonial and postcolonial history, dominant Eurocentric sociopolitical narratives have been pushed as superior and civilised above other forms of knowing, creating a disconnect and looking down upon indigenous or non-'mainstream' ways of knowing. Additionally, such narratives seem particularly incapable of providing nuanced and multi-layered understandings of complex phenomena, such as intergenerational trauma experienced by British Muslims that has left a legacy on minds and bodies resulting in and from painful experiences (this topic itself would require an entire chapter).

It is important to recognise and understand the historical impact of colonisation, especially in thinking about implications on health and health services, and to consider the need to 'decolonise' how we look at health psychology especially for diaspora communities. The open-ended inquiry requires ongoing reflection on what we are decolonising from and what decolonisation really means and involves, including limitations and benefits of movements in this area. We may question the relevance, appropriateness and usefulness of existing health research methods and ask if there is space for an authentic emergence of decolonised, non-mainstream, dominant Western experiences to be considered, included or even centred. For me, it was critical to situate myself as a researcher in a positionality that was able to think beyond the Eurocentric and centre multiple ways of knowing, drawing on the pluriversity of knowledge traditions, in order not to perpetuate and merely reproduce orientalist and limiting ways of knowing. Furthermore, there are serious concerns with how Muslim women's expression of pain and suffering is responded to derogatorily, such as what is known as the 'Begum syndrome':

> You may know a typical Begum. She is an Asian woman suffering from non-specific pains and weakness. When questioned, pains change places. On examination, nothing is apparently wrong . . . Doctors become irritated. Students are perplexed. Twenty years ago, someone wrote her up: 'The Begum syndrome.' (Dosani 2001)

Ali (2020), a neurology registrar, writes about a similar deeply problematic and racist term, 'bibi-itis', stating that 'The term serves as an example of casual clinical stereotyping that can cause unrecognised bias leading to missed diagnoses, delayed treatment, and preventable unwanted outcomes'. In another response to an article in the *BMJ*:

> There are well known stereotypes such as Bibi syndrome or Begum syndrome which are often colloquially used to describe South Asian patients with non-specific complaints. These only serve to undermine patients and as this article points out contribute to health inequality. (Kmietowicz et al. 2019)

Instead of disregarding and devaluing experiences Muslim women may present with, it is crucial to enquire what is actually going on, and after excluding physical illness, to think beyond the physical manifestation, to think about the meaning of that communication of pain. One possibility of enquiry may be to think in terms of unconscious trauma that is stored in the body that can be hard to name. Labelling suffering with derogatory devaluing phrases perpetuates original wounds that may be located in colonial and postcolonial trauma, discrimination and their multifaceted fallouts psychosocially. Knight et al. (2019) highlight a very specific example where research is urgently needed to understand why Black women are five times more likely and Asian women twice as likely to die in childbirth compared to White women. It is necessary to critically enquire into the multifactorial aetiology of this, including the role of discriminatory practices, and how intergenerational and postcolonial traumas may contribute to such outcomes. As such, it may be necessary to draw on alterative research methodology which may not fit easily into the standard 'evidence-based medicine' paradigm. Lack of research and evidence base is also arguably a point requiring critical reflection: why and where resources go, and why some issues and some communities' experiences are lacking or not being supported with resources and funding to carry out critical research on the diverse and complex nature of health and psychological issues being experienced.

There is an urgent need to think about how discrimination and other factors including trauma more generally – in all its forms, be they racial, postcolonial, intergenerational or other – are understood and represented while conducting research in health psychology. With regard to British Muslims in particular, it is important to explore non-Eurocentric ways of understanding and to think about the relevance of Islamic knowledge production about health, the self and the body. For example, there was a time when psychology was understood to be the study of the soul, although later through the secularisation of knowledge this came to be known as study of the mind, which impacts the scope of interpretation and understanding. There are narratives and explanations of health and illness lacking in much of mainstream research. One of the questions we may ponder is how we can conceptualise (and actualise) non-Eurocentric and non-secular ways of knowing and making sense of experiences.

Critical Medical Humanities (CMH) provide a useful framework as a complementary critique within the decolonising methodology approach when thinking about Muslims' experiences of health. Furthermore, drawing on CMH allows a critical look through the research world and practice in Britain. The diversity and plurality expected of CMH have been considered a strength for encouraging creativity and epistemological innovation (Viney et al. 2015):

> [CMH is] intended as an invitation to keep the field of medical humanities open to new voices, challenges, events, and disciplinary (and anti- or post-disciplinary) articulations of the realities of medicine and health; to be adventurous in its intellectual pursuits, practical activities, and articulation with the domain of the political. (ibid.)

This fits well with the decolonising methods approach and lends itself to multiple narratives, ideas and possibilities. CMH has allowed for resistance to positivist biomedical 'reductionism' and is sensitive to narrative-based interventions and their limitations vis-à-vis experiences of health inequalities of British Muslims.

Thinking about Philosophy, Paradigms and their Relevance

Each paradigm and philosophy will have its underpinnings contested. The most important issue is relevance and appropriateness, and that the fit should be right for the group or phenomenon being studied. Concepts in research paradigms, philosophy and methodologies need to be deconstructed, adapted and reconstructed considering ontology, epistemology, methodology, methods and analysis that take the context of British Muslims into account. Furthermore, it is necessary to explore, acknowledge and learn from non-Eurocentric ways of knowing, i.e. ways of knowing prevalent among British Muslims and Muslims in general, particularly those that could support and improve health outcomes, for example. The psychological and historical contexts and roots of theories or philosophies used must be thought about, recognised and reflected upon in reaching an understanding of the chosen approach with British Muslims, with flexibility and creativity in approach and development of new ideas.

Creativity became the starting point for the 'patchwork quilt', where I, as a British Muslim academic researcher, tried to piece together a relevant approach and guiding philosophical enquiry for researching Muslims' experiences:

> Creativity is a crucial issue in science. Scientific research should not be restricted to the logical development and application of known ideas but

should promote new ideas to expand knowledge beyond the existing frontiers. Stimulating scientific creativity means not only giving a boost to creative thinking, but also taking into account the factors that put a brake on creativity. (Grégoire 2018)

Grégoire's (2018) ideas are supported in the context of an Islamic understanding of what constitutes knowledge. God has endowed humans with potentials of creative and conceptual knowledge (Azram 2011). These faculties are used to enhance and further our understanding through various methods of enquiries. This links to ideas about embodiment and the creative nature of the research process itself, whereby research conversations can lead to a 'positive creative transformation of some change' (Gilliat-Ray 2010).

Decolonising Methodologies: the Impact of Colonialism and Epistemicide

It is critical to understand the root of the dismantling of knowledge structures alongside political destabilisation in the Muslim world, during the colonial period and its impact on British Muslims' heritage and the subsequent impact on knowledge, education, science and research. Epistemicide refers to the intellectual genocide that occurred as a result of colonialism (Grosfoguel 2013; Malik 2019). Some important historical context:

> In the late 15th century, Al-Andalus/Muslim Spain was in the final stages of conquest by the Catholic Monarchy and accompanying the physical genocide of the population of Al-Andalus was intellectual genocide, or what Grosfoguel has referred to as epistemicide. Along with murdering and suppressing an entire population of Muslims and Jews, mass burning of libraries was undertaken. (Grosfoguel, in Malik 2019)

Sadly, the above is not the only case of intellectual genocide. Inevitably, this had a significant impact on society and particularly the communities on the receiving end of this aggressive and violent act of intellectual colonisation that ran in tandem with the physical conquest. This is why it can be useful to frame research studies with British Muslims being mindful of Islamic ontology and epistemology as part of the process of empowerment, restoration and healing. For some second- and third-generation children of migrant heritage from countries and communities that were colonised, there is dissociation from, and lack of knowledge of aspects of history because it has been erased. Many immigrant parents faced complex traumas which redirected their focus to survival and being able to establish a secure base. In fact, 'immigrants who are not classified as refugees, especially those with low socioeconomic status and those who migrate to a country without authorization, can experience some of the same traumas experienced by refugees' (Perreira and Ornelas 2013).

With so much to contend with at that time, many Muslim migrants from newly independent ex-colonies under the British Empire could not necessarily prioritise preservation of knowledge or knowledge systems. The majority of Muslim migrants to Britain were from working-class backgrounds. They built their systems and preserved values through mosques and community spaces. Much literature, poetry, ideas, philosophies and (especially tragic) stories have been wiped or are lesser preserved in some sections of Muslim communities and in the memories of forthcoming generations, producing an intergenerational disconnect from the place of origin (Malik 2019).

Grosfoguel (2013) discusses the epistemic racism/sexism that is foundational to the knowledge structures of the 'Westernised University'. He proposes that the epistemic privilege of 'Western Man in Westernised Universities' structures of knowledge is the result of four genocides/epistemicides in the sixteenth century against Jewish and Muslim origin populations during the conquest of Al-Andalus (ibid.). Further, he outlines these epistemicides as the conquest of the Americas in relation to three other world-historical processes such as ethnic and religious cleansing, the enslavement of Africans in the Americas and, significantly, in relation to the point about standardised imposition of research methods: 'the killing of millions of women burned alive in Europe accused of being witches in relation to knowledge structures'. Grosfoguel (2013) proposes a question:

> How is it possible that the canon of thought in all the disciplines of the Social Sciences and Humanities in the Westernized university is based on the knowledge produced by a few men from five countries in Western Europe (Italy, France, England, Germany and the USA)?

He goes on to question the nature of how is it possible for these few men to have achieved epistemic privilege to such a degree that this knowledge is seen as superior to that of the rest of the world. How did they monopolise the authority of knowledge? And why is it that what we know today of the social, historical, philosophical and other disciplines is based on the sociohistorical experience and worldviews of men from these five countries? (ibid.).

This raises critical questions around power and control, oppression and injustices within health and social sciences and how research methodologies and analytic interpretations are applied in relation to exploring lived experiences of British Muslims. What does it mean for students, researchers and academics if the 'canon of thought' that is learned from and the legacy it has left in the health and social sciences and humanities is based entirely on the 'white privilege' and 'whitewashed' worldviews in five Western countries that he refers to? Grosfoguel (ibid.) talks about how this is guised under the notion of 'universality' of knowledge production. As a consequence, other non-Western forms of inquiry are viewed as anecdotal and inferior in scope and application. This highlights the urgency for critical engagement at all levels of research, science, knowledge, theory formation and policies.

Western Domination of Science and its Application

The normalisation of Eurocentric and liberal secular application of research ontology, epistemology and thus methodology have been taken for granted as a standard way of knowing that is systemically entrenched within academia. This can be difficult to notice, certainly for the novice student researcher or academic not previously exposed to a critical line of thinking and the need for thinking about other ways of knowing than what are presented to us. In a globalised world, these dominant so-called 'superior and civilised' methods have been problematically internalised by, and historically exported to, other societies. The projection of dominant Eurocentric ideas, ontologies and customs becomes the normative culture and anything outside of that is viewed as 'foreign' or inferior, including that of health practitioners who do not embody colonial mindsets and develop approaches with holistic goals in mind, becoming marginalised. As Chilisa (2011) states:

> When any group within a large, complex civilisation significantly dominates other groups for hundreds of years, the ways of the dominant group (its epistemologies, ontologies and axiologies) not only become the dominant ways of that civilisation, but also these ways become so deeply embedded that they typically are seen as 'natural' or appropriate norms rather than as historically evolved social constructions.

There is little recognition of, and much obliteration of, the vast and complex exchange of learning that occurred over centuries between the Muslim and Western worlds. There is a rich tradition and heritage of excellent scholarship, in ethics and medicine for example, with the first mental health hospital being established in Basra around the ninth century, the first university, known as al-Qarawiyyin University, being established in 859 by a Muslim woman – Fatima al-Fihri – in the Moroccan city of Fez. Today it is recognised as the oldest existing university in the world. There are numerous inventions, ideas, disciplines and philosophies originally contributed by the Muslim world that the public conscience remains unaware of. For example, Ibn Khaldun, one of the earliest sociologists and an associate of al-Qarawiyyin University, is rarely discussed in the context of sociology subjects in Britain, and nor are numerous other leading figures in many disciplines. In obliterating various knowledge traditions, there are wider implications; what is lost has immeasurable value that all of humanity could benefit from.

Alternative approaches to Eurocentric methodologies have created a space of their own within knowledge production systems. However, in practice they are arguably still not seen as equal in academia, and are often labelled condescendingly as 'soft approaches'. Similarly devalued are indigenous research methods and theories, which are often not considered valid or worthy, as is evident from the lack of wide availability of examples in academic texts or published articles (Martin and Mirraboopa 2003). The application of Eurocentric hierarchical systems that miss the voices of women and people of other worldviews and a consideration of divine knowledge and reality beyond rationality will have limited scope in inquiries about bodies and health in documenting and understanding experiences of British Muslims and others.

The 'Crisis' of Values?

In developing my ontological position, I drew on some ideas argued in Davutoğlu's discussion of Husserl's *Crisis of European Sciences* (Morrison 2014). Initially when I set out on this path of researching a methodology, I did so within what I would now refer to as taken for granted and commonly drawn upon methodologies within health and social sciences. This was not something I would have questioned in the way I ultimately ended up doing. I started by looking at phenomenology, as that was a well-trodden path in my field. In my quest to look at sources of knowledge and theories I drew on my Islamic education that centres the importance of considering chains of narration, and context; narrators/authors and what influenced them is an inherent part of Islamic intellectual tradition. I explored the three philosophers Heidegger, Husserl and Merleau-Ponty, considered the main 'founding fathers' of Western phenomenology. Reading about their logic, theory and conclusions raised multiple questions. Ideas of phenomenology were not fully aligned with my positionality and I found them to be limiting, one reason being bracketing out the self as researcher in a space where embodiment was essential.

My engagement with the debates on ontologies and methodologies became about locating them within historically and currently relevant contexts. Morrison (2014) discusses Ahmet Davutoğlu's understanding of Husserl's *Crisis of European Sciences* that draws on commonality and divergence on philosophical issues. The commonality for Husserl and Davutoğlu was that they both 'perceive a crisis in humanity and identify its causes in scientism and logical positivism, against which they develop their respective phenomenological alternatives' (in Morrison 2014). Morrison illuminates for the reader Davutoğlu's

> putatively comprehensive interpretation of Islam, diagnosis of the ills of secularism, modernisation, and crisis of values he finds in Muslim societies; and his prescribed treatment for those ills: the privileging of ontology over epistemology, and the full unfolding of core theological concepts of revelation, monotheism, and prophecy. (ibid.)

This exploration of the 'ills' of secularism and the 'crisis of values' in Muslim societies invoked my quest for positionality by virtue of being a Muslim academic and a researcher in health psychology, I wanted to explore what this meant.

For example, the concern I had with Husserl's key concept of 'bracketing out' the self as researcher could not work in a study that is fundamentally about embodiment of experience, rooted in *tawhid* (oneness and unity) and cognisant of Islamic ontology, and it felt too reductionist. Engaging with the concept of bracketing out critically was a significant intellectual dissonance in the formation of my ideas. This helped shape the argument for my methodology as well as an awareness that applying bracketing out would create a split and be the opposite of the constituting elements of my ontological positionality that includes connection, embodiment and oneness.

It became particularly critical to question my own ideas based on Western education which at times felt limited, irrelevant and creating a disconnect from my positionality. Davutoğlu (in Morrison 2014) addresses the need to recognise 'the actual or attempted imposition of the Western worldview onto Muslim peoples, whether at the insistence of Western people engaged in (neo-)imperialist enterprises, or Muslims themselves in misguided modernisation efforts'. There is a distinction being made regarding the origin of the differences being from the 'philosophical, methodological, and theoretical background rather than institutional and historical differences' (Morrison 2014).

Research Models Alien to the Socioreligious Realities of British Muslims

The dogma of colonisation and secularisation of knowledge has been that it considered anything 'Eastern' or non-Western as inferior and uncivilised:

> Throughout the last two centuries the standard thesis has been that classical science is originally European, emanating directly from Greek philosophy and science. Economic discourse justifies a superior power over the world, which then becomes economically dependent on an international division

of labor. All forms of social organization and political management outside the West are considered inferior and incapable of renewal and development. This resulting dogma justifies imperialism and Western hegemony in its worst forms. (Hussein 2013)

The dominance of the Eurocentric knowledge production system has led to a dangerous erasure of history and experiences. Elmessiri (2013) describes the widespread neglected academic issue of the adoption and acceptance of paradigms, terminologies and research models which are alien to the realities and context of the Muslim world. He highlights that despite the cultural paradigm being different, academics in some Muslim countries encounter a foreign Western paradigm in the form of research and science methodologies as permeating their thought processes. Arguably, this is due to ignorance of the process and awareness of their own epistemologies and to the fact that without critical thinking it is easy to take for granted mass notions of education and what constitutes valid knowledge. His point rings true outside Muslim countries for Muslims in the West and Global North who may not have come across discourses around decoloniality, critical thinking and the issues associated with dominant discourses. I can attest to this journey of starting from a default position of not knowing and using whatever was available and presented to me through the education system. Ultimately, reality becomes distorted through the lens of the other, when one sees one's own self and community through the eyes and models and frameworks of others. The paradigms, ontologies, epistemologies, methodologies and theories may have advantages in their own context in the West. However, trying to transpose them onto a different cultural context can be seriously problematic and have a distorting effect. Elmessiri (2013) highlights the process where any community that adopts an imported alien paradigm and – often without awareness of the epistemological implications of such paradigms – ends up becoming threatened. This trend is visible in the Western portrayal of Islam and Muslims as terrorists or the longstanding trope of oppressed women that need liberating. There are long-term psychological and practical implications of this on research, on scholars and on practice, and how this translates to application in the real world such as policy implications or clinical practice. Elmessiri (2013) suggests a remedy by 'establishing a new science with its own mechanisms, methodologies, and points of reference to address epistemological biases and invite "ijtihad" (interpretation)'.

Many epistemological metaphors come biased and limit freedom of research and thought. Other realities are overlooked, missed or not even conceptualised at all due to the bias of the prevalent and dominant Western models of research. New methodologies will help express new paradigms. It is not necessary that these new paradigms replace existing ones but they may function as more relevant and useful and be wider in their parameters, allowing more nuanced means to study Muslim societies (Elmessiri 2013). For example, many cultures and worldviews emphasise life in circular and cyclical ways of knowing, not just in linear ways which much of the Eurocentric system is based on. Islamic philosophy highlights the interdependence of God's creation, including cyclical relationships between creation – there are several passages in the Qur'an that detail the cycles of day and night, light and dark, the moon and the sun as metaphors. Cyclical ways of knowing also connect to feminine ways of knowing and embodying spiritual-biological experiences which work on the cyclical. This is an area to research further in terms of health experiences of women that would offer new insights. Linear frameworks remain dominant in virtually every aspect of life in the Western world and are adopted globally. Pope (2012) focuses on female leadership through embracing the cyclical nature of menstruation as the central guiding force in a woman's life and argues against the domination of the unhelpful linear model of living and working as being detrimental not just to women but to all of society. In expressing new paradigms, working with a cyclical understanding may offer new insights missed on a linear plane. The bio-psycho-spiritual elements of women's health and psychology and female ways of knowing are an essential area to further explore; they are, however, beyond the scope of this chapter.

Ibn Khaldun, a prominent social scientist from the fourteenth century, wrote extensively on education and processes of social transformation (Hozien 2010). Writing centuries before European colonialism, he observed that it is

> in the nature of conquest that the conquered imitate those who conquer them. This occurs because the conquered are either impressed by the conqueror or erroneously attribute their own subservience to the perfection of the conqueror, failing to analyze the nature of their defeat. (Malik 2019)

This is an example of where psychological and ego factors which are not kept in check (as is encouraged in Islam) supersede higher realms of functionality and wisdom considered as 'ilm' knowledge, leading to destruction and significant losses in history to date (Malik 2019). Epistemology, from the Greek *episteme*, is an enquiry into the nature of knowledge. Knowledge in Islam is often expressed using the Arabic word *ilm*, however the English translation of the word falls short of the all-embracing term covering theory, action, education and wisdom (Azram 2011). In looking at the application and need for understanding the context and reality of experiences in relation to how Muslims' minds and bodies are researched and/or documented, the below example is used for illustrative purposes.

A Historical Example of the Legacy of Colonisation on Muslim Women's Bodies

One example of the legacy of colonialisation on Muslim women's bodies is that of the horrific experiences of the Partition of the Indian subcontinent and subsequent migration in Punjab in 1947 along religious lines. The violence against South Asian Muslim and other women and the resultant trauma, including how it impacts bodies and minds across generations, is often a missing part of the significant cultural history of these communities in Britain. It is rarely talked about openly. The period of the Partition of the subcontinent was a dark era of history during which multiple massacres, ethnic cleansing, rape and kidnapping of Muslim women occurred (Kiran 2017). This was about power and domination, and women were targets of violence; systematic rape was used as a weapon of mass violence and destruction that left legacies of trauma on the female body, in particular the pelvic area. This relates directly to the experiences I am studying and working with in everyday clinical private practice as a therapist with Muslim women. I have spoken to many people in my generation, fellow British Muslims, who are completely unaware of this tragedy and other violent events like the massacre at Jalianwala Bagh in Amritsar, Punjab in 1919. Has the cultural memory of second- and/or third-generation British South Asian Muslims been wiped in relation to this and other events as a result of a postcolonial epistemicide of the knowledge of our own histories? I noted through my therapeutic work that remnants of these experiences can sometimes be located in anxieties, fears, sensations and feelings that are difficult to name but are experienced as a felt sense in the body through the manifestation of intergenerational transmission of trauma. This includes, for example, issues manifesting around chronic unexplained body pains, difficulties relating to menstruation, fertility and trauma around pregnancy and birth. Others do have some knowledge of these stories where their grandparents or others managed to share these horrific experiences which, for some, are loaded with dishonour, shame and humiliation, as well as their not having the appropriate language to talk about such horrors and traumas. For many it was and remains unspeakable.

There has been some preservation of these experiences. Kiran (2017) talked to women and sought out archives to bring to light their stories. In many languages there are no equivalent words for trauma or depression – how could they even begin to relay their horrific experiences in a way that would be understood? There were many Muslim women who had been abducted and, due to shame, did not subsequently feel ready or able to go back and join their families in Pakistan (Kiran 2017); the loss was unimaginable. This is significant because these women who were carrying grave traumas imprinted on their bodies and minds went on to have children whilst retaining this trauma within, and some were pregnant as a result of rape and went on to give birth to and raise those children without the child ever being told about that painful legacy. What might be the psychological and health outcomes for these families? Some of these women were 'recovered', as Kiran (2017) states, and brought back to their families in Pakistan. Some of them, or the next generation, eventually migrated to Britain. Papers such as Kiran's (2017) are absolutely critical as the minority-within-minority voice bringing light to such events using primary source material. Kiran (ibid.) highlights the epic tragedy and how it 'changed the destiny of thousands rather millions of women who had not been given centric position in the historical analysis', one reason being, as she further expounds, the 'unwillingness of female victims to share their traumatic experiences with the strangers' (ibid.). Kiran (2017) also talks about the attempts of a male researcher, Ishtiaq Ahmed, and a female Western researcher, Pippa Virdee, to produce works on the experiences of Partition. However, Virdee cites that women were not ready to share their traumatic experiences and while acknowledging the excellence of his work Kiran (2017) highlights that Ahmed's attempts to document these experiences were through 'men's eyes' and there was no space for the female experience. This highlights the importance of having a female researcher from within the community in studies of this nature to ensure a shared safe space and allow for these stories to be told and represented mindfully and accurately with a great deal of sensitivity and compassion. These traumas are significant because they provide a historical backdrop to the context of Muslim women in Britain. The divide, rule and conquer that came with the colonial agenda to Asia created a religious ideology-based divide among communities. The sacrifices women made to achieve independence were far greater than has ever been recognised, validated, acknowledged or accepted. It remains unrecognised in cultural and colonial memory.

The Neurobiology of Trauma – a Colonised People

The above was one example from the course of history, though sadly there are countless examples of women, men and entire communities experiencing trauma through critical historical events that are difficult to remember and name, or that, for whatever reason, are actively erased. These events have deeply impacted physical and mental health, particularly in a cultural context when women are often expected to keep quiet and not bring 'shame' to the family. It is useful to think about this in terms of the neurobiology of trauma and how violence and fear shapes an individual. Bruce Perry (1997) posits that it is crucial to understand both origins and impact of violence, including interpersonal violence, and how it affects development and health. Experiencing terror and violence on the body, whether adult or child, situates a person in a position of vulnerability. Perry describes that the major 'modifier of all human behavior is experience. Experience, not genetics, results in the critical neurobiological factors associated with violence.' This is another reason why I feel documenting experiences of British Muslim research participants in health psychology and health sciences research is critical to capture latent meanings of personal experience. It is also crucial that measures are taken by researchers to critically question their own role, as well as to acknowledge structural socio-politico-legal systems of discrimination and Islamophobia, including the profiling and securitisation of British Muslims (Younis and Jadhav 2019), alongside historical factors that may hinder and deter British Muslims from being part of research processes. Trust needs to be established; healing and reparative work needs to be done.

Employing narrative analysis or reflexive thematic analysis (RTA) as research methods can potentially be useful and can be adapted to analyse Muslim experiences. Narrative methods recognise growth, change and development. Rosenweld and Ochberg (2008) suggest that

> narrative analysis disrupts the traditional social scientific analysis, which has realist assumptions and a focus on information collection. Instead the focus shifts to look at the very construction of narratives and likewise the role they play in the social construction of identity.

This provides a useful space for holding complex, nuanced, multi-layered stories and allowing them to be told and heard, whilst bearing in mind the sociocultural dimensions of the construction of meanings. An event such as the 1947 massacre, violence, ethnic cleansing and rape of Muslim women occurred within the past century; there are people still alive today who witnessed it or were direct victims. So how do we make sense of all of the violence that surrounds us, especially that enacted on the body of women – Muslim women? Can we conduct meaningful reflexive, engaging, reconnecting, empowering research that can lead to making sense of unexplained pains, for example? Perry (1997) states that there are many different types of violence – institutionalised violence, violence in behaviours, violence in ideas, violence in words – that manifest in behaviours and stress on the body. Here we can see how the application of neurobiological science – the affects of trauma – meets the impact of intellectual genocide – epistemicide, the destroying of stories and knowledge – as well as the terror imprinted on the physical and mental lives of individuals and the collective consciousness of particular communities (Malik 2019).

The Colonised Mind and Empowerment through Relational Interconnectedness

Malik (2019) states that Western scientists became as integral to the colonial project as the military official, paving the way for intellectual genocide. This has left a lasting imprint in the individual and collective bodies and minds of

Muslims for generations: 'Decolonization, once viewed as the formal process of handing over the instruments of government, is now recognized as a long-term process involving the bureaucratic, cultural, linguistic and psychological divesting of colonial power' (Pihama 1993, in Ritchie 2014). It is all too easy for researchers to ignore or be ignorant of the underlying impacts of the legacy of colonisation and its discourse within research contexts, thus inadvertently perpetuating these effects.

While knowledge production and science from other cultures and societies were being 'mythologised', science coming from the West was being claimed as universal; hence, 'science' became a means of intellectual colonisation. The minds of the non-Western world were being colonised beyond physical borders. The loss for the Muslim world includes how this intellectual colonisation process gradually led to the replacement of the integrative and holistic approach to knowledge that was traditionally inherent within Islamic ontology, being replaced with a secularised knowledge system that was 'fragmented, reductionist, and materialistic' (Malik 2019). This has led to multiple problems but is particularly relevant to research ontologies and methodologies when considering, for example, what methodologies could be used in health psychology research that may be relevant to research of British Muslims' experiences.

My attempt to highlight the importance of integrating an awareness of the role of epistemicide in the research process (which deeply impacts, informs and feeds into healthcare services) has come from my experience as a Muslim female researcher, one who struggled to find an appropriate guiding philosophy and method that felt relevant as a Muslim researcher and working with Muslim participants. For its relevancy and appropriateness in application to research with British Muslims and Muslim narratives, it is essential to reclaim the lost heritage of an Islamic ethos within health sciences and health psychology research. As a Muslim researcher I was disheartened to discover there were virtually no writings accessible and preserved that were the works of Muslim female philosophers or social scientists/psychologists that I could draw on in the English language. I am still left wondering what happened to the potential body of work of Muslim female philosophers and psychologists of times gone by: did they exist? If they did, were they preserved? If so, where are they? Were they not preserved? If not, why not?

There is an increasing consciousness to how our histories have been influenced and distorted, and narratives falsely shaped; some academics and researchers are increasingly wary of importing the intellectual dependency of Western social theories (Hussein in Elmesseri 2013). For Zavala (2013) decolonising research strategies are 'less about the struggle for method and more about the spaces that make decolonizing research possible'. This is a crucial point to think about for any researcher: how and where I do my research and what space that occupies and what it means for the participants of the study. For many indigenous people, knowledge is also seen as spiritual, to be exercised in service of survival of both human and 'more than human co-habitors', the purpose of gaining knowledge being 'to nurture and regenerate the world' (Kincheloe and Steinberg 2008, in Denzin et al. 2014). This is in alignment with Islamic ontology and the Muslim psyche which at its essence is a model of unity, one that recognises the place of humans in connection with the wider creation where there is a delicate balance of rights and responsibilities in line with one's *fitra* (innate sense of self). Though there are different needs, experiences and challenges, there are also parallels and connections between indigenous experiences and those of Muslims. There is a critical focus on justice and equity as Muslims are taught in Qur'anic teachings to continually be striving for balance despite the battle of the mind, egos and desires. One is encouraged to seek justice 'even if it be against the self' which means to hold oneself to account in the wider ecosystem. Indigenous onto-epistemologies are a potential source for restoring our damaged relationship with the more-than-human world, as Ritchie (2014) states. 'Their knowledge about respecting and healing the Earth can be used to counter the destructive effects of Western science on the Earth' (Denzin et al. 2008). The centrality of spiritual interconnectedness at the heart reinstates focus or direction in our relationality with, as Ritchie (2014) phrases it, 'the more-than-human world'. This is a process of decolonisation that

> transcends interrelated individual and collective, personal, professional and political realms. It is also intensely emotional, since extending one's paradigmatic interface to embrace (an) Indigenous onto-epistemology/ies require(s) the intimacy of an emotional connectedness that allows empathic passion to enter one's relationships. (Kincheloe and Steinberg 2008, in Ritchie 2014)

Perhaps we can question ourselves as scholars, researchers, academics: do we have an ethical obligation to share the responsibility for bringing back and helping to restore knowledge systems and their wisdoms that can benefit all of humanity? Can we go beyond the discourse and implement something that looks like meaningful transformation? Tuck and Yang (2012) state that 'Decolonization is not a metaphor' and 'the too-easy adoption of decolonizing discourse is just one part of that history and it taps into pre-existing tropes that get in the way of more meaningful potential alliances'. What actions can we take to affect outcomes in healthcare? This may be difficult, as we are required to shift our worldviews in seriously challenging ways: away from individualistic, linear, hierarchical, authoritarian, patriarchal, compartmentalised, white-privileged complacency, to an unsettled, contingent, relational, spiritual and emotional space, to work within a 'cultural interface' (Martin Nakata in McGloin 2009, in Ritchie 2014).

If we are to be agents of social, cultural, cognitive and ecological justice, we need to understand the dynamics of local/global indigenous movements (Kincheloe and Steinberg 2008, in Ritchie 2014). It is crucial to position ourselves as being in service (*khidmah* in Arabic) repairing the world, and recognising and utilising local and indigenous knowledge as integral to this process (Kincheloe and Steinberg 2008, in ibid.).

Indigenous research and the dire need for non-Anglo Northern and Western mainstream approaches to research are part of much broader struggles for decolonisation, for equity in healthcare and all spheres of life. Despite all the discourse surrounding decolonisation, it is important to keep in mind that this has far from been achieved as much as is required. We must remain mindful so as not to be overcome by the illusion that discussions and events talking about decolonisation are the same as effective, meaningful change. There are many layers to ensuring social and cognitive justice; it is important to recognise cognitive, micro- and neo-colonisations and the multiple other layers that exist in subtle and overt forms.

Islamic Ontology

The process of trying to make sense of phenomena and experiences can be particularly anxiety-inducing, especially in the context of a lost or robbed intellectual heritage; perhaps there are no words, no narrative that can be drawn upon, perhaps languages fail to capture what the body, mind and soul hold. Şentürk et al. (2020) used the term 'multiplexity' to 'refer to the multiple levels of existence (physical, metaphysical and divine), knowledge (acquired via reason, sense perception, intuition, and divine revelation) and truth (relative and ultimate)'. In his holistic perspective of social research, multiplexity encapsulates the concept of human ontology as consisting of multiple levels: body, mind and soul, and includes social action of that which is observable and unobservable. It is useful and necessary to have an understanding of one's positioning in ontology to provide a container for the messy art of thinking, all the while remaining open to constructive and thoughtful reflections about that knowledge and what it means relationally. Martin and Mirraboopa (2003) discuss the importance of this awareness:

> It is through ontology that we develop an awareness and sense of self, of belonging and for coming to know our responsibilities and ways to relate to self and others". Barbara Thayer-Bacon refers to this as relational ontology and writes: A relational (e)pistemology, which is supported by a relational ontology, helps us focus our attention on our interrelatedness, and our interdependence with each other and our greater surroundings. (Martin and Mirraboopa 2003).

Unfortunately, there is no neatly designed existing methodological framework with a pre-prepared map or guide for researching British Muslims, from ontology through to methodology, methods and analysis in health, psychological and social sciences. It is not as simple as selecting and using a single process, for example phenomenology or narrative theory. At present, it requires a piecing-together approach which requires creativity in drawing different parts together to create a whole along with courage and openness to create new methods. It is helpful to think about these cognitive barriers; Grégoire (2018) highlights the pressures in research as 'obstacles' in the researchers' mind and 'outside obstacles':

> The most important obstacles inside the researcher's mind are epistemological obstacles and cognitive bias (e.g., confirmation bias). While the most impor- tant obstacle outside are the social norms, i.e. the pressure for the scientific community and, sometimes, the whole society, to conform to the dominant scientific model, which is called 'normal science' by Kuhn (1962) . . . Sci- entific norms are too often supported by the current assessment system of scientific projects and productions, i.e. the peer review procedure.

For too long the idea that quantitative research – the 'objective' and 'measurable' – is superior to qualitative research has been dominant, and it arguably remains so. In various academic circles and in the media, it seems to be numbers that still count most. Ideas of rationality, objectivity and positivism as being superior sys- tems of thought rule much of science and academia, particularly health research influenced historically by the upper echelons of a male-dominated imperial- ist society, which have subsequently become ingrained as mass application in research education. To limit and narrow thinking, research and application to a few known comfortable, acceptable models is akin to robbery. Some knowl- edge or information has been missed out about the world, people and phenom- ena, whether observable or unobservable by the limitations of the human mind, and that loss is felt or experienced, even if not consciously recognised. Arguably some of these limitations of the human mind are more cognitive blind spots and unconscious defences than the capacity of what the mind can do if allowed to be creative and to think entrepreneurially, hence the need to re-evaluate scientific norms and 'assessment systems' (Grégoire 2018).

The Islamic understanding of knowledge ('ilm) is understood as two forms: revealed and derived knowledge. Azram (2011) elaborates on these two forms. Revealed knowledge, also known as al-wahy in Arabic, has two main attributes: 'instinctive' (fitra – the innate pure disposition that one is born with, i.e. what one innately knows, similar in nature to 'gut-sense' and 'revelation' – that which was revealed through divine revelation, immortalised in the Qur'an and hadith (tacit sayings, approvals and actions of the Prophet Muhammad's lived embodiment of the Qur'an). Part of this divine knowledge are two important concepts known as *fikr* (reflection) and *dhikr* (contemplation and remembrance of God and the signs of God in Creation). In *dhikr*, Muslims remember and contemplate God and the miraculous signs of nature, which cause us to naturally be in a state of *fikr* – reflection, thinking, pondering, wondering about the nature of things, which can then lead to searching or 'research'. This is illustrated in the following Qur'anic verses:

> Verily, in the creation of the heavens and the earth, and in the succession of night and day, there are indeed messages for all who are endowed with insight . . . [and] who remember God when they stand, and when they sit, and when they lie down to sleep, and [thus] reflect on the creation of the heavens and the earth: 'O our Sustainer! Thou hast not created [aught of] this without meaning and purpose. Limitless art Thou in Thy glory! Keep us safe, then, from suffering . . .' (Qur'an 3:190–1)

Human beings are implored to reflect, to think, to continuously be seeking knowledge. The process of creation, the womb and knowledge are deeply intertwined:

> And God has brought you forth from your mothers' wombs knowing nothing – but He has endowed you with hearing, and sight, and minds, so that you might have cause to be grateful. (Qur'an 16:78)

It can be understood from this verse that though a baby is born in a pure form (*fitra*) without 'knowledge', it is by the grace (*rahmah* – also related to the root word for womb, *rahm*) of God that humans are given faculties to understand and engage with the signs of creation, and to be in a state of gratitude for what has been provided. In Islamic tradition, humans are encouraged to 'seek knowledge from the cradle to the grave'.

The second type of knowledge is 'derived' or acquired knowledge. It is understood that this knowledge, as with all knowledge, is ultimately from Allah, as the human mind and faculties are God given. However, humans use methodologies inspired by Islamic ethics and their faculties through their senses, research and deep thinking to acquire 'worldly' knowledge (Azram 2011). Hence all knowledge is connected to the sacred. Ogunnaike (2019) elaborates on this connection:

> In traditional systems of education knowledge was always connected to the sacred, was connected to piety, to know more was to be more and to be better and so piety and the development of virtue and ethics was always a part of

education. Teaching someone without training them in virtue is like selling a soul to the thief . . . knowledge is powerful and connected to virtue and teaching someone without it is dangerous. (Ogunnaike 2019)

Education and all forms of learning and knowledge seeking are processes of developing and cultivating virtue. It is a divinely connected and driven endeavour. Azram (2011) expounds on the notion that humans are placed as vicegerents of God on Earth. With this comes a great sense of responsibility and duty of care to all of creation, and a duty to make use of knowledge to achieve a greater understanding of the physical and spiritual realms.

Therefore, as a Muslim researcher, it is incumbent upon me to be seeking knowledge and to use the most appropriate research methods and methodologies in the process of discovery and knowledge seeking. This is the case even when I am not pursuing formal academic studies. These are in themselves rules or methods of knowledge seeking. As Dhaouadi (2013) states, 'A Muslim researcher would logically consult the Quran . . . to further explore the transcendental nature of human intelligence'. It is therefore part of the natural process that a conscious Muslim academic rooted in their tradition may seek to contextualise their research paradigm and methodology within a worldview that they embody.

Conception of Methodology

Bakar (2012) calls for our special attention to the question of methodology, stating that there are fundamental differences between the conception of methodology of science in Islam, or for that matter in every other traditional civilisation such as Chinese or Indian, and that of the conception of methodology in modern science. He states that even the way we look at Islamic sciences in the modern world is through the lens of the modern 'scientific method' as if it is a universally applicable 'yardstick' of the scholarly community (Bakar 2012). Islamic sciences have always been pluralistic and not exclusive in the adoption and application of different methods in 'accordance with the nature of the subject in question and modes of understanding that subject' (Bakar 2012). Bakar talks about the history of the single methodology of science having been demolished over the preceding decade, with the idea of a pluralistic methodology gaining currency amongst contemporary historians and philosophers of science to the extent where some have begun to accept sacred scriptures to be 'an integral component of this pluralistic methodology'. One attempt to decolonise disciplines has been through 'Islamisation' processes in an attempt to reclaim, redefine and re-own concepts and sources that may have been distorted through history, colonisation movements, 'ethnic' cleansing and/or lost concepts, such as the renewed interests in Islamic finance and Islamic psychology, where Muslims are looking for answers to questions and problems within the context of their worldviews. The idea is to look at the disciplines from within an Islamic ontology, to apply or reapply, or go back to the roots of the founding principles and ethics of, for example, Islamic finance, or attempting to understand the human psyche through an Islam-based ontological view. For research with Muslims, this may mean looking at what is meaningful for British Muslims and encouraging the emergence of non-Eurocentric ways of knowing as being just as valid and acceptable. Furthermore, this means acknowledging that being rooted in Islamic tradition, these will and should be very different from orientalist ways of thinking about Muslims and will add significant value and different dimensions of learning and knowing.

Reflexivity and Soul Searching

> To be reflexive is to have an ongoing conversation about experience while simultaneously living in the moment. (Etherington 2010)

In my search for methodologies, I came across work on indigenous communities decolonising and reclaiming their spaces through reflexivity, which is useful to connect with as a Muslim researcher:

> Reflexivity in research design affords the 'space' to decolonise western research methodologies, then harmonise and articulate Indigenist research. Reflexivity is a process that allows us to work . . . with relatedness of self and Entities. Reflexivity challenges us to claim our shortcomings, misunderstandings, oversights and mistakes, to re-claim our lives and make strong changes to our current realities. Being reflexive ensures we do not compromise our identity whilst undertaking research. (Martin and Mirraboopa 2003)

I found support and much-needed validation in the struggle of fellow researchers trying to work authentically to reclaim narratives within a frame that was representative of their worldview and that of the communities they work with. This was a crucial and necessary element of my research process.

In that research process as a Muslim woman looking at Muslims' experiences, much soul searching and exploration was required to discover what would be the best, accurately representative and 'authentic fit' methodology currently available to work with. This required thinking creatively, looking for pieces of a jigsaw that I was not sure even existed in the first place, much less of how or where to find them. I could not see myself or my community, and our worldviews and ontology represented in the field of health research I was engaging with. Thus, the enquiry into the nature of knowledge became a pivotal one in an attempt to re-search and re-present our worldviews and realities as the basis for an authentic academic endeavour.

Any scholarly endeavour is defined by its values and processes which are inherent in the researcher. It is worth constantly checking in with ourselves regarding our biases, how open-minded or not we are, and how willing and able we are to engage with concepts and knowledge systems that may not be familiar to us. In this reflexivity it is important not to be restrictive and to continuously consider unconscious thought processes that shape the research and potentially the outcomes. Two common paradigms in research are often drawn on: inductive and deductive. However, when conducting studies that require stepping into the unknown it may be worth drawing on abductive reasoning: the idea that there may not necessarily be a conclusion and that the research process starts with 'puzzles' and is devoted to their explanation (Business Research Methodology 2019). Grégoire (2018) posits that abductive reasoning is essentially creative since it involves guessing and risk taking, in contrast to inductive and deductive reasoning. He extrapolates that since guessing is more frequently wrong than right, researchers prefer building projects on deductive or inductive reasoning than on abductive reasoning. He further highlights the capitalist nature of the process by stating that

> a research project based on deduction from a well-known theory is less risky than a project based on an original theoretical framework and can be more easily approved and financed. As a consequence, a lot of research projects are not very creative, following the rules of the dominant theories. (Grégoire 2018)

These ideas have far-reaching consequences and societal impact; they influence available funding, investments, what and who is considered important to study and policies implemented, and creates a bias in itself for what is valuable to research and what is not. In light of all this, it is critical for researchers to develop 'intellectual independence' (Şentürk 2020) or what Cutcliffe (2003) refers to as 'intellectual entrepreneurship', which effectively implies conscious and deliberate actions by researchers to make bold decisions and take risks in exploring the world of research (ibid.). Şentürk et al. (2020) advise that researchers engage with what he refers to as the 'art of theory building rather than passively applying conventional theories and methods in social sciences that are coloured with Eurocentrism'.

Conclusion

This chapter has explored ideas around underpinning philosophical enquiries relevant for studying British Muslims in health psychology through the need to employ a creative approach, exploring the role of CMH as a helpful starting point to provide context. I have considered the historical context, decolonising methodologies and the impact of colonialism and epistemicide on the application of knowledge and its reproduction. Furthermore, I have touched upon differences in values in Western science and in the Islamic knowledge systems, with a historical example of the legacy of colonialisation of Muslim women's bodies, the neurobiology of trauma of a colonialised people. I went on to look at the concept of the colonised mind and empowerment through relational interconnectedness, discussing research models alien to socioreligious realities of the Muslim world, reflexivity and the idea of an Islamic ontology frame where connection and unity, the immaterial and divine (non-observable phenomena) are equally important to draw upon when researching Muslim experiences. It is essential to critically explore multiple lenses of history away from a colonising perspective, and to actively encourage new possibilities in knowledge systems and research methodologies. This will provide relevant, authentic, rooted and meaningful contextual paradigms for health research with Muslims. I ended by considering reflexivity, soul searching and the need for intellectual entrepreneurship. Researchers considering studying British Muslims' experiences need to be mindful of the historical backdrop against which their research is situated. There needs to be acknowledgement of both historical and ongoing intergenerational, collective and individual traumas that deeply impact health and engagement with health services and research. There is also a need to consider decolonising methodologies and the research process itself. Reflexivity of researchers, and ethical practice which questions structural and systemic injustices is required. Integrating and allying with researchers, medical practitioners, nurses and psychologists who do not embody colonial, Eurocentric, Western or Global North mindsets of healthcare as being the only and exclusive way of knowing, and who are open to the diversity of untapped knowledge systems would be a way to develop more holistic goals around services, provisions and even medical procedures. We need more Muslims to invest in (and be invested in), lead and produce research in health science and health psychology, and to work collaboratively with the community and in partnership with organisations that can support authentic innovative research into the specific issues impacting the health and wellbeing of Muslim individuals and communities and contribute to new knowledge in the wider community. There is a desperate need for improvement and advancement in this field for any social and cognitive justice to occur in research with Muslim populations and to meaningfully understand their needs, and to improve therapeutic cultures, services and provisions in the healthcare disciplines. As researchers we must go boldly as 'intellectual entrepreneurs' into the research terrain if we are to discover new solutions to healing the ill and recover from 'intellectual genocide'. The potential rewards and new insights make it a challenge worth pursuing.

References

Ali, F. (2020). 'Don't call me Bibi – or anybody else, for that matter'. *BMJ*, 368, m535.

Azram, M. (2011). 'Epistemology – an Islamic perspective'. *IIUM Engineering Journal*, 12(5).

Bakar, O. (2012). *The History and Philosophy of Islamic Science*. Cambridge: Islamic Texts Society.

Business Research Methodology (2019) 'Abductive reasoning (abductive approach)'. Available at: https://research-methodology.net/research-methodology/research-approach/abductive-reasoning-abductive-approach/#_ftn1 (last accessed 4 May 2022).

Chilisa, B. (2011). *Indigenous Research Methodologies*. Thousand Oaks, CA: SAGE Publications Inc.

Cutcliffe, J. R. (2003). 'Reconsidering reflexivity: introducing the case for intellectual entrepreneurship'. *Qualitative Health Research*, 13(1), 136–48.

Denzin, N. K., Lincoln, Y. S. and Smith, L. T. (eds) (2008). *Handbook of Critical and Indigenous Methodologies*. Thousand Oaks, CA: SAGE Publications Inc.

Dhaouadi, M. (2013). 'Inside Muslim minds'. *Contemporary Sociology*, 42(1), 83–4.

Dosani, S. (2001). 'How to practise medicine in a multicultural society'. *Student BMJ*, 323, 0110380.

Elmessiri, A. M. (ed.) (2013). *Epistemological Bias in the Physical and Social Sciences*. Herndon, VA: The International Institute of Islamic Thought. Available at: https://iiit.org/wp-content/uploads/2018/07/books-in-brief_-_epistemological_bias.pdf (last accessed 4 May 2022).

Etherington, K. (2017). 'Personal experience and critical reflexivity in counselling and psychotherapy research'. *Counselling and Psychotherapy Research*, 17(2), 85–94.

Gilliat-Ray, S. (2010). 'Body-works and fieldwork: research with British Muslim chaplains'. *Culture and Religion*, 11(4), 413–32.

Grégoire, J. (2018). 'Overcoming obstacles to creativity in science'. *Estudos de Psicologia (Campinas)*, 35(3), 229–36.

Grosfoguel, R. (2013). 'The structure of knowledge in Westernized universities: epistemic racism/sexism and the four genocides/epistemicides of the long 16th century'. *Human Architecture*, 11(1). Available at: http://scholarworks.umb.edu/humanarchitecture/vol11/iss1/8 (last accessed 4 May 2022).

Hozien, M. (2010). 'Ibn Khaldun: studies on his contribution in economy'. Available at: https://muslimheritage.com/ibn-khaldun-contribution-economy (last accessed 4 May 2022).

Hussein, A. (2013). 'Bias in Western schools of thought: our heritage as the starting point for development', in A. M. Elmessiri (ed.), *Epistemological Bias in the Physical and Social Sciences*. Herndon, VA: The International Institute of Islamic

Thought. Available at: https://iiit.org/wp-content/uploads/2018/07/books-in-brief_-_epistemological_bias.pdf (last accessed 4 May 2022).

Kincheloe, J. L. and Steinberg, S. L. (2008). 'Indigenous knowledges in education. Complexities, dangers, and profound benefits', in N. K. Denzin, Y. S. Lincoln and L. T. Smith (eds), *Handbook of Critical and Indigenous Methodologies*. Thousand Oaks, CA: SAGE Publications Inc., pp. 135–56.

Kiran, N. (2017). 'Punjab migration 1947: violence against Muslim women and the settlement'. *South Asian Studies*, 32(1), 161–76. Available at: http://pu.edu.pk/images/journal/csas/PDF/13_v32_1_17.pdf (last accessed 4 May 2022).

Kmietowicz, Z., Ladher, N., Rao, M., Salway, S., Abbasi, K. and Adebowale, V. (2019). 'Ethnic minority staff and patients: a health service failure'. *BMJ*, 365, l2226.

Knight, M., Bunch, K., Tuffnell, D., Shakespeare, J., Kotnis, R., Kenyon, S. and Kurinczuk, J. J. (2019). 'Saving lives, improving mothers' care: lessons learned to inform maternity care from the UK and Ireland confidential enquiries into maternal deaths and morbidity 2015–17'. MBRRACE-UK. Available at: www.npeu.ox.ac.uk/downloads/files/mbrrace-uk/reports/MBRRACE-UK%20Maternal%20Report%202019%20-%20WEB%20VERSION.pdf (last accessed 4 May 2022).

Malik, F. (2019). 'All that we lost: the colonized mind and the decline of the Islamic education system'. Yaqeen Institute. Available at https://yaqeeninstitute.org/faisal-malik/the-colonized-mind-and-the-decline-of-the-islamic-education-system (last accessed 4 May 2022).

Martin, K. and Mirraboopa, B. (2003). 'Ways of knowing, being and doing: a theoretical framework and methods for indigenous and indigenist re-search'. *Journal of Australian Studies*, 27(76), 203–14.

McGloin, C. (2009). 'Considering the work of Martin Nakata's "cultural interface": a reflection on theory and practive by a non-Indigenous academic'. *The Australian Journal of Indigenous Education*, 38(suppl.), 36–41.

Morrison, S. (2014). 'Muslim Selbstverständnis: Ahmet Davutoğlu answers Husserl's Crisis of European Sciences'. *The Muslim World*, 104(1–2), 150–70.

Ogunnaike, O. (2019). 'Can we free our minds in a postcolonial world?' YouTube. Available at: www.youtube.com/watch?v=WNndxz7jKF4 (last accessed 4 May 2022).

Perreira, K. M. and Ornelas, I. (2013). Painful passages: traumatic experiences and post-traumatic stress among immigrant Latino adolescents and their primary caregivers. *The International Migration Review*, 47(4), 976–1005.

Perry, B. D. (1997). 'Incubated in terror: neurodevelopmental factors in the 'cycle of violence', in J. Osofsky (ed.), *Children, Youth and Violence: The Search for Solutions*. New York: Guilford Press, pp. 124–48.

Pihama, L. (1993). 'No, I will not be a post. . . .' *Te Pua*, 2(1–2), 35–7.

Pope, R. E. (2018). 'Gender and society', in P. S. Wells, K. Rebay-Salisbury and C. Haselgrove (eds), *The Oxford Handbook of the European Iron Age*. Oxford: Oxford University Press.

Ritchie, J. (2014). 'Counter-colonial research methodologies drawing upon post-colonial critique and Indigenous onto-epistemologies'. Paper presented at 10th Annual Congress of Qualitative Inquiry, University of Illinois at Urbana-Champaign, 21–24 May. Available at: https://hdl.handle.net/10652/3042 (last accessed 4 May 2022).

Rosenwald, G. C. and Ochberg, R. L. (1992). *Storied Lives: The Cultural Politics of Self-understanding*. New Haven, CT: Yale University Press.

Savransky, M. (2017). 'A decolonial imagination: sociology, anthropology and the politics of reality'. *Sociology*, 51(1), 11–26.

Stonebanks, C. (2008). 'An Islamic perspective on knowledge, knowing, and method-ology', in N. K. Denzin, Y. S. Lincoln and L. T. Smith (eds), *Handbook of Critical and Indigenous Methodologies* 2014. Thousand Oaks, CA: SAGE Publications, Inc.

Şentürk, R., Açıkgenç, A., Küçükural, Ö., Yamamoto, Q. N., Aksay, N. K., Özalkan, S., Asadov, A., Naeem, D., Belkız, E., Faytre, L., Taiai, M., Noorata, M. and Kırkarlar, O. (eds) (2020). *Comparative Theories and Methods between Uniplexity and Multiplexity*. Istanbul: Ibn Haldun University Press.

Tuck, E. and Yang, K. W. (2012). 'Decolonization is not a metaphor'. *Decolonization: Indigeneity, Education & Society*, 1(1), 1–40.

Viney, W., Callard, F. and Woods, A. (2015). 'Critical medical humanities: embracing entanglement, taking risks'. *Medical Humanities*, 41(1), 2–7.

Younis, T. and Jadhav, S. (2019). 'Keeping our mouths shut: the fear and racialized self-censorship of British healthcare professionals in PREVENT training'. *Culture, Medicine and Psychiatry*, 43(3), 404–24.

Zavala, M. (2013). 'What do we mean by decolonizing research strategies? Lessons from decolonizing, indigenous research projects in New Zealand and Latin America'. *Decolonization: Indigeneity, Education & Society*, 2(1), 55–71.

PART 2

CLINICAL CARE

5

GENETIC HEALTH IN BRITISH MUSLIM POPULATIONS: ANALYSIS OF CONSANGUINITY, INTERVENTIONS AND SOCIOCULTURAL CONTEXTS

Aysha Divan, Ghazala Mir, Mehrunisha Suleman, Arzoo Ahmed and Ataf Sabir

Introduction

A consanguineous relationship is defined as a union between two people who are descended from the same biological ancestor and, in practice, who are related as second cousins or closer (Bittles 1994). More than 1 billion people globally are estimated to live in societies where consanguineous marriages are common (Bittles 2012), and across the world 15 per cent of babies born are from consanguineous parents (Bittles and Black 2010). The incidence of consanguinity varies by geographical region, with population frequencies of 20 per cent to over 50 per cent in some locations, including the Middle East, North Africa, and South and West Asia (Oniya et al. 2019). In contrast, the UK has a much lower rate of consanguinity (less than 1 per cent). However, transnational migration has resulted in a mix of communities within the UK, for some of whom the practice of consanguinity is customary and remains favoured. These include people of Pakistani, Bangladeshi and Middle Eastern origin (Modell and Darr 2002), communities that are predominantly Muslim.

Parental consanguinity is associated with an increased risk of giving birth to a child with a congenital anomaly, with studies showing that the risk increases from 1–3 per cent in the general population to 2–7 per cent in those practising consanguinity (Becker et al. 2015; Sheridan et al. 2013; Bittles and Black 2010). Much of the risk is attributed to the expression of genes that are inherited from the parents in an autosomal recessive manner. We usually have two 'working' copies of every gene. Should an individual inherit two 'non-working' copies of the same gene, then this may result in a recessive disease. Blood relatives are more likely to carry the same gene variants than unrelated couples; if both parents carry one copy of the 'non-working' gene, then their offspring has a one in four (25 per cent) chance of inheriting that recessive condition.

Congenital anomalies translate into higher infant and childhood mortality rates and increased prevalence of long-term health conditions and disabilities (Bittles 2012; Bittles and Black 2010; Bundey and Alam 1993). However, not all congenital anomalies are genetic in origin and a complex mix of socioeconomic factors interact to influence health outcomes. For example, it is known that consanguineous marriages are more common in lower socioeconomic groups (Bhopal et al. 2013) and there is strong evidence that socioeconomic status plays a significant role in infant mortality and morbidity (Bittles 2012). Women with diabetes and poor glycaemic control are at higher risk of anomalies (Kurinczuk et al. 2010) and this condition is up to six times higher within South Asian communities than in European populations (WHO 2019).

Furthermore, there is evidence that knowledge and genetic service uptake amongst communities at higher risk of recessive conditions due to consanguinity is poor (Darr et al. 2016, 2013; Khan et al. 2010). The need to improve access to genetic testing and counselling amongst minority ethnic groups has been acknowledged by the Department of Health (2012, 2010). However, this has not translated into the development of a national-level policy, guidelines or resources to support service delivery. All of these issues highlight the need to identify, develop and implement best practices for improving healthcare outcomes for families where cousin-marriages remain customary. To contribute to this discussion, we explore the following questions in the context of published literature:

- What cultural, socioeconomic and faith-based perspectives influence choices in relation to consanguineous relationships?
- What interventions have been implemented within the UK and internationally to address the increased genetic risk associated with consanguineous relationships and what is their impact?
- Is there a case for the offer of preconception and/or pre-marital carrier screening for recessive disorders amongst consanguineous populations in the UK to reduce reproductive genetic risk associated with consanguinity?

Socioeconomic Perspectives that Influence Choices around Consanguinity

Often the debate surrounding consanguineous unions is negatively framed, suggesting that the custom is outdated and should be stopped, leaving communities that practise consanguinity feeling stigmatised and disempowered (Ajaz et al. 2015; Qureshi and Raeburn 2011). However, a number of social, economic and health benefits have been associated with consanguineous marriages.

An example of a positive association is demonstrated through a prospective birth cohort study, Born in Bradford. The authors (Bhopal et al. 2013) showed that Pakistani mothers in consanguineous relationships (59.3 per cent of women (n=3038)) were less educated and of lower socioeconomic status than those in non-consanguineous relationships (7.3 per cent of women (n=127)). Despite this disadvantage, the Pakistani consanguineous group's life circumstances were equivalent to, and in some cases better than, women in non-consanguineous relationships, highlighting the potential protective effects of consanguineous relationships. Indicators of life circumstances included capacity to pay bills (similar), divorce (rarer), warmth and trust in the marital relationship (similar) and enjoyment of day-to-day activities (similar).

Whilst this particular study found consanguinity to be associated with lower levels of education and income, other studies have provided contrary evidence suggesting that drivers of cousin marriage may vary by ethnicity and geographical location. For example, consanguineous marriages between wealthy families has been reported as a means of retaining wealth and property within the family and strengthening kinship ties (Shaw 2014; Hamamy et al. 2011). It is therefore critical that any discussions around cousin marriages and associated (genetic) risk to progeny is balanced with the potential benefits and understood in the context of cultural and religious factors.

Despite the prevalence of consanguinity in Muslim communities in the UK, there is no faith-based imperative in Islam, suggesting a more culturally rooted practice. Such patterns are evident globally where consanguineous marriages occur in Christian, Hindu and Muslim communities in India and among Arab populations (Teebi and Farag 1997; Rao et al. 1972). Similar to Biblical teachings, Islamic normative sources neither encourage nor prohibit marriage with cousins. The marriage of the Prophet Muhummad's daughter to her second cousin is used as justification for such marriages (Shaw 2001). There are, however, also teachings within the Islamic tradition that counter consanguineous relationships. For example, Umar Ibn Al-Khattab, the second Calif, on noticing that the tribe of Bani Althaa'b had become weak and unhealthy due to inter-marrying, advised: 'Marry from faraway tribes; otherwise you will be weak and unhealthy' (Al-Bar and Chamsi-Pasha 2015a).

Nevertheless, the relationship between faith and consanguinity is an under-researched area. For example, does the complex interaction between religious and ethnic identity in communities that practise consanguinity play a role in promoting and maintaining this cultural practice and what are the implications of such dynamics for interventions in this area? Given also that the religious teachings are equivocal, is it cultural and/or socioeconomic factors that drive such practices? Understanding the interaction between religious identity, cultural practices and socioeconomic contexts is of pivotal importance when trying to design genetic interventions, education and outreach for communities for whom practices such as consanguinity carry intergenerational significance. Such research and subsequent findings could inform how each of these factors contributes to individual and familial practices, preventing oversimplification and assumptions both at the policy and practice levels.

What Interventions have been Implemented or Tested in the UK and Internationally?

UK-based approach

In the UK, the general approach utilised to address high levels of congenital abnormalities arising from consanguineous relationships is to identify families at risk. This is possible once an affected child is diagnosed, which occurs in most instances after the child is born. On occasion, an anomaly may be detected during pregnancy through routine antenatal healthcare processes. In such circumstances, the reproductive choices open to the couple may be limited to termination of the pregnancy or preparing for the possibility of a disabled child.

Diagnosis of an affected child can lead to the exploration of the parents' genetic status and that of any siblings and may ultimately lead to the identification of an extended family at increased genetic risk for a particular condition. This approach relies on family members cascading information to other family members (immediate and extended) who may be at risk. It also relies on these members taking up genetic counselling and genetic testing where feasible (Darr et al. 2016, 2013). This family-centred approach is recommended by the Eastern Mediterranean Regional Office of the World Health Organization, which recognises that 'consanguineous marriages is an integral part of cultural and social life in many areas' and views 'any attempts to discourage it at the population-level as undesirable and inappropriate' (Modell and Darr 2002; Alwan and Modell 1997).

In line with the recommendations of the WHO, a series of local-level initiatives across England are emerging, focusing on three strands of activity: (1) provision of genetic counselling and testing services for at-risk individuals and families; (2) enhancing genetic literacy amongst communities where consanguinity is customary; and (3) training health professionals to deliver information and services in a culturally competent manner.

A review of these local-level responses shows that interventions are in their infancy and vary hugely in scope, level of investment and longevity (Salway et al.

2016). More recent recommendations from a multi-stakeholder Delphi exercise (Salway et al. 2019) on the development of national policy highlight the need for strong national leadership to ensure efficient sharing of knowledge and promotion of equitable and more consistent responses across the UK.

An example of a local-level approach from which lessons can be learnt is the Enhanced Genetic Service Project (EGSP) established by the Birmingham Primary Care Trust during 2009–12 (Alberg et al. 2014). The project aimed to address excess infant mortality and morbidity in Birmingham linked to autosomal recessive conditions. Previous work in the Birmingham area (Birmingham Birth Study) suggests the prevalence of congenital and genetic disorders is 4.3 per cent in North European children and almost double that (7.9 per cent) among British Pakistani children, with a substantial proportion of these due to recessive-inherited disorders (Bundey and Alam 1993). About a third of the affected children die before the age of five. Most of the survivors suffer chronic disability and are cared for by community or specialist paediatric services. The clinical strand of the project focused on identifying index patients through a review of patients already on the Clinical Genetics department database, and offering them genetic counselling and testing. Where relevant, cascade testing and counselling was offered to other 'at-risk' family members via the index patient or, in cases when the index patient was a child, via the patient's parents. Whilst the offer of genetic counselling was taken up by almost 50 per cent of eligible patients, there was a reluctance to share genetic information with other family members (approximately 10 per cent of family members had known contact with the index patient). Deciding whether to share genetic information is a complex process depending on family relationships, timing with regard to when to share the information and impact on the wider family (Alberg et al. 2014). In families where marriages are arranged, stigma associated with the cancellation of marriages may also prevent individuals taking up testing.

However, not all studies have shown a reluctance amongst families to share genetic information. A study by Darr et al. (2016) involving British Pakistani families reported a willingness to share and use genetic information, but this was dependent on the provision of high-quality and timely information from healthcare professionals. These authors put forward a strictly ordered sequence for communicating genetic information starting with an understanding of recessive inheritance followed by a discussion of the possible consequences of having children with close blood relatives. The study confirmed previous findings that genetic information is difficult to communicate and comprehend. Families can be confused by receiving two different explanations of the cause of recessive disorders: recessive inheritance and cousin marriages. In addition, they can be sceptical of evidence that may link consanguinity with genetic disorders or childhood mortality, as their lived experience indicates that couples in non-consanguineous relationships can also have affected children and that the vast majority of consanguineous relationships (93–98 per cent overall) do not result in congenital anomalies. This creates confusion and leads to mistrust of professional advice. Thus there is a need for health professionals to be trained and supported to provide clear, accurate and culturally competent advice for communities with a preference for consanguineous marriages. In line with this, Khan et al. (2010) identified the input of healthcare workers from the same ethnic background as one of the key factors in the successful uptake of genetic services designed for South-Asian (primarily Muslim) families in Blackburn with Darwen.

Recommendations from the multi-stakeholder Delphi exercise (Salway et al. 2019) also reinforce the need for both cultural knowledge and genetic literacy amongst healthcare and other relevant professionals. Suggestions included the use of standardised resources developed nationally for training purposes, updating of medical and social care curricula to reflect developments in genetics and competencies required to meet the needs of populations practising consanguineous unions, as well as clear guidance on referrals to genetic services.

Targeted reproductive carrier screening programmes – international examples

An alternative approach to identifying at-risk individuals is through targeted reproductive carrier screening programmes. The purpose of these is to test populations whose risk of particular conditions is known to be elevated, prior to conception (first pregnancy) or pre-marriage, to determine whether or not an individual carries a gene that could result in the birth of an affected child. Several countries with a high genetic burden, including Mediterranean countries such as Cyprus and predominantly Muslim countries including Saudi Arabia, Iran, Qatar and the United Arab Emirates, now have mandatory pre-marital genetic and/or haematological screening programmes (El-Shanti et al. 2015; Alswaidi and O'Brien 2009). Screening programmes vary dependent on the disease profile of the country and the availability of tests to effectively detect the disease-causing genotype.

As an example, Saudi Arabia was one of the first Middle Eastern countries to implement a pre-marital screening programme, initially for sickle-cell anaemia and thalassaemia and recently for other genetic conditions with high rates (El-Shanti et al. 2015). This approach can, of course, only be taken where screening tests exist, which is often not the case for rare genetic conditions. The programme includes mandatory pre-marital medical testing of couples with the provision of genetic counselling where required. This allows genetically at-risk couples to make informed decisions on marriage with full knowledge of the risks and options available to them. Compliance with the counselling recommendations are voluntary and not enforced.

A six-year review of the national pre-marital screening and genetic counselling programme for sickle-cell anaemia and thalassaemia (Memish and Saeedi 2011) showed that prevalence of β-thalassaemia dropped from 32.9 per cent to 9.0 per cent following the implementation of mandatory pre-marital screening. In addition, there was a 60 per cent reduction in the number of at-risk couples and a 51.9 per cent cancellation rate of at-risk marriages. Similar reductions have been observed in other countries where mandatory pre-marital screening programmes have been implemented. In Turkey, cancellation of 53 per cent of at-risk marriages and an 80 per cent reduction in at-risk births has been reported, while in Bahrain a 58 per cent cancellation rate of at-risk marriages was observed (Saffi and Howard 2015). These studies indicate that pre-marital screening programmes can be successful in reducing marriages between carriers and hence reducing the number of individuals with hereditary disorders. However, a substantial proportion of at-risk couples will choose to go ahead and marry, highlighting that reasons for marriage are often complex and multifaceted and that couples may have diverse approaches to risk-taking, as in other areas of health behaviour (Shaw 2015). Depending on the legal and sociocultural environment, reproductive options may be available to carrier couples such as undergoing pre-implantation genetic diagnosis prior to in vitro fertilisation to eliminate the risk of having a sick child (Al-Bar and Chamsi-Pasha 2015a).

A number of studies have explored the attitudes of men and women towards pre-marital screening in countries where such programmes are mandatory. A large-scale community-based study conducted in Qatar (Bener et al. 2019), highlighted that knowledge of the objectives of the programme was low and that it was not viewed favourably, with the respondents indicating low agreement with government intervention. In contrast, studies in other countries have reported a positive attitude (Cousens et al. 2010), particularly amongst university students. For example, a study of female university students in King Saud University, in Saudi Arabia, showed that 86 per cent of them responded positively about pre-marital testing (Awatif 2006), as did 94 per cent of participants in a study involving university students and people attending scientific meetings and health centres (El-Hazmi 2006).

Pre-conception Carrier Screening in a UK Context

The Enhanced Genetic Service Project (Alberg et al. 2014) recommended identifying at-risk families (immediate and extended) through affected children and providing members with information on individual genetic risk. This model aims to inform the reproductive options for subsequent children that a couple with an affected child may have. It also aims, through cascade screening, to inform the wider family and thus facilitate informed reproductive decision making amongst at-risk individuals.

Is there a case, however, for offering carrier testing for recessive disorders to consanguineous populations either pre-marriage or pre-conception (first child) as is offered in some countries? In the UK, voluntary carrier screening is offered for certain conditions where there is a heightened genetic risk but this differs between population groups, highlighting a fragmented policy approach. For example, routine screening is offered where a family history of sickle cell or thalassaemia is identified (Dormandy et al. 2010). Additionally, increasing average maternal age is highlighted as a specific target for work to reduce risk factors in the Maternity Transformation Programme (NHS England 2016). However, risk factors relating to consanguinity are not mentioned and the extent to which this issue will be taken up in implementation of the programme remains to be seen. Similarly, antenatal screening for all pregnant women in England for Down's syndrome takes account of maternal age but, in contrast, consanguinity is not highlighted as a risk factor for any of the listed conditions (Public Health England 2016).

Gaps in current UK screening opportunities have been met by charities within the Jewish community. In 2016, the GENEius programme (2019) was launched by the Jewish charity, Jnetics. The GENEius programme is an education and screening initiative that aims to eliminate severe recessive Jewish genetic disorders (JGDs) from the UK Jewish community. Carrier screening for nine common recessive conditions (including cystic fibrosis and Tay-Sachs) is undertaken for Ashkenazi Jews, who make up 90–95 per cent of the UK Jewish community (Burton et al. 2009). Three groups are targeted: students aged 16–17 in predominantly Jewish colleges or sixth forms, young engaged couples (predominantly through the synagogue pre-marriage system) and university students. The cost of the screening (£250 per person) is fully subsidised by Jnetics for all Jewish 16–17-year-olds and university students. The charity has a regular carrier screening clinic in Barnet hospital (London) and a university outreach programme. The latter involves running a clinic every three years at major universities, with its first clinic at the University of Birmingham having seen over 140 individuals in March 2019 (GENEius 2019).

Would such an approach work for the British Muslim community? The British Muslim community is much larger than the British Jewish community and more ethnically diverse, with communities represented from the Indian subcontinent, Africa and the Middle East. Thus targeted screening is more challenging to implement for a number of scientific and economic reasons. Firstly, high-quality data on carrier frequencies is required. Whilst this is available for some conditions and some ethnic communities, the majority of genetic studies have been conducted on individuals of European ancestry (Gurdasani et al. 2019) and therefore data specific to UK ethnic minority populations is not always available. Secondly, a comprehensive health economics evaluation of such programmes is needed. Typically, carrier screening is performed for one or a few relatively common recessive disorders associated with significant morbidity and reduced life expectancy. Some conditions may occur at a high carrier frequency but the 'relatively limited' severity of the condition is such that it would not satisfy the Wilson and Junger WHO criteria for the implementation of a screening programme (Andermann et al. 2008).

These limitations could be overcome through the use of whole exome and whole genome sequencing. These technologies are able to screen the whole exome (or genome) of the patient for very many genetic conditions relatively quickly and cost-effectively. Recent studies show that whole exome sequencing can identify couples that are at risk of having a child with a recessive inherited disorder where disease-causing variants have been identified, and can be used across multiple ethnic groups (Sallevelt et al. 2017). A recent study explored the acceptability and perceived utility of reproductive carrier exome screening in consanguineous couples (Josephi-Taylor et al. 2019). Semi-structured interviews with twenty-one consanguineous couples from diverse ethnic backgrounds were conducted. All practised a religion and fourteen of the couples were Muslim. Almost two-thirds of the couples, representing all the religious backgrounds, said they would use the information of their carrier status to inform reproductive choices, although they acknowledged that the decision to terminate a pregnancy would be difficult. All choices made by couples were based on consideration of their values, their current family situation and on test reliability and incidental findings.

Screening at the pre-conception or pre-relationship stage has the key advantage in that carrier individuals are informed before pregnancy. This increases the number of options available to them and provides more time to reflect on their decision making. The rapid expansion of genetic testing technologies that enable screening for multiple recessive conditions at a much reduced cost could facilitate earlier detection of at-risk individuals. However, the use of such tests also raises significant technical, ethical, legal and social questions that need to be addressed before they are implemented into public healthcare provision (Antonarakis 2019; HCSTC 2018; Henneman et al. 2016). It is also important to bear in mind that detection of carrier status alone is insufficient for genetic counselling regarding the risk to affected individuals. Other factors such as knowledge of the exact variants in both carriers (i.e. the couple) is necessary to provide accurate genetic counselling.

Case Study 1

Miriam and Dawud are both aged twenty-seven, are first cousins and recently got married. They are both healthy, keen to have their first child and are aware of the increased risk of congenital anomalies (birth defects) to any future pregnancy for couples who are related (compared to unrelated couples).

They are keen to find out what the risk is of congenital anomalies for their future pregnancy and what their options are. Miriam asks her midwife, Jo, to explain the risk.

Jo: *The risk of having a child with birth anomalies is between 1 and 3 per cent for an unrelated couple. This increases to 2–7 per cent for related couples, which means 93–98 per cent of related couples will have a child without birth anomalies. The risk figures are modified for individual circumstances, such as age (the older you are the higher the risk in general terms) and medical problems (maternal diabetes, especially if poorly controlled, is a risk factor).*

Currently there are no specific NHS screening programmes targeted at consanguineous (related) couples (who are at increased risk of having offspring with recessive conditions). There is however specific NHS screening for some recessive genetic disorders during pregnancy (sickle cell disease and thalassaemia).

Routine NHS antenatal screening (screening in pregnancy) for all women in the UK will include ultrasound scans and blood tests for specific genetic conditions, for example Trisomy 21 (Down's syndrome), Trisomy 13 and Trisomy 18. If abnormalities are detected such as on the ultrasound scan then further genetic testing may or may not be offered.

Miriam mentions that they are Jewish, and asks if there is anything else available?

Jo: *There is currently no additional specific screening for Jewish couples in this scenario on the NHS but there is a charity called Jnetics who offer additional screening for nine significant genetic conditions that are commonly seen in certain parts of the Jewish community.*

Jo directs Miriam and David to the Jnetics website for more information.

Reproductive Options, Faith-identity and Health Inequalities

Increased reproductive options include choices around selection of marriage partners, IVF followed by pre-implantation genetic diagnosis, use of donor sperm and/or eggs from those that are non-carriers, refraining from pregnancy, adoption or choosing to proceed with a pregnancy. Muslim identity can be a key influence on health behaviours and decision making in relation to these issues and may intertwine with other social factors affecting parental choices.

A recent study by Verdonk et al. (2018) exploring Dutch Moroccan and Turkish women's perspectives on pre-conception carrier screening and reproductive choices revealed that a complex mix of religious, cultural and gender logics frames the women's perspectives on these topics. Although the sample size interviewed was small (ten women in consanguineous marriages and seven group discussions (n=86)), the women welcomed pre-conception carrier screening. Knowing about the health of their future child was paramount. They spoke openly of not marrying or even divorcing if both partners were carriers. Whilst some reproductive options (termination of pregnancy and IVF with a donor egg or sperm) were not acceptable to the participants, IVF combined with pre-implantation genetic diagnosis were considered to be valuable interventions.

Information and support that fits with the cultural and religious norms of a particular community is an essential component of any programme where people are tested for a genetic condition. This becomes even more important where testing may increase the number of people identified as being at risk and where the reproductive choices are increased. However, reports show that a family's need for information, and the opportunity to discuss the faith implications of their clinical choices, are rarely met in a clinical setting. A small-scale study exploring the experiences of faith group members in the UK using new reproductive and genetic technologies found that participants reported a lack of awareness of, or sensitivity to, faith issues in their clinical encounters (Scully et al. 2017). Both Christian and Muslim interviewees reported difficulties in obtaining information on their respective faith teachings or found that relevant faith organisations had not yet crafted a formal position on the use of new reproductive or genetic technologies. This is one of very few studies that have attempted to look at the implications of faith group membership and experiences of faith communities in clinical settings in the UK, relating to new reproductive and genetic technologies.

Historically, research and policy have considered birth outcomes and health or social inequalities in the context of ethnicity, rather than religious identity (Modood 2006; Department of Health/HM Treasury 2002). This focus overlooks particular issues for Muslim populations in the UK, in which religion, as distinct from ethnicity, is a prime aspect of identity (Modood 2006; Modood et al. 1997). Muslim faith identity can be a personal resource for health but also a trigger for discrimination in healthcare settings (Mir and Sheikh 2010), exposing Muslim communities to additional layers of exclusion. Muslims experience the highest levels of racism in the UK (Nazroo and Bécares 2017) and their religious identity can impact on the quality of health services they receive, regardless of their level of religious observance (Elahi and Khan 2017). Muslims experience particular disadvantage in areas affecting poor birth outcomes, such as long-term illness and unemployment (ONS 2013, 2004) and are over-represented in infant mortality statistics (ONS 2013; Department of Health 2007). Explanations for poorer outcomes in this area have focused on consanguinity as well as low antenatal attendance and socioeconomic position. However, the social structures within which individuals live are crucial to understanding such health inequalities (Karlsen and Nazroo 2002). An important issue raised in this literature is that observed ethnic inequalities in health can be attributed to the processes of racism, including Islamophobia, that lead to social and economic inequality (Nazroo and Bécares 2017) and poorer-quality healthcare (Knight et al. 2009).

It is evident that there needs to be a greater acknowledgement of the impact of faith identity on patients. In terms of parental decision making, healthcare professionals may find it helpful to know that Islamic theological and ethical perspectives are still emerging on issues pertaining to genetic and reproductive health. Families may therefore seek to include other interlocutors, such as scholars and other family members, in their decision-making process. An awareness of an extended model of decision making and differing religious and cultural values may help to facilitate clinical conversations, enrich trust building and prevent conflict.[1] In relation to the relationship between quality of care, discrimination and Muslim faith identity, recognising Islamophobia as a form of racism and incorporating this within institutional and policy initiatives to reduce discrimination could help address structural inequalities associated with poor health outcomes (Elahi and Khan 2017).

Islamic Perspectives on Interventions to Improve Genetic Health

At an international level, a body of work has been undertaken to examine the biomedical issues that have arisen as a result of technological advances in the past few decades and the impact of these on Islamic legal-ethical rulings including issues pertaining to genetic health. Within mainstream Islamic scholarship, the protection of the health of an individual and his/her progeny are key objectives (*maqasid al-Shariah*, objectives of the Shariah). Interventions that support protection of lineage or prevent harm to future generations are encouraged. Such

---

[1] See Malcom et al. (2019), Khushf (2019), and Benbenishty and Biswas (2015) for examples on the role of religion and spirituality in decision making in clinical settings and the different ways in which cultural and religious competence and awareness can facilitate the experience of patients and families.

interventions, however, are evaluated alongside other key objectives, such as the protection of life. Although genetic screening, counselling and testing would not only be acceptable but encouraged by such Muslim scholars, the identification of a genetic risk or genetic disease would have to be carefully evaluated before an intervention would be acceptable. Muslims adhering to such guidance, therefore, would generally welcome interventions that offer identification of harms and may prefer prevention that is afforded by pre-marital screening programmes, as established in Saudi Arabia and other countries in the Middle East. If, however, pre-marital screening is unavailable or unsuccessful at mitigating genetic disease, then Islamic law allows for such abnormalities to be identified and, if considered extremely severe, for the pregnancy to be terminated. 'Termination due to genetic defects' has undergone significant Islamic juridical scrutiny, and there is broad consensus that such termination is acceptable if the condition is severe, untreatable and unmanageable and if conducted prior to 120 days of gestation (Al-Bar and Chamsi-Pasha 2015b). The severity of a genetic disease, however, is open to interpretation and Muslim families would therefore be keen to understand more fully the extent of the underlying risk as well as the severity of the condition, due to their theological commitments to preserve life. Diagnostic uncertainty may therefore lead to anxiety in consultations (Al-Odaib et al. 2003).

In the UK, there is an emphasis on individual autonomy, and a couple may or may not choose to share information with wider family members. For many Muslims, however, decision making is undertaken with extended family members. Interventions, such as counselling, may need to be extended beyond the couple to wider family units such that these interventions can be more reflective of religio-cultural norms. Marriage in such contexts is considered a union of the couple, their families, extended families and often entire communities. Understanding and respect for such relationships may require recognised best practice to be flexible and adaptive to shared decision making and consultation, whilst being mindful of key ethical concerns around privacy and consent. Such extended decision-making units are also seen among families from East Asia, and some experts have suggested to clinicians and counsellors that they ought to

> encourage aunts, parents, grandparents, or other important elders to attend the genetic counselling sessions and let them express their views or encourage your patients to go home and discuss the relevant genetic counselling issues with other family members as they see fit. (Biesecker et al. 2019: 51)

By recognising and enabling the presence of such relationships within the shared decision-making model, the clinical setting will be better adapted for people who deeply rely on such values to inform their practices.

Case Study 2

Amina and Faisal had a daughter with a rare lethal genetic disorder called Raine syndrome, who sadly died a few days after birth. The version of Raine syndrome in their family results in death within the first few weeks of life, and is recessively inherited. This means both parents are healthy carriers of the altered gene that causes Raine syndrome, and have a one in four risk of having another child with the condition.

Amina and Faisal are worried about having another child with Raine syndrome and have heard about embryo screening to prevent the condition occurring in future pregnancies. They ask their genetic counsellor, Susie, for more information about 'embryo screening'.

Susie: *Since Amina and Faisal have a high risk – more than 10 per cent – of having another child with a serious genetic condition they can be offered PIGD (pre-implantation genetic diagnosis), sometimes thought of as 'embryo screening', on the NHS.*

PIGD is a new genetic technology whereby embryos are conceived in the laboratory (an IVF technique), in this case using 'eggs' from Amina and sperm from Faisal. The embryos are then screened to check for the specific genetic condition, for example Raine syndrome. If a suitable embryo, unaffected by the condition, is identified, it can be implanted in Amina for pregnancy.

Amina and Faisal are both Muslim. They are amazed by the technology but are concerned about the process, especially the discarding of embryos, and wonder if this is allowed from an Islamic perspective. They know Susie is not Muslim but ask if she has any experience and/or advice.

Susie: *Some Muslim couples have been in similar circumstances before and taken up PIGD. There are ethical articles by Muslim health professionals that explore the Islamic position on PIGD freely available on the internet.*

Susie signposts the couple to further information and suggests that Amina and Faisal could speak to the hospital chaplain who may know a good religious scholar who is versed in such matters.

Concluding Comments

The risk of birth defects arising due to consanguinity is currently estimated to increase from 1 to 3 per cent in the general population to 2 to 7 per cent in consanguineous couples. The consequences of this risk, including shortcomings in preventative services and the care of children and their families where there is a child with a birth defect, can be affected by a number of factors that interact: cultural, ethnic, religious and socioeconomic. As such, any discussions around genetic risks associated with consanguinity need to be understood within the socioeconomic contexts in which they occur.

In the UK, no national-level policy aimed at improving birth outcomes for those in consanguineous relationships currently exists. However, the need for such a policy is recognised and recommendations have been put forward to improve and standardise provision within the Maternity Transformation Programme. These still need to be approved at policy level but include, among others, providing appropriate training for health professionals and co-design of initiatives that empower parents in consanguineous relationships.

What is not highlighted in the recommendations, however, is the role of faith identity. Whilst rarely considered in health policy, it can be an important trigger for social exclusion and so linked to health inequalities experienced by Muslims. As such, development of policy and practices that attempt to address genetic risk associated with Muslim consanguineous couples should take account of the impact of faith identity on health behaviour in Muslim communities and on healthcare interactions.

In the UK, couples at risk of giving birth to offspring with recessive inherited disorders are currently identified at the prenatal or post-natal stage through targeted screening. We would advocate that individuals at risk should be identified at an earlier time-point (pre-conception or pre-relationship) so that reproductive options available to them are maximised. To facilitate this, more effort should be made to learn from international examples and national initiatives (e.g. the Jnetics GENEius programme) where earlier testing is being trialled or implemented.

The lack of knowledge of disease-causing genetic variants amongst the ethnically diverse Muslim population in the UK may at this time limit the implementation of multi-gene carrier screening of the type utilised by the Jnetics programme. However, as genome testing technologies develop, these could facilitate earlier testing for those in, or considering, consanguineous relationships and as such their integration into healthcare should be explored. Earlier testing and increased choices around reproductive options could reduce the expression of recessive disease genes in future generations and hence lead to a decline in the prevalence of specific recessive disorders.

Evidence suggests that Muslim couples are open to the use of new reproductive and genetic technologies that align with their faith values. However, these studies tend to be small-scale and limited to specific geographical locations (e.g. Australia, Netherlands) and groups (e.g. post-first pregnancy in a consanguineous relationship). To understand more fully user acceptability relating to these areas, larger, multi-regional, multi-ethnic studies involving participants defined as pre-first pregnancy are required.

Reproductive and genetic technologies are evolving rapidly and there is often a long time lag before Islamic scholarly responses are made to the new technologies. Therefore further research is also required to address questions raised as a result of new reproductive and genetic technologies from an interdisciplinary perspective. By combining Islamic philosophy, law, ethics and anti-racist practice appropriate guidance could be constructed to facilitate decision making by members of Muslim communities.

References

Ajaz, M., Ali, N. and Randhawa, G. (2015). 'UK Pakistani views on the adverse health risks associated with consanguineous marriages'. *Journal of Community Genetics*, 6(4): 331–42.

Al-Bar, M. A. and Chamsi-Pasha, H. (2015a). 'Ethical issues in genetics (premarital counseling, genetic testing, genetic engineering, cloning and stem cell therapy, DNA fingerprinting), in M. A. Al-Bar and H. Chamsi-Pasha, *Contemporary Bioethics*. Cham: Springer, pp. 187–207.

Al-Bar, M. A. and Chamsi-Pasha, H. (2015b). 'Abortion', in M. A. Al-Bar and H. Chamsi-Pasha, *Contemporary Bioethics*. Cham: Springer, pp. 155–72.

Alberg, C., Kroese, M. and Burton, H. (2014). 'Enhanced Genetic Services Project: Evaluation Report'. PHG Foundation. Available at: www.phgfoundation.org/report/egsp (last accessed 5 May 2022).

Al-Odaib, A. N., Abu-Amero, K. K., Ozand, P. T. and Al-Hellani, A. M. (2003). 'A new era for preventive genetic programs in the Arabian Peninsula'. *Saudi Medical Journal*, 24(11), 1168–75.

Alswaidi, F. M. and O'Brien, S. J. (2009). 'Premarital screening programmes for haemoglobinopathies, HIV and hepatitis viruses: review and factors affecting their success'. *Journal of Medical Screening*, 16(1), 22–8.

Alwan, A. and Modell, B. (1997). 'Community control of genetic and congenital disorders'. WHO Regional Office for the Eastern Mediterranean. Technical Publication Series, 24. Available at: https://apps.who.int/iris/handle/10665/119571 (last accessed 5 May 2022).

Andermann, A., Blancquaert, I., Beauchamp, S. and Déry, V. (2008). 'Revisiting Wilson and Jungner in the genomic age: a review of screening criteria over the past 40 years'. Bulletin of the World Health Organization. Available at: www.who.int/bulletin/volumes/86/4/07-050112/en (last accessed 5 May 2022).

Antonarakis, S. E. (2019). 'Carrier screening for recessive disorders'. *Nature Reviews Genetics*, 20(9), 549–61.

Awatif, A. (2004). 'Perception of female students of King Saud University towards premarital screening'. *Journal of Family & Community Medicine*, 13(2), 83–8.

Becker, R., Keller, T., Wegner, R.-D., Neitzel, H., Stumm, M., Knoll, U., Stärk, M., Fangerau, H. and Bittles, A. (2015). 'Consanguinity and pregnancy outcomes in a multi-ethnic, metropolitan European population'. *Prenatal Diagnosis*, 35(1), 81–9.

Benbenishty, J. and Biswas, S. (2015). 'Developing cultural competence in clinical practice'. *Journal of Modern Education Review*, 5(8), 805–11.

Bener, A., Al-Mulla, M. and Clarke, A. (2019). 'Premarital screening and genetic counseling program: studies from an endogamous population'. *International Journal of Applied & Basic Medical Research*, 9(1), 20–6.

Biesecker, B. B., Peters, K. F. and Resta, R. G. (2019). *Advanced Genetic Counseling: Theory and Practice*. New York: Oxford University Press.

Bhopal, R. S., Petherick, E. S., Wright, J. and Small, N. (2013). 'Potential social, economic and general health benefits of consanguineous marriage: results from the Born in Bradford cohort study'. *European Journal of Public Health*, 24(5), 862–9.

Bittles, A. H. (1994). 'The role and significance of consanguinity as a demographic variable'. *Population & Development Review*, 20(3), 561–84.

Bittles, A. H. (2012). *Consanguinity in Context*. Cambridge: Cambridge University Press.

Bittles, A. H. and Black, M. L. (2010). 'The impact of consanguinity on neonatal and infant health'. *Early Human Development*, 86(11): 737–41.

Bundey, S. and Alam, H. (1993). 'A five-year prospective study of the health of children in different ethnic groups, with particular reference to the effect of inbreeding'. *European Journal of Human Genetics*, 1(3), 206–19.

Burton, H., Levene, S., Alberg, C. and Stewart, A. (2009). 'Tay Sachs Disease carrier screening in the Ashkenazi Jewish population'. PHG Foundation. Available at: www.phgfoundation.org/report/tay-sachs-disease-carrier-screening-in-the-ashkenazi-jewish-population (last accessed 5 May 2022).

Cousens, N. E., Gaff, C. L., Metcalfe, S. A. and Delatycki, M. B. (2010). 'Carrier screening for beta-thalassaemia: a review of international practice'. *European Journal of Human Genetics*, 18, 1077–83.

Darr, A., Small, N., Ahmad, W. I. U., Atkin, K., Corry, P., Benson, J., Morton, R. and Modell, B. (2013). 'Examining the family-centred approach to genetic testing and counselling among UK Pakistanis: a community perspective'. *Journal of Community Genetics*, 4(1), 49–57.

Darr, A., Small, N., Ahmad, W. I. U., Atkin, K., Corry, P. and Modell, B. (2016). 'Addressing key issues in the consanguinity-related risk of autosomal recessive disorders in consanguineous communities: lessons from a qualitative study of British Pakistanis'. *Journal of Community Genetics*, 7(1), 65–79.

Department of Health (2007). *Implementation Plan for Reducing Health Inequalities in Infant Mortality: A Good Practice Guide*. Health Inequalities Unit. London: Department of Health.

Department of Health (2010). 'Tackling health inequalities in infant and maternal health outcomes: report of the Infant Mortality National Support Team'. Available at: www.gov.uk/government/publications/tackling-health-inequalities-in-infant-and-maternal-health-outcomes-report-of-the-infant-mortality-national-support-team (last accessed 5 May 2022).

Department of Health (2012). 'Building on our inheritance: genomic technologies in healthcare'. Human Genomics Strategy Group. Available at: https://assets.publishing.service.gov.uk/government/uploads/system/uploads/attachment_data/file/213705/dh_132382.pdf (last accessed 5 May 2022).

Department of Health/HM Treasury (2002). *Tackling Health Inequalities: Cross Cutting Review.* London: Department of Health.

Dormandy, E., Gulliford, M., Bryan, S., Roberts, T., Calnan, M., Atkin, K., Karnon, J., Logan, J., Kavalier, F., Harris, H. J., Johnston, T. A., Anionwu, E. N., Tsianakas, V., Jones, P. and Marteau, T. M. (2010). 'Effectiveness of earlier antenatal screening for sickle cell disease and thalassaemia in primary care: cluster randomised trial'. *BMJ,* 341, c5132.

Elahi, F. and Khan, O. (2017). 'Introduction: What is Islamophobia?', in F. Elahi and O. Khan, 'Islamophobia: still a challenge for us all. A 20th-anniversary report'. The Runnymede Trust. Available at: www.runnymedetrust.org/publications/islamophobia-still-a-challenge-for-us-all (last accessed 5 May 2022).

El-Hazmi, M. A. (2006). 'Pre-marital examination as a method of prevention from blood genetic disorders: community views'. *Saudi Medical Journal,* 27(9), 1291–5.

El-Shanti, H., Chouchane, L., Badii, R., Gallouzi, I. E. and Gasparini, G. (2015). 'Genetic testing and genomic analysis: a debate on ethical, social and legal issues in the Arab world with a focus on Qatar'. *Journal of Translational Medicine,* 13, 358.

GENEius (2019). The GENEius programme. Available at: www.geneius.org (last accessed 5 May 2022).

Gurdasani, D., Barroso, I., Zeggini, E. and Sandhu, M. S. (2019). 'Genomics of disease risk in globally diverse populations'. *Nature Reviews Genetics,* 20(9), 520–35.

Hamamy, H., Antonarakis, S. E., Cavalli-Sforza, L. L., Temtamy, S., Romeo, G., Kate, L. P., Bennett, R. L., Shaw, A., Megarbane, A, van Duijn, C, Bathija, H, Fokstuen, S, et al. (2011). 'Consanguineous marriages, pearls and perils: Geneva International Consanguinity Workshop report'. *Genetics in Medicine,* 13(9), 841–7.

Henneman, L., Borry, P., Chokoshvili, D., Cornel, M. C., van El, C. G., Forzano, F., Hall, A., Howard, H. C., Janssens, S., Kayserili, H., Lakeman, P., Lucassen, A. et al. (2016). 'Responsible implementation of expanded carrier screening'. *European Journal of Human Genetics,* 24(6), e1–e12.

House of Commons Science and Technology Committee (2018). 'Genomics and genome editing in the NHS'. Third Report of Session 2017–19. Available at: https://publications.parliament.uk/pa/cm201719/cmselect/cmsctech/349/349.pdf (last accessed 5 May 2022).

Josephi-Taylor, S., Barlow-Stewart, K., Selvanathan, A., Roscioli, T., Bittles, A., Meiser, B., Worgan, L., Rajagopalan, S., Colley, A. and Kirk, E. P. (2019). 'User acceptability of whole exome reproductive carrier testing for consanguineous couples in Australia'. *Journal of Genetic Counseling*, 28(2), 240–50.

Karlsen, S. and Nazroo, J. Y. (2002). 'Relation between racial discrimination, social class, and health among ethnic minority groups'. *American Journal of Public Health*, 92(4), 624–31.

Khan, N., Benson, J., Macleod, R. and Kingston, H. (2010). 'Developing and evaluating a culturally appropriate genetic service for consanguineous South Asian families'. *Journal of Community Genetics*, 1(2), 73–81.

Knight, M., Kurinczuk, J. J., Spark, P. and Brocklehurst, P. (2009). 'Inequalities in maternal health: national cohort study of ethnic variation in severe maternal morbidities'. *BMJ*, 338, b542.

Kurinczuk, J. J., Hollowell, J. Boyd, P. A., Oakley, L., Brocklehurst, P. and Gray, R. (2010). 'The contribution of congenital anomalies to infant mortality'. Inequalities in Infant Mortality Project Briefing Paper 4. National Perinatal Epidemiology Unit, University of Oxford. Available at:www.npeu.ox.ac.uk/infant-mortality (last accessed 5 May 2022).

Khushf, G. (2019). 'When religious language blocks discussion about health care decision making'. *HEC Forum*, 31, 151–66.

Malcolm, H. V., Desjardins, C. M., Ferrara, B., Kitamura, E. A., Mueller, M., Betz, J., Ragsdale, J. R. and Grossoehme, D. H. (2019). 'Parental use of religion and spirituality in medical decision-making', *Journal of Health Care Chaplaincy*, 27(3), 146–58.

Memish, Z. A. and Saeedi, M. Y. (2011). 'Six-year outcome of the national premarital screening and genetic counseling program for sickle cell disease and β-thalassemia in Saudi Arabia'. *Annals of Saudi Medicine*, 31(3), 229–35.

Mir, G. and Sheikh, A. (2010). '"Fasting and prayer don't concern the doctors . . . they don't even know what it is": communication, decision-making and perceived social relations of Pakistani Muslim patients with long-term illnesses'. *Ethnicity & Health*, 15(4), 327–42.

Modell, B. and Darr, A. (2002). 'Genetic counselling and customary consanguineous marriage'. *Nature Review Genetics*, 3, 225–9.

Modood, T. R. (2006). 'British Muslims and the politics of multiculturalism', in T. Modood, A. Triandafyllidou and R. Zapate-Barrero (eds), *Multiculturalism, Muslims and citizenship*. London: Routledge.

Modood, T., Berthoud, R., Lakey, J., Nazroo, J., Smith, P., Virdee, S. and Beishon, S. (eds) (1997), *Ethnic Minorities in Britain: Diversity and Disadvantage*. London: Policy Studies Institute.

Nazroo, J. and Bécares, L. (2017). 'Islamaphobia, racism and health', in F. Elahi and O. Khan, 'Islamophobia: still a challenge for us all. A 20th-anniversary report'.

The Runnymede Trust. Available at: www.runnymedetrust.org/publications/islamophobia-still-a-challenge-for-us-all (last accessed 6 May 2022).

NHS England (2016). National Maternity Review. Available at: www.england.nhs.uk/mat-transformation (last accessed 6 May 2022).

Office for National Statistics (2004). 'Focus on religion'. Available at: https://webarchive.nationalarchives.gov.uk/ukgwa/20160128144717/http://www.ons.gov.uk/ons/rel/ethnicity/focus-on-religion/2004-edition/index.html (last accessed 8 July 2022).

Office for National Statistics (2013). 'Pregnancy and ethnic factors influencing births and infant mortality: 2013'. Available at: www.ons.gov.uk/peoplepopulationand-community/healthandsocialcare/causesofdeath/bulletins/pregnancyandethnicfac-torsinfluencingbirthsandinfantmortality/2015-10-14#ethnicity (last accessed 6 May 2022).

Public Health England (2016). 'Fetal anomaly screening programme (FASP): pro-gramme overview'. Available at: www.gov.uk/guidance/fetal-anomaly-screening-programme-overview#screening-test-downs-edwards-and-pataus-syndromes (last accessed 6 May 2022).

Qureshi, N. and Raeburn, S. (2011). 'Risks to offspring of consanguineous marriage: we need straight, not crooked thinking'. *Journal of the Royal College of Physicians of Edinburgh*, 41(3), 194–5.

Rao, S. S. P., Inbaraj, S. G. and Jesudian, G. (1972). 'Rural-urban differentials in consanguinity'. *Journal of Medical Genetics*, 9(2), 174–8.

Saffi, M. and Howard, N. (2015). 'Exploring the effectiveness of mandatory pre-marital screening and genetic counselling programmes for ß-thalassaemia in the Middle East: a scoping review'. *Public Health Genomics*, 18(4), 193–203.

Sallevelt, S. C. E. H., de Koning, B., Szklarczyk, R., Paulussen, A. D. C., de Die-Smulders, C. E. M. and Smeets, H. J. M. (2017). 'A comprehensive strategy for exome-based preconception carrier screening'. *Genetics in Medicine,* 19(5), 583–92.

Salway, S., Ali, P., Ratcliffe, G., Such, E., Khan, N., Kingston, H. and Quarrell, O. (2016). 'Responding to the increased genetic risk associated with custom-ary consanguineous marriage among minority ethnic populations: lessons from local innovations in England'. *Journal of Community Genetics*, 7(3), 215–28.

Salway, S., Yazici, E., Khan, N., Ali, P., Elmslie, F., Thompson, J. and Qureshi, N. (2019). 'How should health policy and practice respond to the increased genetic risk associated with close relative marriage? Results of a UK Delphi consensus building exercise'. *BMJ Open,* 9(7), e028928.

Scully, J. L., Banks, S., Song, R. and Haq, J. (2017). 'Experiences of faith group members using new reproductive and genetic technologies: a qualitative inter-view study'. *Human Fertility*, 20(1), 22–9.

Shaw, A. (2001). 'Kinship, cultural preference and immigration: consanguineous marriage among British Pakistanis'. *Journal of the Royal Anthropological Institute*, 7(2), 315–34.

Shaw, A. (2014). 'Drivers of cousin marriage among British Pakistanis'. *Human Heredity*, 77 (1–4), 26–36.

Shaw, A. (2015). 'Cousin marriages: between tradition, genetic risk and cultural change', in A. Shaw and A. E. Raz (eds), *British Pakistani Cousin Marriages and the Negotiation of Reproductive Risk*. New York: Berghahn Books, pp. 113–29.

Sheridan, E., Wright, J., Small, N., Corry, P. C., Oddie, S., Whibley, C., Petherick, E. S., Malik, T., Pawson, N., McKinney, P. A. and Parslow, R. C. (2013). 'Risk factors for congenital anomaly in a multiethnic birth cohort: an analysis of the Born in Bradford study'. *The Lancet*, 382(9901), 1350–9.

Teebi, A. S. and Farag, T. I. (1997). *Genetic Disorders among Arab Populations*, 1st edn. New York: Oxford University Press.

Verdonk, P., Metselaar, S., Storms, O. and Bartels E. (2018). 'Reproductive choices: a qualitative study of Dutch Moroccan and Turkish consanguineously married women's perspectives on preconception carrier screening'. *BMC Women's Health*, 18(1), 79.

World Health Organization (2019). Diabetes: Data and statistics. Available at: www. euro.who.int/en/health-topics/noncommunicable-diseases/diabetes/data-and-statistics (last accessed 6 May 2022).

6

CARING FOR MUSLIM PATIENTS AND FAMILIES AT THE END OF LIFE: EMPIRICAL RESEARCH ANALYSING THE PERSPECTIVES OF SERVICE USERS AND PROVIDERS

Mehrunisha Suleman

Introduction

Before beginning an investigation into the particular needs of Muslim patients at the end of life, it is important to acknowledge what all people share in common. A defining characteristic of the human condition is to be faced with the knowledge that each of us will die. Death brings suffering, both because of the severance of relationship it inevitably entails, but also because of the physical and psychological challenges that individuals face as the body declines (Salinsky 2002). Although medicine has done much to ease this suffering, it cannot prevent all suffering. Furthermore, as technology advances, so choices increase, and more questions without simple answers are generated, such as whether or not to artificially hydrate or sedate patients at the end of life (Steinhauser et al. 2000), or whether or not to allow suffering individuals to be assisted to end their own lives by choice (Warnock and Macdonald 2009).

The challenges and choices faced at the end of life bring a person's values into sharp relief. For Muslims, Islam's normative sources (the Qur'an and the tradition of the Prophet Muhammad) are the source of ultimate authority from which the values that guide the end of life choices and behaviour derive. Muslims carry these commitments within not just their private sphere, but also the public space, including the healthcare setting. Understandings about death and dying, within the palliative and end-of-life care context, require Muslim patients and families to carefully consider their religious and cultural values. For others within that context, such as healthcare professionals with varying sources of ultimate authority, their deliberations will be influenced by other faith values and/or other sources. In the predominant secular model of democratic society, this authority lies with individuals and the laws and guidelines that their communities create.

From here a paradox arises. Humans are the same; all face suffering and death. All need values to navigate the difficult choices and events that are faced at the end of life. However we are also different. We live within different paradigms, from which values emerge, and at least some of those values differ from one another. Sometimes those values, with their associated choices and behaviours, will be contradictory and will become sources of disagreement or conflict.

Negotiating differing values and commitments, within the healthcare setting, is wrought with moral and emotional difficulty. Training and education of healthcare professionals has been transformed to include syllabi on clinical ethics, the social context of health and illness as well as cultural literacy and competency. National guidelines (NICE 2011) are also emphasising that care at the end of life 'should be sensitive to personal preferences' and that 'treatment and care, and the information given about it, should be culturally appropriate'. There is, however, very little guidance offered on the particularities of such preferences and the needs of different faith and cultural groups. Reports have shown that there are unmet needs and disparities in access to palliative and end-of-life care services, including religious and cultural needs, of minority groups in the UK. Challenges raised by providing care for such groups is also resulting in uncertainty and stress among healthcare professionals who are trying their utmost to provide the best possible care (Calanzani et al. 2013).

Although healthcare professionals are recognising the need for cultural competency and training, when providing palliative and end-of-life care, there are few resources offering them insights into the deliberations carried out by Muslim patients and families, the complexities that they encounter and negotiate in relationship with a healthcare system that exists within a secular paradigm. The aim of this study was to address this knowledge gap by first assessing whether and how the religious commitments of Muslims and the teachings of Islam influence deliberations in the context of end-of-life care in the UK. Through an analysis of stakeholder deliberations we also sought to study patients' and families' 'personal preferences' and 'spiritual needs', as well as investigating what the barriers, challenges and facilitators may be for healthcare professionals seeking to ensure that treatment, care and information provided at the end of life is culturally appropriate.

Despite the amorphous nature of any community, there are tendencies and values that many Muslims have in common as they reach the end of life. A key aim of this study was to gain insight into what values and subsequent experiences, behaviours and choices were most prominent for Muslim patients and families as they negotiated the complexities of doing this in relationship with a healthcare system that exists within a secular paradigm, and to understand better the challenges that they and those providing care for them face when different sources of authority and ethical reasoning are relied upon.

As shall be shown, for healthcare professionals care for Muslims is in many respects no different from care for any patient: the professional approaches all patients with respect and with the understanding that individuals will come with specific needs to be cared for and treated. As will become apparent, there are notable issues that arise for Muslim patients, their families and the healthcare professionals that care for them at the end of life. The themes include ethical challenges raised by the reconciliation of beliefs and practices in Muslim communities when they encounter the health service, and in particular religio-cultural commitments in the understanding and articulation of values around death and dying such as sacred duties to care and the elevated status of the mother within the Islamic tradition. This chapter will organise these issues into key themes that will distinguish between conflicting values as necessary. From this, suggestions will be made about how policy, training and education might be enhanced to better serve Muslim patients and families who receive end-of-life care and healthcare professionals who provide these services in the UK.

Methodology

To better understand the beliefs, values and practices of Muslims pertaining to end-of-life care decision making in the UK, an empirical qualitative study was carried out.

Sampling

Sampling was carried out in London and Birmingham, to maximise the opportunity to study Muslim values in end-of-life care decision making, as these two cities have the highest population of Muslims in the UK (MCB 2015). Sampling was also carried out in Cambridge, despite the small population of Muslims, to include narratives of stakeholders in a varied sociodemographic profile.

Given the aim of the study, the following types of key stakeholders were identified as important and included in recruitment:

- Muslim patients and family members
- healthcare professionals (doctors, nurses, physiotherapists, psychologists etc.) – Muslim and non-Muslim
- bereavement staff, funeral service staff, mortuary staff and coroners – Muslim and non-Muslim
- chaplains (multifaith and/or Muslim)
- imams and/or Islamic scholars involved in end-of-life care decision making

The rationale for sampling these five types of interviewees was because they constitute the five groups most likely to be able to provide insight into the role of Islam and the beliefs, values and practices of Muslims as pertaining to decision making within end-of-life care. The reason for interviewing diverse actors, at multiple levels and throughout the pathway of patient and family care, was to allow for an assessment of the multiple relevant perspectives within end-of-life care in the different contexts. It was also to enable a deeper understanding of the interaction between different stakeholders, such as the complex dynamics concerning healthcare professionals, patients and family members, and the interplay of faith-based and secular values in such encounters. A purposive sampling method was employed to capture a range of experiences.

Emails were sent systematically to all hospices in London, Birmingham and Cambridge that were listed on the Hospice UK website to recruit hospices and individual participants into the study. An email including a brief of the study was sent via the Hospice UK mailing list. Emails were also sent to chaplaincy offices at hospital trusts in the three cities. Once interviews began, further recruitment was carried out via internet searches (purposive sampling) and emailing of suitable participants as well as recruitment based on the advice of interviewees (snowballing).

A total of seventy-six interviews were conducted. This number was based on our being able to interview a sufficient number of suitable individuals within each of the participant categories such that data saturation was achieved, i.e. until a point was reached beyond which it was judged the addition of new themes was unlikely.

Ethical review

As the study involves direct participation involving human subjects, it has undergone review by the University of Cambridge School of Humanities and Social Sciences Ethics Committee as well as the NHS Health Research Authority (IRAS number: 220682).

Semi-structured interviews

As one of the objectives of the study was to investigate whether and how Islam and the beliefs, values and practices of Muslims influence their understanding and approaches to end-of-life care, the semi-structured interview presented the ideal means of probing and also challenging participants' views to better understand their reasoning and experiences. Green et al. (2013) describe the interview as 'a conversation that is directed, more or less, towards the researcher's particular needs for data'.

For in-depth interviews with participants, an open-ended thematic topic guide was developed to ensure that the same themes were covered in each of the five interview tiers. The guide did, however, provide flexibility to ensure that questioning could occur freely and to allow the interviewer to choose the questions appropriate to the context and enable suitable probing of topics and issues that were pertinent and that arose within the interview.

Framework analysis

A framework approach has been used to analyse the data, as it is a flexible method of analysis in allowing for both inductive and deductive contributions to analysis. Concepts and themes from the literature were used as pre-existing theoretical constructs during the analysis of the data (deductive analysis), alongside an inductive approach, whereby themes were identified directly from the qualitative data before revisiting the literature (Gale et al. 2013). This method also has the advantage that although in-depth analysis can take place across the entire dataset, the process of coding and charting ensures that the views of each participant remain connected within a matrix (ibid.). The data analysis in this study employs the thematic framework analysis method that was devised by Ritchie and Lewis (2003). Semi-structured interviews were audio recorded and transcribed. Using data from notes taken at the interviews and transcriptions of the audio recordings, a framework analysis approach was employed (Green et al. 2013; Pope et al. 2000). The method I used reflects the framework analysis requirements described first by Ritchie and Lewis (2003) who suggest that the framework should ensure the investigator:

1. remains grounded in the data
2. permits captured synthesis – this is reflected in the charting process where verbatim text is reduced from its raw form
3. facilitates and displays ordering – again this is reflected in the charting process
4. permits within and between case searches – the charting process allows for searching and comparisons to be made within and between datasets

Such a method ensures that the data analysis process is systematic, comprehensive and flexible to enable new ideas to be generated. It also enables refinements and ensures transparency to others. Ritchie and Lewis's method of analysis is one that involves an 'analytical hierarchy' which begins with familiarisation of the data or data management followed by the generation of descriptive accounts and finally abstraction through the development of explanatory accounts (ibid.). The following sections describe how I carried out these steps of analysis:

Familiarisation with the data

This first step was employed to ensure that, as primary investigator, I remained close to the data and involved immersion in the data with repeated reading of field notes, summaries and transcripts, in order to list key ideas, recurrent themes and patterns. I did not code at this stage and instead summarised the key points participants made via a summary sheet for each interview. A selection of the transcripts were discussed with my research team at the Centre of Islamic Studies during the early stages of the interview period, to enable me to develop an initial systematic reflection of the data.

Generating themes

A coding scheme was developed by identifying all the key issues, concepts and themes. This was carried out by drawing on a priori issues and questions derived from the aims and objectives of the study and the literature review, as well as emergent issues raised by the participants. The coding framework was discussed and reviewed with research colleagues at the Centre of Islamic Studies, as well as at research meetings with key stakeholders. During the coding process, inductive codes, or those emerging from the data, were added to the coding framework if they described a new theme or expanded a predetermined code.

Indexing

The themes in the data were then used as labels for codes, which were subsequently applied to the whole dataset. This was done systematically to ensure all the data was accurately coded using NVIVO version 10. The process of generating themes and indexing continued until the point of data saturation. Data saturation was assessed at the point where 'no new information or themes' (Guest et al. 2006) were observed in the data. After this point only indexing continued until all of the data had been coded.

Charting (descriptive accounts)

After the data was coded according to the identified themes, it was then charted to assist in the generation of descriptive accounts where verbatim text was reduced from its raw form. This involved a rearrangement of the data according to the thematic content by comparing data within and between interviews. Once judged to be comprehensive, each main theme was charted by completing a matrix where each interview had its own row and columns representing the subtopics. These charts contain summaries of data that can be referenced back to the original transcript. This enabled a presentation of the range and diversity of views. Key quotes were recorded and certain themes were listed in the participants' own language. This was then followed by a refinement of categories to address overlap and to develop typologies that assisted in the collation of the related themes helping to divide and unite the participants' views.

Mapping and interpretation (developing exploratory accounts)

The charts were then used to examine the data for patterns and connections. This stage was influenced by the original aims and objectives of the study as well as emergent issues from the data. Here patterns in the data were identified to then derive explanations of participants' experiences and views. An account was developed to explain reasons behind the differences and similarities captured between and within participant accounts to arrive at an understanding of Muslim perspectives on end-of-life care. For example, recurrent themes were identified and the reasons for these were explored. Explanations and reasoning given by participants were also studied in order to distinguish these from my own analysis as the investigator (reflexivity).

Data analysis and the process of developing the main themes for this chapter

Having analysed the literature and studied the transcripts using a framework analysis, I identified two main themes and four subthemes that helped me organise the insights emerging from the data pertinent to Muslim values and end-of-life care decision making. Although the data could have been presented in multiple ways and I drafted several versions of the data tables, the themes outlined below ultimately functioned best as organising concepts for the data I gathered from the participants I interviewed. The themes are as follows:

1. End-of-life care decision making in modern healthcare systems: values, norms and ontologies:
   a. encountering cultures and traditions at the bedside
   b. ensuring patient-centred care – beyond rituals
2. Values, beliefs and practice in end-of-life care decision making: sources, languages and authorities:
   a. lack of trust in healthcare institutions and individuals
   b. understanding and interpreting values – need for 'trusted people and trusted spaces'

Whilst these themes emerged as being important from my analysis of participant accounts, they also provided a framework through which the data and discussion from this chapter could be related back to the broader discussion and aims of this volume in addressing whether and how faith commitments are encountered within the palliative and end-of-life care context (Chenail 1995; Sandelowski 1998).

Analysing the role of faith

As the focus of the study was on Muslim perspectives on end-of-life care, participants were chosen and asked about their experiences and understandings of the impact of Islam and the beliefs, values and practices of Muslims within end-of-life care decision making. Discussions with some participants who were not Muslim (for example, doctors, nurses and multifaith chaplains) did inevitably include descriptions of their own faith commitments and how these manifest in their deliberations and understandings of end-of-life care. Although such accounts were incredibly rich and helpful in providing an important backdrop to participants' narrative accounts, I did not employ such descriptions to develop a comparative analysis of different faith accounts. The latter would be highly valuable, but was outside the scope of this study. Thus, within the presentation of the data, the faith of a participant is only listed in cases of Muslim participants as all other participant accounts were analysed primarily on their role (as nurses or multifaith chaplains) and not their religious background.

Presenting the data – how quotes were chosen

For evidencing the findings and illustrating perspectives of participants (San-delowski 1994), quotes were carefully chosen for presentation in this chapter. However, in keeping with the 'aesthetics and ethics' (ibid.) of qualitative research reporting, as some of the participant explanations were lengthy, quotes had to be selected that were relevant for each section and sometimes edited further for brevity. I was careful however to select and edit quotes that retained the over-all message of each transcript from which they were extracted. I kept detailed memos during the coding process to assist in the selection of appropriate quotes.

Limitations of the methodology

There were numerous limitations in relation to the methods employed for the empirical study. Sampling was restricted to sites in London, Birmingham and Cambridge. There are a significant number of Muslims in other cities across the UK including Leicester and Bradford. Future studies in such areas will help to add to the findings elucidated through this dataset. In addition, interviews with more than 75 participants cannot be representative of all the myriad views and complexities encountered within end-of-life care, which does limit our ability to generalise the findings from this study.

Another limitation was that participants were not sent the topic guide before the interviews. The information sheet provided a broad outline of the research objectives and methods; however, the precise questions and topics were not included. This was to enable me to document participants' own description and analysis of events and an explanation of the practical deliberations they under-take in a more organic, unrehearsed manner. It was also to encourage partici-pants to offer a more diverse range of issues than was included in the interview guide. In addition, I was concerned that sending the topic guide in advance may have led to bias in the data collection. However, this approach meant that, given the time constraints of the interview, it took some participants a long time to connect the questions they encountered with the underlying ethical problems. Although many of the participants were doctors, nurses and chaplains and had had some training in ethics, few were ethicists and so some found it difficult to articulate an account of the ethical problems they encountered and how they addressed these. However, in such cases, topics from the interview guide were used to first ascertain whether the participants had faced a similar problem and, if so, to provide them with the opportunity to elaborate on the experience. Often, this method was successful in drawing out participants' own views and values that emerged from carefully disentangling the challenges they had faced. Future research may combine blinded topics or questions as well as some questions that participants may reflect on prior to the interview so they feel less pressured by the time constraints.

Findings

End-of-life care decision making in modern healthcare systems: values, norms and ontologies

An analysis of more than seventy interview transcripts has revealed the prominence of healthcare professionals' encounters with the Islamic tradition and Muslim values, beliefs and practices at the bedside. Many spent a significant amount of time describing the individuals and communities they provide care for, the learning they have acquired in recognising and meeting diverse needs, and the persisting challenges they face.

Encountering cultures and traditions at the bedside

Many healthcare professionals talked about encountering patients of different faiths, ethnicities, and cultural and linguistic heritages and how, at the bedside of the dying patient, they encounter the myriad elements of family members' lives. Some healthcare professionals talked about the sensitivities and responsibility their role confers when patients and/or families confide in them. They may encounter values and commitments that they are unfamiliar with, or unable to fully understand or respond to:

> it was with reticence and reluctance that she came in, to be honest. And when she did, she talked a lot about the family . . . so the sense of a responsibility and role within the context of culture in caring for the dying person. It was her husband that was dying. A lot of what we did was unpicking that a little bit and helping her to . . . I felt that that had to be very delicately done, because

I'm not a religious figure in any way or equipped or able to advise on any of those things. I feel that quite often the issues that the family were facing were quite interwoven with spiritual and religious issues, actually. *(Interview 10, clinical psychologist, London)*

A senior nurse also described the challenges of recognising and respecting Muslim patients' and families' paradigmatic views, whilst trying her utmost to provide the best possible care:

I would give the mum an opportunity to ask questions, but I was sort of respectful of their wishes, and the sons and I had long conversations about it's different, Western and Eastern, that they give up hope, and this is said to me a lot. If you tell them they are dying, then they give up hope and we shouldn't be doing that, and the more Eastern philosophy that you have to keep trying right until the end, which I think doesn't always meet the Western philosophy of there is a point where you say, 'No more' and we want quality of life. *(Interview 3, palliative care nurse, London)*

The perception of palliative care for some Muslim patients I think is very difficult. From a social perspective I think they feel they need to be seen doing everything possible for their relative and it's a sign of love and it's what's expected of them by their wider family. It's hard for them to say do the Western thing and that it's all going to end now. Some of them do, I'm not saying that you can generalise can't you? But that's something I come across quite a lot. *(Interview 3, palliative care nurse, London)*

Her experience and the views of other participants in the research highlight that for Muslim patients and families, their understandings and commitments at the end of life are deeply rooted in Islamic theological and ethical teachings. Whereas there is a focus within the secular medical paradigm of knowing when you are going to die and to focus on quality of life, within the Islamic tradition there is an emphasis on the 'sanctity of life' (Al-Shahri 2016) and, concurrent with other Eastern traditions, the giving and sustaining of hope to the dying (Searight and Gafford 2005; Turner 2002). Although death is considered a part of life, and integral to the human biography, within Islam and for many Muslims there is a delicate balance between accepting death and not hastening it (see Box 6.1). Muslims consider death a necessary transition to an afterlife that is a means of reuniting with God. They are therefore mindful of decisions at the end of life as their present carries a metaphysical weight in the hereafter. The data points to a need to foster better understandings around palliative and end-of-life care services among different communities who are unfamiliar with such services and for whom religious and cultural values are weighted towards sustaining life.

In practice, the data shows that the juxtaposition of different traditions and values raises challenges for healthcare professionals trying to understand better the needs and choices of patients at the end of life and to carry out normative practices such as advanced care planning. In many ways, healthcare professionals consider caring for Muslim patients as no different from any other patient: the professional approaches all patients with respect and with the understanding that individuals will come with specific needs to be cared for and treated. The data shows that these specific needs and preferences do, however, raise ethical challenges and questions for healthcare professionals.

Box 6.1 Excerpts from Islam's normative sources (the Qur'an and tradition of the Prophet Muhammad). Understandings of these underlie commitments that Muslim patients and families display when making end-of-life care decisions.

'It is God who creates you and takes your souls at death; and of you there are some who are sent back to a feeble age, so that they know nothing after having known (much): for Allah is All-Knowing, All-Powerful' (Qur'an 16:70).

'Do not express your wish to die, and do not pray for death before it comes on you, because death will terminate your good deeds, while prolonged living will further increase the good deeds of the faithful' (Sahih Muslim Book 48 Hadith 15).

'Every soul shall taste death, and you will only be given your [full] compensation on the Day of Resurrection. So he who is drawn away from the Fire and admitted to Paradise has attained the object (of Life): For the life of this world is but goods and chattels of deception' (Qur'an 3: 185).

'It is He who created death and life to test you [as to] which of you is best in deed – and He is the Exalted in Might, the Forgiving' (Qur'an 67:2).

'Say, "Indeed, the death from which you flee – indeed, it will meet you. Then you will be returned to the Knower of the unseen and the witnessed, and He will inform you about what you used to do"' (Qur'an 62:8).

Ensuring patient centred care – beyond rituals

One participant reflected deeply on the issue of providing care for diverse communities. She described her extensive nursing career in palliative care and explained that more recently she has faced challenges when ensuring 'patient-centred care', particularly for patients from minority faith and ethnic groups. She emphasised how healthcare professionals' understandings of the needs and preferences of these groups ought to extend beyond the recognition, documentation and fulfilment of ritualistic requirements alone:

> In your nurse training, and even at quite a high level of specialist pallia-tive care training, when you are discussing religion, and religion sensitivities and things, everyone gets caught up in the tasks and practicality. When does somebody want to be washed after they've died? What way do they want to be laid out? What food do they want brought in? That's the easy stuff. You ask the patient and the family, or you read it somewhere. Somebody will know. The much more subtle things of how to have a conversation, around this stuff. *(Interview 6, senior palliative care nurse, London)*

The question of understanding the 'subtle things' within Muslim patients' and families' deliberations around end-of-life care requires a careful consideration of underlying values and relationships. Many healthcare professionals described the challenges of initiating and sustaining a conversation and rapport with patients and families about end-of-life decision making. One focus of this study was to better understand the underlying reasons for such challenges.

The views and experiences presented in this and subsequent sections enable us to sketch the contours of the changing face of death and dying in the UK. The multicultural and multi-ethnic social fabric of British society reveals that prefer-ences and needs around death and dying ought to be reflected through more diverse practices and services. In London and Birmingham, the demographic profile from the 2011 census reveals that the population of Muslims is as high as 1 in 10 and 1 in 5 respectively (MCB 2015). The recognised normative models of care delivery within palliative and end-of-life care may need to be adapted to ensure services are fair in how they resonate with the variegated practices and values that underlie our communities.

Values, beliefs and practice in end-of-life care decision making: sources, languages and authorities

A recurring barrier reported by participants was lack of trust or difficulties in building and sustaining trust between patients, families and healthcare profes-sionals. This section provides evidence of the challenges of trust encountered by healthcare professionals and the types of 'trusted people and trusted spaces' that Muslim patients and families may rely on when deliberating end-of-life care decision making. Chaplaincy is key to this concept of 'trusted people and trusted spaces'. Although not covered here, it is dealt with in depth in Suleman (2022). Given the evidence, policy makers and healthcare providers ought to recognise such trends to ensure that the needs of different communities can be better understood and met.

Lack of trust in healthcare institutions and individuals

Healthcare professionals of differing roles, levels of seniority and specialism described facing suspicion, lack of trust and wariness on the part of Muslim patients and families when trying to negotiate or administer end-of-life care:

> I also feel there's that clash still where some of the Muslim community still don't have that trust for the medical system . . . 'cause I already feel where sometimes you do get a family where there is that split with the medics, they don't have that trust. It's always like they don't have that trust. (Interview 23, hospital chaplain, Muslim, London)

The participant explained that there may be myriad reasons for this institutional level of distrust. He explained his context in East London where many Muslim patients and families encounter similarly fraught relationships with other institutions due to their socioeconomic status, poor access to education, barriers to accessing services and prejudices:

> I think a lot of it is the second, third generation who might have seen racism towards their parents and are determined that they are going to get the best. These second, third generations might be doctors themselves, you know what I mean? Or training to be. I think there is a lot of that goes on. (Interview 11, hospice nurse, Birmingham)

Some of the participants explained how a lack of trust in individuals and teams is expressed as demands for additional interventions and services:

> And sometimes to deal with relatives' distress and lack of trust, you will explain to them that if that is what you want, we will provide it as long as it does not cause any harm. And you explain to them that in the dying phase, the body will not be able to process excess fluids and it's likely to cause problems in the form of oedema, fluid retention, pulmonary oedema, difficulty of breathing, bubbliness in the breathing in the final stages . . . in layman's terms it's called

a death rattle which will develop most likely in dying patients who are given IV fluids or any fluids in the dying phase. And you explain that if that were to happen, that is harm that we have caused from putting up fluids, and in that situation we'd want to take it down. *(Interview 59, hospice palliative care consultant, London)*

One healthcare assistant described a case in extremis of a Muslim family, mainly comprising healthcare professionals, installing cameras around the house before agreeing to nursing care for their mother.

We're working in the community then so the family were very vocal the whole time. They had cameras all other things that . . . even when you did the personal care everything was watched. It was almost like we weren't trusted. I can understand you've gotta be very careful who you're . . . to look after your loved ones. You just never know how they're going to be treated. We didn't have a problem with it. But when you encounter it's almost like there isn't enough trust in the work that we're coming in to do, because I think people don't always realise that when you're in palliative and end-of-life care it's a different kind of care that you're giving. *(Interview 46, healthcare assistant, community hospice team, London)*

In addition to the institutional challenges pertaining to trust mentioned above, the data reveals key Islamic values related to the 'role of the family', the 'duty to care', and the 'status of parents' and especially the 'status of the mother in Islam' that contribute to underlying anxieties and tensions about end-of-life care decision making, access and acceptability of services. The following section will explore these concepts further, pointing to a need for such trends to be recognised and embedded within training, education and practice.

Understanding and interpreting values – need for 'trusted people and trusted spaces'

A recurrent theme within the data is the role of the family within the Islamic tradition. Muslim patients and family members reiterate the importance of relationships and community. Healthcare professionals spent a lot of time describing their encounters with Muslim families, the different individuals involved, the various dynamics, whether and how such encounters impacted their ability to communicate effectively with the patient and if there were specific challenges and reflections.

I think they're more together as families . . . often living locally, which is really supportive. They've got strong bonds, and . . . they respect. We might think we are very important, that we are very clever, but they might be getting advice from other areas as well, there is that going on.

I feel that I don't know what my patients want because the family are in charge. If they aren't speaking English and they won't let me bring an interpreter then I have a slight concern sometimes.

Just that I might be missing something from the patient's perspective and it's what they want. If I'm really nervous I will get an interpreter in. They may be too weak or too poorly to actually talk about the point as well. *(Interview 11, hospice nurse)*

Many participants described how the family of Muslim patients plays a key role in communications around diagnosis, prognosis, decision making, access and acceptance of advice, interventions and services. Palliative care teams described the additional challenge of building trust with patients and families whilst negotiating barriers such as English proficiency, particularly when encountering Muslim female patients at the end of life:

This is where religion crosses into other cultural stuff, crosses into gender stuff, doesn't it? I found it very difficult sometimes where Muslim women, perhaps older Muslim women, aren't allowed to be part of the conversation, or it seems to me that they're not allowed to be part of the conversation. Whether it's with me, or whether it's within the family, or whether it's all together. Not allowed to hear the information, to hear the options and then to make an informed decision about the options . . .

[It was] a lady in and out [because of] bowel obstruction . . . she was in her last few weeks . . . [she was] symptomatic of that, in terms of pain and vomiting. Looked very frightened, non verbal cues, spoke a little English, but not fluent for a big conversation.

Wanting to eat and drink, but then being sick, and not knowing if she understood what all that was about. Food and drink seemed very important to her and the family. Loads of pots being brought in. The time had come to say, 'Actually we are now entering the terminal phase. We allow you to eat and drink, but you probably will vomit on it, but we can talk about the options of gastric tubes or not, whatever'. Wanting to talk about a syringe driver, for some pain relief. Wanting to talk about where she wanted to be, in terms of staying in hospital, or the hospice or going home, and what the reality of that might be. The practicalities. Just not being able to get to have that conversation, because the men of the family would be the only ones who wanted to have the conversation . . . they didn't even really want to have the conversation, but they would be the only ones speaking, for the patient. Almost to the point of keeping guard over, I mean that in a kind way . . .

I don't think she had a very good death at all. I wouldn't necessary attribute that . . . It's not because that she's Muslim, that she didn't get what I think is the right care. It was other factors around that . . . Is it that that family didn't want to talk to me because I was a nurse, and not a doctor? Did I have not enough value there? Was it because I was a woman, and not a man? We have had situations where we've changed the role and gender of the person they're dealing with to try and make something more acceptable. We don't do that just because of religion, we do it for various reasons. You think actually somebody might get on with an older person here or whatever . . . I am a great believer of just keeping going sometimes. It would have been very easy, particularly on a busy day to go, 'I just won't go and see her today, because I'm not doing anything.' I would make a point of going every day, and keeping my face there. Perhaps dealing with the things, perhaps on a very simple level about, 'Has the pain got worse today? Can we try some new medicine for the sick feeling', or something like that? Nobody was ever rude to me, I always had those conversations. The outcome was that no decisions really were made. They were made on a day to day basis – 'Let's change this medication', it became a bit, sort of inertia. Let's leave it for another day, let's leave it for another day. By the lack of decision making she did die in hospital. We got her pain controlled, but it just felt she was in a five bedded bay, small ward, with patients having treatments and chemo, and things. She wasn't having treatment. I would have loved to have known what was going on in her mind.

Interviewer: Did you ever get a sense of what the reasons were for the men, was it her husband, was it her son? Did you know who they were or why it was they felt that they had to be the interface of that decision making?

I think it was kindness, protection, please don't tell her bad news. Of course, we see that with all cultures and all families. Now, if that had been a white English Christian family, I would have been more challenging, I think, about the reasons why I thought the patient would need to know. I'd be a bit clearer about, if she asked me any questions. Maybe I wouldn't go in and hit her with the bad news, if she wants to know and ask me questions. I have to professionally be as honest and as gentle as I can. I couldn't, that's where the language thing comes in as well. To arrange an interpreter, perfectly easy to do, we had no problems with resources or anything. That becomes quite a statement in itself. Makes this a big set piece, a big important conversation. If everybody spoke the same language, would be a much more natural and relaxed thing about it.

I think, ignore the language, my impression was that she didn't have a voice. I only see her in a hospital bed, in her nightie, feeling poorly, with her family around her. It might be in her own home, she is very powerful and rules the roost. I just got the impression that even if she and I were converging to the same language, there was something, that certainly may be a public decisions would be made by somebody else. I will never know if that is true, we all know that the tiniest, quietest, oldest person can be the powerful one in the room. I just didn't get that. *(Interview 6, senior palliative care nurse and co-ordinator, London)*

The participant's reflections and views on the above case reveal the different challenges and facets of communication and ethics encountered by healthcare professionals caring for patients of different traditions and cultures. The nurse was keen to know what 'was going on in her [patient's] mind' and felt 'she didn't have a voice'. This was partly due to (1) the patient's inability to converse fluently in English; (2) her being 'guard(ed) over' by male relatives; and more importantly (3) the nurse not knowing whether the situation was acceptable to the patient and what her concept of a 'good death' would be.

This and other cases encountered within the scope of the research reveal that healthcare professionals' ability to assert their professional ethical duties is particularly challenging in the context of end-of-life care but all the more so when encountering patients with limited autonomy. In such contexts deliberations and decision making to ensure that the rights and dignity of the patient are maintained, where an individual's competency is dependent on a degree of literacy and comprehension at a time when the clinical encounter may be very stressful and the patient is commonly also physically and mentally subdued, can be not only challenging but unattainable. Expecting to follow normative practices of informed consent and shared decision making in such cases may be a challenge and raises particular ethical concerns for healthcare professionals in contexts where patients are not literate and therefore may be unable to comprehend their condition and options for care.

Veatch (1995) offers additional challenges to the conventional model of shared decision making and informed consent that may be pertinent to cases like the one outlined above. He argues that clinicians cannot obtain valid consent, as they are unaware of which treatment options will ensure the best interests of the patients. He describes a deliberative challenge that healthcare professionals may encounter when trying to implement best interest standards. Veatch proposes that healthcare professionals must first determine what will serve the patient's medical/healthcare interests. Second, the medical team must balance the latter interests against the patient's other interests. Third, the patient's interests (healthcare and other) ought to be balanced against 'other moral goals and responsibilities, including serving the interests of others' (Veatch 2013). Such concerns are reflected in participant accounts where healthcare professionals note the role of the family superseding their own when Muslim patients are negotiating end-of-life care decisions:

> usually what the patient will want is what the family are asking for. Because the family will trust their own daughter, their own son, their nephew their mother more than they will trust the strange doctor that they don't know. And they are more likely to have faith in the fact that what their daughter wants for them is the right thing and will help them, it's for their benefit, rather than the stranger who they don't know what his agenda is. *(Interview 59, hospice palliative care consultant, London)*

Veatch further notes that meeting standards as outlined by national guidance, which emphasise that patients' preferences are understood and met, is unfeasible, and that in order for healthcare professionals to make better guesses as to what may serve a patient's best interests, patients ought to be paired with providers who share their 'deep values'. The latter would involve pairings on the basis of religious, political, philosophical and social inclinations (Veatch 2013). He understandably highlights that achieving such pairings may be very challenging. Yet his critique of the traditional autonomy-informed consent model does require further reflection, in the context of providing end-of-life care for patients from different faith traditions and cultures. The types of challenges and anxieties shared by participants in this research point to barriers that they themselves highlight, including: being unfamiliar with different value systems; lacking confidence in pushing conversations further to initiate rapport and the building of trust; encountering family members and others at the interface of decision making.

Veatch's analyses call for a more diverse workforce (Calanzani et al. 2013) that can help ensure that 'deep values' are paired. The data however also points to a training and education gap, where healthcare professionals unfamiliar with Muslim values and the Islamic tradition may unnecessarily perceive a lack of trust and failure in providing good care and ensuring a good death.

Many participants explained that what they may perceive as a 'lack of trust' and the 'need to control' from the perspective of Muslim families is in reality their deep-seated need to care:

> It's the family dynamics, it's the people, isn't it? That's across the board, it's just slightly different isn't it? I think we sometimes misinterpret caring for controlling, and then you get into safeguarding and I think sometimes we have to be careful, really think through what we are doing. *(Interview 11, hospice nurse)*

These views suggest that perceptions from healthcare professionals' perspectives may require a shift in understandings about 'control versus care'. Furthermore, involving and relying on family members may not only serve to relinquish the normative model of healthcare professionals having predominance within shared decision making, but also assist in the brokering and building of trust with patients themselves.

The other important feature of the role of Muslim families in caring for the dying that emerges from the data is rooted in their theological and moral commitments to care for their loved ones, especially their parents:

> It's just expected that they will care for them, you know, whatever. You'll have sons who work all day and then will look after their dad all night. Because that is just what they will do and they just don't want any support, they just want advice when they need it. They will do all the personal care, thank you very much. It's very important for them to do that at that time. *(Interview 11, hospice nurse)*

The healthcare assistant quoted earlier as mentioning that the patient's family had installed cameras later explained that this was because the family members were really struggling to hand over the care of their mother. Muslim families are committed to a paradigmatic worldview that relies on metaphysical understandings and theological commitments about life and how one ought to administer to the dying. In particular, teachings from the Qur'an and the tradition of the Prophet are central to their understanding of the duties and compassion owed to parents and especially the mother (see Box 6.2). For families facing the loss of a loved one, especially a parent, there is the additional theological and moral challenge of handing over their care, essentially handing over their sacred duty.

Box 6.2 Excerpts from Islam's normative sources (the Qur'an and tradition of the Prophet Muhammad). Understandings of these underlie commitments that Muslim family members may display when caring for loved ones, especially parents at the end of life.

'Your Lord has decreed that you worship none but Him, and that you be kind to parents. Whether one or both of them attain old age in your life, say not to them a word of contempt (or "uff"), nor repel them, but address them in terms of honour' (Qur'an 17:23).

'They ask you [O Muhammad] what they should spend. Say, "Whatever you spend of good is [to be] for parents and relatives and orphans and the needy and the traveller. And whatever you do of good – indeed, Allah is Knowing of it"' (Qur'an 2: 215).

Status of the Mother in the Islamic Tradition

'And We have enjoined upon man, to his parents, good treatment. His mother carried him with hardship and gave birth to him with hardship, and his gestation and weaning [period] is thirty months. [He grows] until, when he reaches maturity and reaches [the age of] forty years, he says, "My Lord, enable me to be grateful for Your favour which You have bestowed upon me and upon my parents and to work righteousness of which You will approve and make righteous for me my offspring. Indeed, I have repented to You, and indeed, I am of the Muslims"' (Qur'an 46:15).

'Allah's Messenger, who amongst the people is most deserving of my good treatment? He said: Your mother, again your mother, again your mother, then your father, then your nearest relatives according to the order (of nearness)' (Sahih Muslim Book 45 Hadith 2).

'"Do you have a mother?" He said: "Yes". He said: "Then stay with her, for Paradise is beneath her feet"' (Sunan An Nasai Book 25 Hadith 20).

Conclusion

The study shows that healthcare professionals encountering Muslim families dealing with the emotional burden of losing a parent may also be confronted with the additional theological and moral challenge of family members seeking to fulfil their scared duty to care and to preserve the status and dignity of their parents, especially their mother. For Muslim families who may have fraught relationships with institutions or consider the healthcare system as a 'foreign country', with differing values and commitments, it may be all the more pertinent for healthcare professionals and policy makers to think of adaptable and innovative ways of engaging such groups and families. The healthcare institutions (GP surgery, hospital or hospice) may not be the ideal setting to broker trust and initiate conversations about end-of-life care needs. It may be more appropriate to engage patients in conversations about end-of-life care decision making in the community with 'trusted people in trusted spaces' to initiate discussions, foster trusting relationships and to sustain decision making such that it is seamless when patients wish to interface with more formal healthcare institutions.

The views highlighted in the study also point to a need to re-evaluate the 'locus of decision making' (Searight and Gafford 2005) for different groups accessing palliative and end-of-life care services within the NHS. Within the Islamic tradition, there is a higher value placed on beneficence and non-maleficence over autonomy (Sachedina 2009). This is reflected in practice by patients relying on or entirely deferring to family members to carry out 'family-centred decisions'. Here the focus is not only on what the healthcare professionals may consider to be the patient's needs and best interests; rather the family's concern to protect and care for the patients becomes an additional feature of the clinical encounter.

Furthermore, perceptions from healthcare professionals' perspectives may require a shift in understanding of 'control versus care' and that involving and relying on family members may not only serve to relinquish the normative model of healthcare professionals having predominance within shared decision making, but may also assist in the brokering and building of trust with patients themselves.

For Muslim patients and families, being able to develop relationships with healthcare staff where their varying needs are understood is likely to lead to perceptions of receiving good care. Such differences also highlight that end-of-life care ought to be structured around relationship building and not decision making. It is relationships that can accommodate differences whereas decision-making may emphasise differences. Adapting training and education to recognise these differing preferences and models of decision making and care may assist healthcare professionals to be more confident at recognising differing needs but also to face less anxiety and frustration when encountering a mismatch in 'deep values'.

Acknowledgements

I am grateful to Professor Gurch Randhawa, University of Bedfordshire for reviewing transcripts and the data analysis for external validation. I am also indebted to Dr Aileen Walsh (School of Nursing and Midwifery, Faculty of Health, Education, Medicine and Social Care, Anglia Ruskin University) for her advice and guidance in the writing of this chapter.

References

Al-Shahri, M. Z. (2016). 'Islamic theology and the principles of palliative care'. *Palliative & Supportive Care*, 14(6), 635–40.

Calanzani, N., Koffman, J. and Higginson, I. J. (2013). 'Palliative and end of life care for Black, Asian and Minority Ethnic groups in the UK'. Available at:

www.mariecurie.org.uk/globalassets/media/documents/who-we-are/diversity-and-inclusion-research/palliative-care-bame_full-report.pdf (last accessed 9 May 2022).

Chenail, R. J. (1995). 'Presenting qualitative data'. *The Qualitative Report*, 2(3), 1–9.

Gale, N. K., Heath, G., Cameron, E., Rashid, S. and Redwood, S. (2013). 'Using the framework method for the analysis of qualitative data in multi-disciplinary health research'. *BMC Medical Research Methodology*, 13(1), 117.

Green, J., Thorogood, N. and Green, G. (2013). *Qualitative Methods for Health Research*, 2nd edn. Thousand Oaks, CA: SAGE Publications Inc.

Guest, G., Bunce, A. and Johnson, L. (2006). 'How many interviews are enough? An experiment with data saturation and variability'. *Field Methods*, 18(1), 59–82.

Muslim Council of Britain (2015). 'British Muslims in numbers: a demographic, socio-economic and health profile of Muslims in Britain drawing on the 2011 census'. Available at: https://www.mcb.org.uk/wp-content/uploads/2015/02/MCBCensusReport_2015.pdf (last accessed 9 May 2022).

NICE (2011). 'End of life care for adults'. Available at: www.nice.org.uk/guidance/qs13/resources/end-of-life-care-for-adults-pdf-2098483631557 (last accessed 9 May 2022).

Pope, C., Ziebland, S. and Mays, N. (2000). 'Analysing qualitative data'. *BMJ*, 320(7227), 114–16.

Ritchie, J. and Lewis, J. (eds) (2003). *Qualitative Research Practice: A Guide for Social Science Students and Researchers*. London: SAGE Publications Ltd.

Sachedina, A. (2009). *Islamic Biomedical Ethics: Principles and Application*. Oxford: Oxford University Press.

Salinsky, J. (2002). 'The death of Ivan Ilyich by Leo Tolstoy', in *Medicine and Literature: The Doctor's Companion to the Classics, vol. 2*. Abingdon: Radcliffe Medical Press Ltd, p. 119.

Sandelowski, M. (1994). 'Focus on qualitative methods. The use of quotes in qualitative research'. *Research in Nursing & Health*, 17(6), 479–82.

Sandelowski, M. (1998). 'Writing a good read: strategies for re-presenting qualitative data'. *Research in Nursing & Health*, 21(4), 375–82.

Searight, H. R. and Gafford, J. (2005). 'Cultural diversity at the end of life: issues and guidelines for family physicians'. *American Family Physician*, 71(3), 515–22.

Steinhauser, K. E., Christakis, N. A., Clipp, E. C., McNeilly, M., McIntyre, L. and Tulsky, J. A. (2000). 'Factors considered important at the end of life by patients, family, physicians, and other care providers'. *JAMA*, 284(19), 2476–82.

Suleman, M. (2022). 'Muslim values and end of life healthcare decision-making: values, norms and ontologies in conflict?', in A. Al-Akiti and A. Padela (eds), *Biomedicine and Islam*. Cham: Springer.

Turner, L. (2002). 'Bioethics and end-of-life care in multi-ethnic settings: cultural diversity in Canada and the USA'. *Mortality*, 7(3), 285–301.

Veatch, R. M. (1995). 'Abandoning informed consent'. *Hastings Center Report*, 25(2), 5–12.

Veatch, R. M. (2013). 'Abandoning informed consent', in H. Kuhse and P. Singer (eds), *A Companion to Bioethics*. Malden, MA: John Wiley & Sons.

Warnock, M. and Macdonald, E. (2009). *Easeful Seath: Is There a Case for Assisted Dying?* Oxford: Oxford University Press.

7

DEMENTIA AMONGST MUSLIM COMMUNITIES IN THE UK

Mohammed Akhlak Rauf

Introduction

This chapter focuses on dementia in British Muslim communities of South Asian heritage. It touches on faith, immigration, the social construct of dementia and dementia care, awareness of dementia, access to services and intercultural care. Whilst there is a lot that can be said on the subject of dementia and dementia care in British Muslim families, this chapter provides a broad overview of several aspects that impact how these communities are faced with both facilitators and barriers enabling or restricting appropriate support. In this chapter, British Muslim experiences of dementia are mainly grounded on my experience working with South Asian families through Meri Yaadain CiC, a community interest company working to raise awareness of dementia and support for these families.

'Dementia' is an umbrella term used to label many cognitive impairments. It can result in various functional challenges such as memory loss, communication difficulties, trouble with time and spatial recognition, and many symptoms and behaviours (Quinn et al. 2008). The World Health Organization's International Classification of Diseases and Related Health Problems defines dementia as a syndrome occurring as a result of underlying brain diseases (WHO 1993). It adds that dementia is progressive, affecting various aspects of cognition, function and emotion (Sandilyan and Dening 2015).

Given that there is no name for dementia in the five main South Asian languages, the South Asian Muslim community in the UK does not have a translatable word for dementia. Over the next few decades, dementia in Black and Minority Ethnic (BME) communities is expected to increase approximately seven to eightfold in the UK, from the current figures of around 15,000–25,000 BME individuals (Department of Health 2009; All Party Parliamentary Group on Dementia 2013; Botsford and Harrison Dening 2015). In contrast, it is only expected to increase around twofold for the indigenous White British population, with around 800,000–850,000 people currently affected (APPG 2013). However, whilst Alzheimer's disease is one of the better-known forms of dementia, other types such as vascular dementia, dementia with Lewy bodies and frontotemporal dementia may be lesser known. Vascular dementia, for instance, is more common in South Asian and African Caribbean communities as it is related to high blood pressure and stroke (APPG 2013).

There have been Muslim communities in the UK for many years, beginning with small groups such as the Yemeni sailors in Liverpool and Cardiff, followed later by the better-known migration from various countries, notably Pakistan, India and Bangladesh, in the 1950s to 1970s. However, Muslims are not one community, but a diverse range of communities who share their faith as a commonality but have different languages, food, dress, cultural norms and expectations. Other aspects of living with deprivation causing ill health among diverse Muslim communities include societal prejudice and fear of racism, whether Arab, Asian or African. In addition, Muslim communities have been less able to benefit from the availability of information and services at their disposal due to family barriers such as stigma, whilst the lack of culturally appropriate service provision has meant families have been unable to use external services – giving rise to the false impression that 'they look after their own'.

The British South Asian community has a predominantly Muslim population of Pakistani and Bangladeshi heritage and a sizeable population of Indian origin. The nuances related to migration, cultural obligations and expectations to care will impact the willingness of family members in these communities to provide care. Not only is there an impact on caring, but research also argues that the dementia figures for the BME communities may be an underestimate as a result of the greater stigma, lack of awareness, mistrust of service providers and sociocultural factors (Mackenzie 2006; Moriarty et al. 2011; Mukadam et al. 2013). The Muslim community in the UK is much more heterogeneous than the South Asian heritage community – many aspects of this chapter will therefore be of relevance to other Muslim communities and people of diverse ethnic and religious backgrounds, such as the Sikh and Hindu communities of South Asian heritage.

Given that South Asian communities are more likely than the indigenous White British to provide continuing family care (Lawrence et al. 2008), it is essential that this topic is better understood to provide a more profound insight into the complexities being managed by carers. These complexities are grounded in social constructs of health, dementia, care, and filial and familial responsibilities or expectations. The barriers and facilitators likely to influence carers' ability to cope with the changing demands of dementia care are influenced by social determinants, including socioeconomic and religious influences (Mackenzie 2006; Moriarty et al. 2011; Ali and Bokharey 2015).

While there is existing literature that explores the lack of awareness of dementia among South Asian communities, this chapter considers the impact of spirituality in terms of both reward and punishment from God and possession by spirits or jinns. Religion and cultural beliefs may dictate the 'port of call' when seeking clarity (information) or healing (support) from a faith-based practitioner or a place of worship (Regan 2014). South Asian families have generally understood dementia to be a normal part of the ageing process (Blakemore et al. 2018), whilst services assume that family members will look after their elders (Katbamna et al. 2004). The marked absence of these populations at the point of care can also give the impression that there is little need for services until families reach crisis point (Mukadam et al. 2011). Attempting to understand why this may be the case, research points to two main possibilities: first, social norms or constructs that migrant communities bring with them from the country of origin, having grown up there (Jutlla 2015) and second, the impact or influence of migrant communities living in 'racialised' environments (Tribe et al. 2009). This refers to the culture of the society in which the communities came to live. Housing, employment, education and other social needs are a challenge due to discrimination. Tribe et al. (2009) argue that these added to the barriers causing greater social isolation than experienced by the White British population.

Impact of Migration

The Pakistani migrant community that settled in Britain during the 1960s and 1970s were invited labour during the post-war era in Britain. Whilst initially seeking to come as migrant workers, earn a wage and return home, the 'myth of return' was busted due to subsequent immigration legislation. Successive immigration laws forced many to bring their partners and children to the UK before the opportunity could be closed to them in the future (Anwar 1979). Migrant communities therefore brought with them their social norms and values. Having come from a place where the cohesive nature of family structures is valued, care of the elderly was undertaken at home, or at least within the family setting (Brijnath 2012). However, with migrants arriving as young men and women, whilst they brought with them their cultural values and norms, they had little to show the next generation with regard to how older people are looked after by the family. Instead, these social constructs relating to older people's care remained a utopian concept in a world that was more focused on the individual. The rights of individuals, as opposed to the responsibilities of the collective, were paramount – a shift from the 'Asiacentric' paradigm to a 'Eurocentric one', where younger generations are not exposed to the same cultural expectations (Jutlla 2015). However, further complications arose when the communities were faced with racialised environments. Their experiences of racism meant that fear of or prejudice towards institutions and services pushed communities towards a sense of safety within what they knew rather than what might be unfamiliar territory, i.e. access to and use of care services (Anwar 1979; Ahmed et al. 2017).

Being removed from the care of older relatives in South Asia, the British South Asian Muslim community's lacked knowledge of old age health needs and dementia. Instead, family members saw dementia symptoms and behaviours as a normal part of the ageing process, perhaps due in part to the fact that links to traditional village life had been severed (Giebel et al. 2016b). As such, these symptoms and behaviours are seen on the one hand to be normal and inevitable (Blakemore et al. 2018) but on the other, shameful and to be hidden from the wider community due to the associated stigma. Caring for someone with dementia is therefore dealt with in one of two ways: either as something the family has to cope with without wider support, or as something for which faith-based intervention should be sought (Regan et al. 2013), neither of which necessarily alleviates the burden of care.

Impact of Faith and Spirituality

Of further concern are the issues raised in relation to dementia being associated with spiritual possession by jinns. The impact of spirituality is strengthened where the social construct of dementia-related behaviour is seen to be an abnormality due to the 'troublesome' actions of the jinn instead of the individual's physical changes. The resulting stigma associated with dementia-related behaviour most often leads to the person with dementia being labelled *paagal* – crazy or mad, the 'abnormal' behaviour being out of the ordinary and not expected. This forces family members to cope with the caring, often without seeking outside help. The need to care for the person with dementia is seen as coming from God, i.e. an obligation to care imposed by faith. Where dementia-related behaviours are accepted as being caused by spiritual possession, the stigma forces families to seek faith-based support and healing rather than conventional help (Regan et al. 2013). Some carers are thus seen to care from a sense of cultural duty in that they are being tested by God or are being given the opportunity to care for their relative as a payback for their sense of duty to family (Lawrence et al. 2008; Botsford and Harrison Dening 2015). This, however, is closely linked to the cultural expectation to care rather than to seek help from outside (Botsford et al. 2012; Parveen et al. 2013).

There is also a sense of shame among carers with regard to seeking help from outside services; this might suggest the family is failing to look after their elders, which would go against their religious beliefs. There is a sense of religious duty more than cultural expectations, especially when caring for an elderly parent, although this is often born of the social stigma to which much of the existing research refers. There is, however, growing evidence of a generational shift where faith can be seen as a traditional motivator or a barrier (Lawrence 2008). Strength can be derived from one's faith when looking after one's elders and so can be a positive factor that enables the family to cope with caring, but faith can also act as a barrier, as the carer may question their faith with regard to why the individual has been burdened with dementia or needs care. Parveen et al. (2013) make a clear distinction between willingness to care and obligation to care. The notion of traditional or non-traditional caregiving (Lawrence et al. 2008) is more complex for Muslims, where faith plays a significant role. This influence of faith means that carers see dementia either as an opportunity to serve their relative and thereby attain success in terms of worldly and afterlife gains, or as a burden due to the behaviours of the relative they are now caring for.

Whilst faith might be a coping factor for family carers, especially if they are of a 'traditional' mindset (Lawrence et al. 2008), there is little support from the community itself – i.e. the mosques. On the one hand it may be possible to seek solace in the place of worship, on the other hand the fear of doing something wrong can become a barrier for people with dementia. Carers, too, would be hesitant to send their relatives with dementia to a mosque for fear of stigma or embarrassment (Regan 2016). As communities become more aware of dementia, it may be possible for places of worship to become invaluable assets in supporting families coping with dementia by offering spiritual, social and practical support, especially for those more inclined towards their faith-based identity. This would be of particular relevance to carers who are less likely to consult the GP for support, attributing dementia in their relative as being from God (Giebel et al. 2016a). Given that the older generation hold on to faith-based strengths, religion- and family-based resources are felt to be of value to them (Giebel et al. 2016b).

While it may be commendable to care for older relatives, dementia is more often associated with 'mental ill health', leading to associations with religious and spiritual explanations, and meaning that carers do not want to be ostracised by the wider community. Carers will therefore often hide their relative with dementia from others (Mackenzie 2006), especially as the symptoms or behaviours may be seen as embarrassing, especially if they lack inhibition. Building on the faith-based explanations, some carers' willingness to take on their caring duties is influenced by the notion that spirits, or the 'evil eye', are responsible for their relative's erratic behaviours. Carers have little option but to cope with caring without recourse to external support, as the social bearing upon the family would be very negative if the family were seen to have a member who was displaying these erratic behaviours. The implications of such stigma affect the honour of families, including the impact on younger generations and their potential for marriage (Mackenzie 2006). What is not always clear is whether these family carers keep the relative with dementia hidden away from the wider community to protect them from scorn, or whether they are protecting themselves or their family honour.

Former British-born carers of a relative with dementia in British Pakistani Muslim families have felt that faith does not manipulate their thinking or they ways in which they seek the best possible support. However, their coping strategies indicate that faith does play a part in managing the stresses of their role. Some carers are somewhat oblivious to the fact that their faith subconsciously impacts their ability to cope with care tasks, influencing what is best for themselves and the relative they care for. Faith-based teachings and cultural practices have installed in many Muslim communities the need to care for older relatives and attain reward in the next life. However, what needs to be explored is the extent to which this may be discouraging family carers from seeking external support to cope with and care for their relative.

Social Constructs of Dementia and Dementia Care

Just as some carers assume that dementia-related behaviours are synonymous with old age, it is also the case that many carers do not associate mobility issues or a withdrawal from social interactions and engagement with symptoms of dementia (Giebel et al. 2016b). Carers display different attitudes and behaviours concerning their ability to recognise such symptoms. Some attributed forgetfulness in the relative with dementia to falls or a lack of sleep, i.e. physical causes. Others considered that dementia-related behaviour might be hereditary, or might arise from difficulties with social interactions, an increase in isolation and a loss of skills alongside forgetfulness (Uppal et al. 2014; Giebel et al. 2016a).

Depending on the type of carer, traditional or non-traditional, the social construct of dementia care can make it virtuous or a burden. Both have an impact on how the carer may perceive dementia, as well as how this affects the type of care they provide (Lawrence et al. 2008). Where carers have a traditional attitude towards caring, i.e. seeing it as virtuous, they may be less interested in the need to actually understand dementia. They are more concerned with the act of caring rather than the reason to care (Mukadam et al. 2011; Mukadam et al. 2015). This raises an interesting question of whether or not the social construct of dementia is necessary at all, especially for traditional carers. Conversely, it may also be the case that carers see the loss of skills in an older person as a natural process, but may not want to accept the concept of dementia, thereby limiting their understanding of the disease. This raises another interesting question as to whether there are other reasons why family carers choose not to seek help and support (Mukadam et al. 2011). Perhaps it is the fear of what others within the community will think of the carer or their family if they abandoned their loved ones to the care of support services.

Another aspect of the social constructs around dementia is perhaps evidence of how family carers may give more importance to physical health than mental illness. If dementia is seen to be a mental condition it brings with it the challenges of stigma. This, in turn, may lead to a lack of awareness of dementia (Uppal et al. 2014). Unless there are physical symptoms, carers may be less likely to present the dementia symptoms of the relative to the GP. Non-physical symptoms such as behaviours are hidden for fear of stigma and other consequences from the wider family networks in the community (Uppal et al. 2014). This also indicates that some carers are perhaps aware of their relative's dementia as well as their own struggles in coping with it. Not seeking help and support might suggest that they have failed in their responsibilities to the relative with dementia (Lawrence et al. 2008) and so it becomes easier to accept and talk about physical ill health than it is to raise concerns about mental ill health. Migration-related experiences, stigma from the wider family and the community, the carer's own level of education and knowledge are all factors that contribute to the construct of dementia (Uppal and Bonas 2014).

Awareness of Dementia and Support Services

Many Pakistani families are not aware of dementia until there is a diagnosis. However, many carers delay seeking support from outside services, often because of their lack of awareness or understanding of the condition (Purandare et al. 2007; Greenwood et al. 2015). Whilst a recent increase in publicity surrounding dementia may have made an impact and raised awareness among Pakistani families, research still indicates the difficulties of dealing with dementia as a manageable condition due to the stigma and cultural expectations within such families (Moriarty et al. 2011; Mukadam et al. 2013).

Some of this relates back to how communities socially construct dementia, old age and care. Filial responsibility, for instance, is embedded to a large extent in how communities in or from different countries socially construct notions of care and care giving (Parveen and Morrison 2009; Parveen et al. 2011; Parveen et al. 2013). These traditional notions of care from within the family network and the absence of knowledge of dementia mean that families are trying to cope with dementia needs. But there comes a time where they are no longer able to cope with the dementia-related needs of their relative and reach a crisis point (Mukadam et al. 2011).

Organisational Culture of Services

There is a strong correlation between the ability to cope and access to appropriate services, in that coping without support services will be harder for carers. Where support services are available to carers, the service providers' organisational culture may not be conducive or culturally appropriate for people living with dementia from these communities or for their family carers. While carers are encouraged to look after themselves in order to be able to care, there is a need for services to reassure carers that they must remember to take time to look after themselves. Only if carers can access support services will they feel able to regain their physical ability to care and the emotional capability to cope with their relative's care needs (Lawrence et al. 2008). Organisational culture becomes a barrier if support services cannot be mindful of the diversity requirements of service users and become gatekeepers of who accesses their services (Beattie et al. 2005).

However, service providers may also argue that it does not make economic sense to invest in such services where the take-up is low. Instead, services for minority communities tend to be 'bolted on' to other mainstream provision. The concern raised by this behaviour is that services will not be culturally competent, nor will they attract people from minority communities if cultural and linguistic support is not seen to be made available (Beattie et al. 2005). There is also a similar shortfall for people with dementia and their family carers from minority communities to bypass certain gatekeepers. One such gatekeeper is the GP, who often holds the key to accessing or signposting support services in the statutory or voluntary sector. Doctors are often the initial contact through which the specialist dementia services pathway can be accessed (Mukadam et al. 2011). Carers have also often reported that the GP's attitude has been dismissive faced with concerns raised about a relative with dementia, the implication being that the carer should accept their relative is presenting such behaviours due to old age (Downs et al. 2006; All Party Parliamentary Group on Dementia 2013). Other gatekeepers can be social workers, self-imposed community leaders and the wider family members of the cared for.

Access to Services – Hindering or Facilitating Carers' Ability to Cope with Caring

Academic research has evidenced a number of issues that affect carers' ability to access services. The key barriers to accessing support are the availability of appropriate information at the time of need and the fear of prejudice from institutions (Beattie et al. 2005; Mackenzie 2006; Lawrence et al. 2008; Jutlla 2015). Organisational culture can facilitate or restrict this access to services depending on the service provider's flexibility and provision of information on what resources are available to family carers or their relatives with dementia. The older generation is still perceived as accessing information chiefly through leaf-lets, flyers and community events, whereas the younger generation takes a very different approach in seeking access to information through technology (Giebel et al. 2016b). However, being able to access information does not always equate to accessing services. Similarly, just because a service claims to offer support does not mean it is accessible if a lack of information about it restricts informed choice. The popular message 'our doors are open' communicated to the public by services that promote equality and equity in service provision translates in reality as 'our doors are closed' when it comes to reaching out and publicising their services to communities who would otherwise find it difficult to under-stand or to be aware of what is on offer (Ahmed 2017).

Impact of Stress from Family and Community

Whilst stress amongst carers is documented in literature (Katbamna et al. 2004), the ability to manage gender roles, expectations relating to the obligation to care and the willingness to do so are all shifting. Carers may find the lack of support from family and community a source of stress, but more significant frustration can come from relatives and neighbours judging the quality of care they are providing, irrespective of the understanding they have of dementia and demen-tia care needs. Carers do sometimes have to seek outside help. Support from religious scholars can be helpful, but they too need to have an understanding of dementia in order to provide emotional and spiritual assistance to struggling carers. Having families who do not understand the challenges or the burden asso-ciated with caring for someone with dementia, carers can be pushed to adhere to the cultural obligation to care instead of voicing their need for help. When neighbours and communities, including congregations at mosques, have a lack of awareness or an inability to comprehend the challenges associated with demen-tia, it becomes difficult for carers to continue to support their relative should they want to continue with their regular activities – including congregational prayer at the mosque. Both carer and cared-for begin to be constantly challenged and judged by families, neighbours and communities rather than receiving any meaningful support. The carer's strategy is often to withdraw from seeking fam-ily or community support and to hide the need for help as dementia becomes stigmatised and their own caring judged.

Gender and Dementia Care

The impact of caring can be rewarding as well as burdensome. Nevertheless, the gender-based difference may equate to there being a more significant bearing on women as carers. Women caring for someone with dementia experience more anxiety, stress and depression than male carers caring for their partner. Women are more likely to be the carers within the family structure. They are more likely to undertake care duties themselves rather than bring in external helpers or services to assist them, and the fact that women are expected to undertake care because of cultural expectations negates their experiences of caring as a burden.

There remains a gap in knowledge regarding women's experiences of dementia care, although there is growing interest in this field. Muslim women and their experiences of dementia care needs further exploration and research. There is some research, however, that explores the differences and inequalities between men's experiences of undertaking dementia care and those of women. Men are seen to have a lower level of burden (Pöysti et al. 2012). It is very likely that the influence of cultural expectations, obligation to care, power dynamics in families and the fact that faith may encourage a notion of 'reward' through caring can all put greater pressure on Muslim women carers than it does on Muslim male carers of a relative living with dementia.

Is There a Need for Intercultural Care for People with Dementia from Minority Communities and their Carers?

British Muslim families in the UK are generally well established, although there has also been a recent increase in refugees and asylum-seeking families from war-torn countries such as Somalia, Iraq and Afghanistan. Even in established Muslim communities, however, their presence is often subjected to notions of limited integration, being seen as insular and traditional or conservative in their attitudes and practices. Yet Muslim people are found in almost all economic spheres, working in law, education, business, health, food, sport, transport and many other fields. This ought to move the narrative of insular, conservative communities to one where it is accepted that they are no more a homogeneous group than are White British communities, who also have different identities, ethnicities and languages. Literacy, class and disposable income affect all communities and their ability to access support services. However, a number of other areas need to be examined to rebalance the ability to access health and social care initiatives. This includes understanding why communities feel safer among people of a similar culture and how cultural and racial bias can work against people through unconscious bias even when practitioners may be well meaning. Understanding the wider inequalities associated with health and poverty will also impact social constructs and how meaning is given to ill health and seeking support.

Older people from these communities may struggle with language. Even if they were previously fully able to converse in English, dementia may make them revert to their first home language. Services may be deemed culturally inappropriate, but they may not carry the trust that individuals and families would want before accessing them. Before a service can be chosen for care and treatment, there is a need for an appropriate diagnosis with cultural competency to offer the correct outcomes from memory assessments. Given that there is still no single accepted and approved culturally appropriate diagnostic, there appears to be a difficulty in establishing universally accepted practices to assess minority ethnic communities for dementia (Alzheimer Europe 2018).

With limited knowledge and medical awareness of dementia, family carers perhaps give the impression that they look after their own for fear of having to have a relative placed in a care institution. Conversely, services may perceive this lack of engagement as a positive indicator that family carers are happy to look after their relative at home. Evidence exists that many people are desperate to access help and support, but services are either lacking or inappropriate. Regan (2014) highlights her case study findings by reporting a Pakistani Muslim man struggling to access care or support from the wider family, but also finding that provision from services was not appropriate in terms of culture and faith. Research studies have demonstrated the challenges faced by the Muslim community in the UK, whereby family carers are not able to rely on care support from the wider family networks, nor are they necessarily able to adequately care at home without access to external support services. They are often caught between the obligation and willingness to care and the ability to adequately care.

Summary

In summary, we can see that Muslim communities in the UK have been established for many decades. However, generally speaking, they live in poorer socio-economic circumstances and have poorer health outcomes. While dementia is not a mental health condition, it is often perceived to be one or associated with the individual being possessed by jinns or other spirits. Social constructs of dementia and dementia care for a poorly recognised condition mean that faith may have a stronger influence than the need to seek medical intervention in supporting the person with dementia or their carer. In migrant communities, there is also a need to explore whether a generational shift in attitudes to dementia and dementia care is likely to change what these carers expect from their community and faith institutions and the statutory services in place to support their changing needs. With dementia amongst minority ethnic communities expected to rise seven or eightfold in the next thirty years, there is a need for institutions to move their rhetoric of 'English as a second language' to one where equity and equality serve to meet the needs of diverse communities who share a faith-based identity as Muslims. Muslim communities themselves need to have a more apparent distinction between culture and religion regarding what is culturally induced stigma, pressure and obligation, and what is religious. I end this chapter with the words of the Qur'an: 'It is Allah who creates you and takes your souls at death; and of you, there are some who are sent back to a feeble age, so that they know nothing after having known (much): for Allah is All-Knowing, All-Powerful'

(Qur'an 16: 70). To my mind, this can be interpreted as referencing dementia. If this is the case, is there an argument for Muslim communities to accept dementia and be supported from a faith perspective?

References

Ahmed, A., Wilding, M. A., Howarth-Lomax, R. and McCaughan, S. (2017). 'Promoting diversity and inclusiveness in dementia services in Salford'. Project report. Available at: http://usir.salford.ac.uk/id/eprint/42318 (last accessed 10 May 2022).

Ali, S. and Bokharey, I. Z. (2015). 'Maladaptive cognitions and physical health of the caregivers of dementia: an interpretative phenomenological analysis'. *International Journal of Qualitative Studies on Health and Well-being*, 10(1), 28980–9.

All Party Parliamentary Group on Dementia (2013). 'Dementia does not discriminate: the experiences of black, Asian and minority ethnic communities'. Available at: www.alzheimers.org.uk/sites/default/files/migrate/downloads/appg_2013_bame_report.pdf (last accessed 10 May 2022).

Alzheimer Europe (2018). *The development of intercultural care and support for people with dementia from minority ethnic groups*. Available at: www.alzheimer-europe.org/sites/default/files/alzheimer_europe_ethics_report_2018.pdf (last accessed 10 May 2022).

Anwar, M. (1979). *The Myth of Return: Pakistanis in Britain*. London: Heinemann.

Bartlett, R., Gjernes, G. T., Lotherington, A-T. and Obstefelder, A. (2018). Gender, citizenship and dementia care: a scoping review of studies to inform policy and future research. *Health and Social Care in the Community*, 26(1), 14–26.

Beattie, A., Daker-White, G., Gilliard, J. and Means, R. (2005) '"They don't quite fit the way we organise our services" – results from a UK field study of marginalised groups and dementia care'. *Disability & Society*, 20(1), 67–80.

Blakemore, A., Kenning, C., Mirza, N., Daker-White, G., Panagioti, M. and Waheed, W. (2018). 'Dementia in UK South Asians: a scoping review of the literature'. *BMJ Open*, 8(4), e020290.

Botsford, J., Clarke, C. L. and Gibb, C. E. (2012). 'Dementia and relationships: experiences of partners in minority ethnic communities'. *Journal of Advanced Nursing*, 68(10), 2207–2217.

Botsford, J. and Harrison Dening, K. (2015). *Dementia, Culture and Ethnicity: Issues for All*. London: Jessica Kingsley Publishers.

Brijnath, B. (2012). 'Why does institutionalised care not appeal to Indian families? Legislative and social answers from urban India'. *Ageing and Society*, 32(4), 1–21.

Department of Health (2009). 'Living well with dementia: a national dementia strategy'. Available at: www.gov.uk/government/publications/living-well-with-dementia-a-national-dementia-strategy (last accessed 10 May 2022).

Downs, M., Ariss, S. M., Grant, E., Keady, J., Turner, S., Bryans, M., Wilcock, J., Levin, E., O'Carroll, R. and Iliffe, S. (2006). Family carers' accounts of general practice contacts for their relatives with early signs of dementia. *Dementia*, 5(3), 353–73.

Giebel, C., Challis, D., Worden, A., Jolley, D., Bhui, K. S., Lambat, A. and Purandare, N. (2016a). 'Perceptions of self-defined memory problems vary in south Asian minority older people who consult a GP and those who do not: a mixed-method pilot study'. *International Journal of Geriatric Psychiatry*, 31(4), 375–83.

Giebel, C. M., Jolley, D., Zubair, M., Bhui, K. S., Challis, D., Purandare, N. and Worden, A. (2016b). 'Adaptation of the Barts Explanatory Model Inventory to dementia understanding in South Asian ethnic minorities'. *Aging & Mental Health*, 20(6), 594–602.

Greenwood, N., Habibi, R., Smith, R. and Manthorpe, J. (2015). 'Barriers to access and minority ethnic carers' satisfaction with social care services in the community: a systematic review of qualitative and quantitative literature'. *Health & Social Care in the Community*, 23(1), 64–78.

Hooker K., Manoogian-O'Dell, M., Monahan, D. J., Frazier, L. D. and Shifren, K. (2000). 'Does type of disease matter? Gender differences among Alzheimer's and Parkinson's disease spouse caregivers'. *The Gerontologist*, 40(5), 568–73.

Jutlla, K. (2015) 'The impact of migration experiences and migration identities on the experiences of services and caring for a family member with dementia for Sikhs living in Wolverhampton, UK'. *Ageing & Society*, 35(5), 1032–54.

Katbamna, S., Ahmad, W., Bhakta, P., Baker, R. and Parker, G. (2004). 'Do they look after their own? Informal support for South Asian carers'. *Health & Social Care in the Community*, 12(5), 398–406.

Lawrence, V., Murray, J., Samsi, K. and Banerjee, S. (2008). 'Attitudes and support needs of Black Caribbean, South Asian and White British carers of people with dementia in the UK'. *British Journal of Psychiatry*, 193(3), 240–6.

Mackenzie, J. (2006). 'Stigma and dementia: East European and South Asian family carers negotiating stigma in the UK'. *Dementia*, 5(2), 233–47.

Moriarty, J., Sharif, N. and Robinson, J. (2011). 'Black and minority ethnic people with dementia and their access to support and services'. SCIE research briefing 35. Available at: https://kclpure.kcl.ac.uk/portal/files/13501330/SCIE_briefing. pdf (last accessed 10 May 2022).

Mukadam, N., Cooper, C., Basit, B. and Livingston, G. (2011). 'Why do ethnic elders present later to UK dementia services? A qualitative study'. *International Psychogeriatrics*, 23(7), 1070–7.

Mukadam, N., Cooper, C. and Livingston, G. (2013). 'Improving access to dementia services for people from minority ethnic groups'. *Current Opinion in Psychiatry*, 26(4), 409–14.

Mukadam, N., Waugh, A., Cooper, C. and Livingston, G. (2015). 'What would encourage help-seeking for memory problems among UK-based South Asians? A qualitative study'. *BMJ Open*, 5(9), e007990.

Parveen, S. and Morrison, V. (2009). 'Predictors of familism in the caregiver role: a pilot study'. *Journal of Health Psychology*, 14(8), 1135–43.

Parveen, S., Morrison, V. and Robinson, C. A. (2011). 'Ethnic variations in the caregiver role: a qualitative study'. *Journal of Health Psychology*, 16(6), 862–72.

Parveen, S., Morrison, V. and Robinson, C. A. (2013). 'Ethnicity, familism and willingness to care: important influences on caregiver mood?'. *Aging & Mental Health*, 17(1), 115–24.

Pöysti, M. M., Laakkonen, M. L., Strandberg, T., Savikko, N., Tilvis, R. S., Eloniemi-Sulkava, U. and Pitkälä, K. H. (2012). 'Gender differences in dementia spousal caregiving'. *International Journal of Alzheimer's Disease*, 162960.

Purandare, N., Luthra, V., Swarbrick, C. and Burns, A. (2007). 'Knowledge of dementia among South Asian (Indian) older people in Manchester, UK'. *International Journal of Geriatric Psychiatry*, 22(8), 777–81.

Quinn, C., Clare, L. and Woods, B. (2008). 'The impact of the quality of relationship on the experiences and wellbeing of caregivers of people with dementia: a systematic review'. *Aging & Mental Health*, 13(2), 143–54.

Regan, J. L. (2014). 'Redefining dementia care barriers for ethnic minorities: the religion–culture distinction'. *Mental Health, Religion & Culture*, 17(4), 345–53.

Regan, J. L. (2016). 'Ethnic minority, young onset, rare dementia type, depression: a case study of a Muslim male accessing UK dementia health and social care services'. *Dementia*, 15(4), 702–20.

Regan, J. L., Bhattacharyya, S., Kevern, P. and Rana, T. (2013). 'A systematic review of religion and dementia care pathways in black and minority ethnic populations'. *Mental Health, Religion & Culture*, 16(1), 1–15.

Sandilyan, M. B. and Dening, T. (2015). 'Diagnosis of dementia'. *Nursing Standard*, 29(43), 36–41.

Tribe, R., Lane, P. and Heasum, S. (2009). 'Working towards promoting positive mental health and well-being for older people from BME communities'. *Working with Older People*, 13(1), 35–40.

Uppal, G. and Bonas, S. (2014). 'Constructions of dementia in the South Asian community: a systematic literature review'. *Mental Health, Religion & Culture*, 17(2), 143–60.

Uppal, G. K., Bonas, S. and Philpott, H. (2014). 'Understanding and awareness of dementia in the Sikh community'. *Mental Health, Religion & Culture*, 17(4), 400–14.

World Health Organization (1993). *The ICD-10 Classification of Mental and Behavioural Disorders Diagnostic Criteria for Research*. Geneva: World Health Organization.

8

DOMESTIC VIOLENCE AND ABUSE: IMPACT ON HEALTH OF BRITISH MUSLIM WOMEN AND FACTORS AFFECTING ACCESS TO HEALTH

Parveen Ali and Zlakha Ahmed

Introduction

Domestic violence and abuse (DVA) is a major public health and social problem that affects people in every community, culture and country. It is associated with severe physical and psychological consequence and victims/survivors need help and support from appropriate professionals and services. When it comes to faith-based communities such as Muslims (including migrant Muslims), the situation becomes further complicated as, in addition to experiencing the usual barriers such as those related to gender, ethnicity and marginalisation, victims may experience further issues affecting their ability to disclose DVA and seek appropriate support. Islamophobia and overt or covert racism further impact their experiences as they are stigmatised, blamed for their situation and 'otherised' by institutions and systems (Chantler et al. 2019; Younis and Jadhav 2019).

Muslims make up the second largest religious group in the UK. Although the Muslim population in the UK is ethnically diverse, 68 per cent are of South Asian origin, 8 per cent are from a White background and the remainder are from other backgrounds (MCB 2015). A large majority of British Muslims live in deprived areas and face poverty. Access to health and social care services for the deprived population is an important concern and therefore understanding what affects provision, accessibility and acceptability of healthcare services to this group is imperative. While we know that healthcare professionals (HCPs) can play an important role in the identification and management of DVA, they are often ill prepared (Po-Yan Leung et al. 2018; Renner et al. 2019). If the victim is Muslim, the situation becomes even more difficult as HCPs are often affected by misconceptions, prejudices and bias (Milani et al. 2018). The service providers and professionals often assume culture or religion are underlying the problems patients present with (ibid.; Saleem and Martin 2018) and therefore may be reluctant to address the issue.

This chapter aims to explore the issue of DVA with regard to British Muslims. To provide appropriate context, an overview of DVA, its various forms, prevalence and health impact is presented. The chapter then explores factors affecting the provision of services to Muslim victims of DVA and strategies to overcome barriers.

Domestic Violence and Abuse: What Is It?

Gender-based violence (GBV) refers to

> any act of gender-based violence that results in, or is likely to result in, physical, sexual or mental harm or suffering to women, including threats of such acts, coercion or arbitrary deprivation of liberty, whether occurring in public or in private life. (UN 1993)

While GBV can affect anyone, women appear to be the main victims subjected to various forms of abuse such as female infanticide, female genital mutilation (FGM), child marriage, grooming, trafficking, forced marriage, dowry-related abuse, 'honour'-based violence, rape, sexual assault, stalking, harassment, street violence, DVA and intimate partner violence (IPV). Worldwide, more than one third (35 per cent) of women who have been in a relationship report experiencing some form of physical and/or sexual violence by their intimate partner in their lifetime (WHO 2014a). This phenomenon, identified as DVA in the UK, is defined as

> any incident or pattern of incidents of controlling, coercive, threatening behaviour, violence or abuse between those aged 16 or over who are, or have been, intimate partners or family members regardless of gender or sexuality. The abuse can encompass, but is not limited to psychological, physical, sexual, financial or emotional. (NICE 2016)

The definition also covers acts of honour-based violence, FGM and forced marriage. DVA encompasses a range of forms of abuse and violence occurring within a domestic context and can include child abuse, elder abuse and IPV. In this chapter, the term DVA is used as a broader term to refer to various abusive acts, and the terms violence and abuse are used interchangeably.

The most common forms of DVA include physical, sexual and psychological abuse (WHO 2002) although it can also present as financial abuse, social abuse or coercive control. Individuals may be exposed to one or more forms of abuse at any one time (Devries et al. 2013; WHO 2013). The various types of DVA as identified by NICE's definition are described thus:

Physical violence or abuse

This refers to the use of physical force to inflict pain, injury or physical suffering to the victim. Example acts include slapping, beating, kicking, pinching, biting, pushing, shoving, dragging, stabbing, spanking, scratching, hitting with a fist or something else that could hurt, burning, choking, threatening or using a gun, knife or any other weapon (García-Moreno et al. 2005).

Sexual violence or abuse

This denotes

> any sexual act, attempt to obtain a sexual act, unwanted sexual comments or advances, or acts to traffic, or otherwise directed, against a person's sexuality using coercion, by any person, regardless of their relationship to the victim, in any setting, including but not limited to home and work. (Jewkes et al. 2002)

It also includes physically forcing a partner to have sexual intercourse, to do something that they find degrading or humiliating (García-Moreno et al. 2005), harming them during sex or forcing them to have sex without protection (WHO 2014b).

Psychological violence or abuse

This refers to the use of various behaviours intended to humiliate and control another individual in public or private. Examples include verbal abuse, name calling, blackmailing, constantly criticising, embarrassing the victim by saying or doing something, threats to beat women or children, monitoring and restricting movements, restricting access to friends and family, restricting economic independence and access to information, assistance or other resources and services such as education or health services (Follingstad and DeHart 2000; WHO 2002).

Financial or economic abuse

This refers to controlling a person's ability to acquire, use and maintain their own money and resources. A victim may be prevented from working to earn money (by not letting them go to work, sabotaging job interviews, taking the welfare benefits the victim is entitled to), using their money without consent, building up debts in their name, damaging their property and possessions, and withholding maintenance payments (Ali and McGarry 2020).

Coercive control

This is defined as any act or a pattern of acts of assault, threats, humiliation and intimidation or other abuse that is used to harm, punish or frighten the victim (Home Office 2013). This is now a criminal offence in the UK and if the abuser is found guilty of coercively controlling the victim, they can be sentenced to up to five years in prison, made to pay a fine or both.

* * *

It is important to recognise that victims often experience more than one form of DVA. It is rarely a one-off incident, but a pattern of abusive and controlling behaviour used by one person against another. All forms of DVA can be found in IPV, honour-based violence, forced marriage and FGM as explained below.

Intimate Partner Violence

Evidence suggests that 35 per cent of women worldwide experience physical and/or sexual IPV at some point in their life. More specifically, the IPV prevalence estimates suggest that the figure ranges from 23.2 per cent in high-income countries and 24.6 per cent in the World Health Organization (WHO) Western Pacific region to 37 per cent in the WHO Eastern Mediterranean region, and 37.7 per cent in the WHO South-East Asia region (García-Moreno et al. 2013). However, some national studies mention that up to 70 per cent of women have experienced physical and/or sexual IPV in their lifetime (ONS 2015). According to the Crime Survey for England and Wales (CSEW) (ONS 2020), an estimated 2.4 million adults aged 16 to 74 experienced DVA in the year ending March 2019, equating to a prevalence rate of 6 per cent. Women were twice as likely to have experienced DVA than men (8.4 per cent compared with 4.2 per cent). A comparison of the prevalence of DVA between 2005 and 2019 (Figure 8.1) clearly highlights a slight decrease over time. However, it should be interpreted cautiously as, due to potential limitations of current measurement and reporting of DVA, the impact of harm is difficult to capture accurately (Myhill 2017). While specific information about the ethnicity and religion of those affected is not readily available, it is safe to assume that the DVA prevalence among British Muslims is comparable to that among the general population.

IPV happens in marital, cohabiting, heterosexual and same-sex relationships (Ali et al. 2016; Baker et al. 2013). Whilst it should be acknowledged that both men and women can perpetrate and experience IPV, most victims

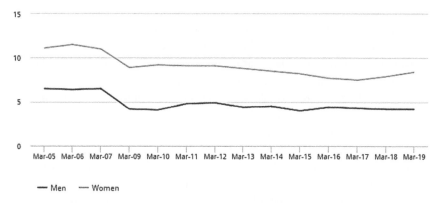

Figure 8.1 Prevalence of domestic abuse for adults aged 16 to 59, by sex: England and Wales, year ending March 2005 to year ending March 2019.

(Source: Crime Survey for England and Wales, Office for National Statistics.)

No data point is available for the year ending March 2008 because comparable questions on stalking, an offence that falls within the domestic abuse category, were not included in that year.

remain women and most perpetrators remain men, with women experiencing repeated, systematic and more severe abuse. In addition, the number of women experiencing injuries or losing their life is much greater. IPV is often considered a private matter and therefore victims, and especially Muslim women, are often encouraged to keep quiet and endure the abuse to maintain the relationship, as exemplified in Case Study 1.

Case Study 1: Intimate Partner Violence

I am Mayra and I came from Pakistan after marriage. There is a significant difference in how things are done in Pakistan and how they are done in the UK. If you ask me my thoughts 10 years ago were much different, how was it? I felt that I was a survivor, that I was surviving, but I had not got out of the situation. I was treated badly by my husband, who I thought was my protector. But I used to get scared when he was home as I didn't know when he will lash out and throw something at me, beat me, kick me or when will he decide to throw me out of 'his' house. I thought I was trapped and there was nowhere to go. The first time I told my family what was happening to me in my marriage, my parents said, 'Darling, things happen in in-laws' families, if your in-laws are raising their voices at you, you just need to keep quiet, don't answer back'. I could not understand why this should be so. I felt that if someone treated me badly, I should be clearing it with them to say why are you doing this/saying this, as I haven't done anything, or done anything to give you a reason to treat me like this.

There was a time in my life when I did feel that 'actually this is how a woman's life should be after marriage' i.e. she has to learn to be quiet in order to survive, for her parents' sake, to save her honour, to save her marriage, and especially when you have had a child, in order to survive, so that your child can have a home. At that time that was my thinking. My feeling was that women who have arguments in their marital homes and they go to their parents, leaving their husbands, shouldn't do this. They should remain in their marital homes. This is what I used to think. I started becoming more involved in religion and it was then that I realised that I was thinking wrong. Patience and *sabur*, as taught in Islam, doesn't mean that I should stay quiet and put up with violence and abuse and forgive. It also means standing up for your rights.

I learned that my religion has given me far more rights than I thought. I learned that as a Muslim I have an Islamic duty to be active and take yourself out of an oppressive situation. But I also know it's not that easy.

Honour-based Violence

HBV has become an increasingly visible problem in the UK since 2000 (Bacchi 2009; Begikhani and Gill 2016; Brandon and Hafez 2008; Mulvihill et al. 2019) and is often wrongly associated with Muslims. HBV refers to acts committed to protect the honour of a family or community. It is defined as a 'collection of practices used predominantly to control the behaviour of women and girls within families or other social groups in order to protect supposed cultural and religious beliefs, values and social norms in the name of "honour"' (HMIC 2015). The Iranian Kurdish Women's Rights Organisation (IKWRO 2014) defined HBV as

> a collective and planned crime or incident, mainly perpetrated against women and girls, by their family or their community, who act to defend their perceived honour, because they believe that the victim(s) have done something to bring shame to the family or the community.

HBV has distinct characteristics as it is deliberate, planned as a collective action, committed to preserve social, cultural or religious norms, condoned by respective communities or groups and involves multiple perpetrators, mainly male members of the family (though women may also be involved) (Eisner and Ghuneim 2013). It is often committed against people who become involved with a boyfriend or girlfriend from a different culture or religion, want to get out of an arranged or forced marriage, or wear clothes or take part in activities not considered appropriate within a culture or religious community.

Unsurprisingly, victims of HBV are usually girls and women, though in some cases, men and boys can be victims too, particularly if they come out as gay. Perpetrators are typically men, and female-on-male incidents remain rare (Bhanbhro et al. 2016). Case Study 2 provides an example from an actual case of HBV committed in the UK.

Case Study 2: Honour-based Violence

Shafilea Ahmed, 17, the elder of two sisters, was killed by her parents for bringing 'dishonour' to the family. In September 2003, the couple pinned their daughter down on the sofa and stuffed a carrier bag into her mouth until she turned blue and suffocated. Her father then put her body in the back of his car and dumped it seventy miles away from their home.

Shafilea's parents would often call her a 'whore' and a 'prostitute' and beat her if they believed she was misbehaving, and would lock her in the garden. Shafilea's fault was that she wanted to be fashionable. As she got older, she adopted a more Western way of living, taking an interest in fashion and wearing make-up and false nails. Her parents tried to curb her 'rebellious' nature, one year arranging a holiday to Pakistan, where they intended to marry her off to a cousin. Shafilea refused to go and so her father drugged her with sleeping pills. After waking in Pakistan, the teenager was so terrified about what would happen she drank bleach in a suicide attempt, severely burning her throat and oesophagus. She was rushed to hospital and was kept there for two months, while her father and siblings flew back home to the UK.

During a furious row over her short-sleeved top, her parents killed her in the living room and made the younger sibling watch. Shafilea's body was found five months after her death in the River Kent near Sedgwick, Cumbria.

In September 2011, her parents were arrested and charged on suspicion of murder. They were found guilty and in August 2012 were sentenced to a minimum of twenty-five years in prison with no parole (The Asian Today, 2019).

HBV can manifest in many forms, including psychological, physical and sexual abuse, withdrawal from school, isolation, imprisonment, kidnapping, acid attacks, forced marriage, forced suicide, forced abortion, blackmail, disfigurement, being held against one's will and even murder (Schlytter and Linell 2010). Killing girls and women in the name of honour is an extreme form of HBV. Every year approximately 5,000 girls and women are killed in the name of honour, but the number may well be much higher (Al Gharaibeh 2016). HBV is often associated with South Asian Muslims (Khan et al. 2018), but these crimes are reported from many populations, including South Asian, African, Middle Eastern, Turkish, Kurdish, Afghan, European, American, Canadian and Australian (HMIC 2015). The practice has also been reported among various religious groups, including Hindus, Sikhs and Christians (Chesler and Bloom 2012; Shafak 2012).

There is no separate criminal offence of HBV in England and Wales and so cases may be flagged under a range of legislation, including injury with assault or harassment (Mulvihill et al. 2019). In the UK, the first HBV-related statistics were collated in 2010, with 2,823 cases reported from 39 police forces (BBC 2011). An inspection of UK police forces revealed that there were 251 HBV referrals made between 2014 and 2015. Another independent examination of police HBV recordings showed that 11,000 cases were recorded between 2010 and 2014 in thirty-nine of the fifty-two forces (IKWRO 2014). Young South Asian women are often identified as HBV victims (Dyer 2015); this does not necessarily mean that HBV is more common in South Asian communities but simply that the size of South Asian communities in the UK is relatively large.

Forced Marriage

Forced marriage is where 'one or both people do not (or in cases of people with learning disabilities, cannot) consent to the marriage and pressure or abuse is used' (Home Office 2013). Under UK law, it is a criminal offence to take someone overseas to force them to marry (whether the marriage takes place or not) and for someone who lacks mental capacity to consent to the marriage (whether they are pressured to or not). It is a form of DVA, and victims can be subjected to physical, sexual, emotional and/or financial abuse, as described in Case Study 3.

Case Study 3: Forced Marriage

Meena is a 20-year-old woman from Afghanistan who was brought to the UK two years ago to care for her husband, Osama. Osama is 30 years old and has lived in the UK all his life. He has a learning disability and requires support with his daily living needs.

Everyone in his family thought that his condition would improve after marriage and that he simply needed someone to look after him long term. Meena didn't know about her husband's learning disability before coming to the UK; in fact, she had not met him nor spoken to him before her wedding day. Learning about the circumstances of the situation came as a big shock to her, and she has no one to talk to. She is expected to meet all Osama's personal care needs and be responsible for him like a 'good wife'. She lives with Osama's parents and siblings and is obliged to cook and clean for the whole family. The family expects Meena to have children with Osama and keeps asking about this.

Meena, while responsible for all the housework, is not allowed to eat with the family. She cannot contact her parents as there is no phone in the house. She speaks little English and is not allowed to leave the house unaccompanied. Meena doesn't know where to go to get help. She is scared because of her visa status and thinks that if she tells anyone about her situation, her marriage will break down and she will be deported to Afghanistan. She is also concerned that her parents would blame her for the breakdown of the marriage and would not accept her back into the family.

Forced marriages are different from arranged marriages, which are organised by the families of both parties with their full and informed consent. The distinction between the two can be blurred and it is often difficult to establish the degree of pressure put on individuals. However, an arranged marriage where both parties have consented and are free to decline should not be a cause for concern. Forced marriage can be a cause or a consequence of HBV, although there are many other motives, including strengthening family links, financial gain, ensuring the retention of family-owned land or wealth, caring for adults or children with special needs, and helping with claims for citizenship and residency. It is therefore important to remember that, whilst some forced marriages will be motivated by honour, the relationship between HBV and forced marriage is complex.

The Home Office (2018) reports that the forced marriage unit has provided support in 1,200–1,400 cases every year since 2012. In 2017 alone, the unit dealt with 355 cases (29.7 per cent) involving victims under the age of 18 and 353 cases (29.5 per cent) involving victims aged 18–25. In 2017, 930 cases (77.8 per cent) involved women and 256 (21.4 per cent) involved men. In 2018, support and advice was provided for 1,196 cases. Since 2005, the forced marriage unit has handled cases relating to over ninety countries across Asia, the Middle East, Africa, Europe and North America. The prevalence of this practice is much higher among South Asian Muslim populations involving Pakistan, Bangladesh, Somalia, India, Afghanistan, Egypt, Iraq, Nigeria, Romania, the UK and Saudi Arabia (Home Office 2018). However, it is also found among Hindus and Sikhs (Gill and Mitra-Kahn 2012).

Girls and women appear more commonly to be victims of forced marriages. While men can also be forced to marry, the ultimate victim even in that situation remains the woman, as the man forced to marry may not be happy with his spouse; he may struggle to develop and maintain a loving relationship with her and move on to another marriage or relationship. Young gay men and women may also be forced into marriages and may face HBV due to their sexuality.

Female Genital Mutilation

FGM – also known as female genital cutting or female circumcision – refers to the cultural practice of cutting off parts of the external female genitalia without any medical purpose. The WHO classifies FGM into four types, listed in Table 8.1. The procedure is usually performed on very young girls, often by traditional circumcisers who do not have any medical training. It is carried out using knives, scissors, scalpels, pieces of glass or razor blades, and without any anaesthesia or antiseptic. It is abundantly clear that FGM is a harmful practice which is related to significant morbidity and mortality of young girls. Despite this, many people feel pressured into maintaining the practice, as indicated in Case Study 4.

Table 8.1 Types of female genital mutilation.

Type	Description
I: Clitoridectomy	Removing part or all of the clitoris
II: Excision	Removing part or all of the clitoris and the inner labia (the lips that surround the vagina), with or without removal of the labia majora (the larger outer lips)
III: Infibulation	Narrowing the vaginal opening by creating a seal, formed by cutting and repositioning the labia
IV	Other procedures, including piercing, incising, cutting, scraping or burning the area

> ### Case Study 4: Female Genital Mutilation
>
> Maryam and Asad are seeking asylum in the UK. They have a 3-year-old daughter, Aisha. Maryam knew that she had been cut as a child and as a result found sex and childbirth painful. Maryam and Asad had only become aware that the cutting was classed as FGM within the UK and against the law when interacting with maternity services. They did not want to return to their country of origin as their family had already begun to put pressure on them to return so that their daughter Aisha could go through the cutting ceremony before she got too old.

The global prevalence of FGM is estimated to be over 200 million, with around 3.3 million girls at risk each year (Khosla et al. 2017; Waigwa et al. 2018). According to estimates, 137,000 women and girls subjected to FGM live in the UK and another 60,000 girls are at risk (Macfarlane and Dorkenoo 2015). Following years of awareness efforts and campaigns, national data for FGM is now collected in more than twenty-nine countries worldwide. The practice is particularly concentrated in certain African, Asian and Middle Eastern countries such as Indonesia, Malaysia, India, Oman, Saudi Arabia and the United Arab Emirates, although migration has resulted in the spread of FGM around the world, including the UK (Muteshi et al. 2016).

The practice is illegal in many countries including the UK, where it carries a penalty of up to 14 years' imprisonment. It has been a serious criminal offence since the passing of the Prohibition of Female Circumcision Act (1985). The Female Genital Mutilation Act (2003) tightened this law to include FGM carried out overseas by UK nationals or permanent residents, and more recently the scope has been extended by the Serious Crime Act (2015). Since 31 October 2015, all regulated health and social care practitioners and teachers in the UK are required to report known and suspected cases of FGM to the police as soon as possible and ideally within 48 hours. They are held personally accountable for this as the responsibility cannot be transferred to anyone else. However, despite this legislation, reporting of FGM and successful prosecutions remain low (Plugge et al. 2018).

Islam and Domestic Violence and Abuse

While all the above forms of DVA are prevalent in various countries and communities, popular misconceptions mean these are often associated with Muslims and Islam. For instance, people often quote verse 4:34 from the Qur'an, confusing it with the issue of *nushuz* (contentiously translated as a wife's disobedience, flagrant defiance or misbehaviour). There is no accurate tranlstion of this word and it is often misinterpreted as supporting domestic violence (Ibrahim and Abdalla 2010). However, violence against women is not encouraged or allowed in Islam in any form or under any circumstances. Instead, according to Islamic teaching, the relationship between husband and wife should be one of mutual love, respect and kindness. For example, 'O believers treat women with kindness even if you dislike them; it is quite possible that you dislike something which Allah might yet make a source of abundant good' (Qur'an 4:19).

Similarly, forced marriage and HBV are often associated with Islam. However, Islam gives both men and women the freedom to choose their partner and clearly prohibits anyone else from making decisions for them (Munir and Akhter 2018). The Qur'an explicitly states that men cannot keep women against their will and any marriage that is forced is considered to be *batil* or void. Further evidence that forced marriage is against Islam can be found in hadith traditions based on reports of the sayings and actions of the Prophet Muhammad (PBUH), such as 'A virgin came to the Prophet (PBUH) and mentioned that her father had married her against her will, so the Prophet (PBUH) allowed her to exercise her choice' (Sunan Abu-Dawud, Marriage (Kitab Al-Nikah), Book 11, Number 2091).

In some countries, there is a widespread view that FGM is a religious requirement, especially in Muslim communities (Ahmed et al. 2019); however, in a number of countries, especially African countries, FGM is practised by members of different religious groups including Muslims, Jews and Christians (Ahmed et al. 2019; El-Damanhoury 2013; Hayford and Trinitapoli 2011). There is no mention of FGM in any religious scriptures including the Qur'an (Ahmed et al. 2019; El-Damanhoury 2013; Hayford and Trinitapoli 2011). Some Muslim scholars, however, believe that FGM is at least permissible as the Prophet Muhammad did not prohibit it and it is mentioned in at least five hadiths (Al-Awa 2019; Kelleher 2019). The authenticity of these hadiths is questioned by other scholars 'who disagree about whether Islam requires, encourages, permits, or discourages the practice' (Hayford and Trinitapoli 2011).

The confusing relationship between religion and culture and a lack of understanding of this relationship may result in health and social care practitioners turning a blind eye to DVA especially when feeling ill equipped to challenge individuals or groups. It is therefore important to raise awareness among the population that these practices are not supported by Islam and that people who present them as such should always be challenged.

The Impacts on Health of DVA

DVA is associated with serious psychological as well as physical impacts. Evidence suggests that approximately 42 per cent of women who experience physical or sexual IPV endure injuries as a result (WHO 2013). Examples of physical impacts include cuts, punctures, bruises and bites. Victims may also be subjected to severe injuries resulting in permanent disability in the form of loss of limb, hearing loss, damage to teeth. Victims of DVA also experience higher rates of ill health, compromised ability to walk, pain, vaginal discharge, loss of memory and dizziness and self-harm. The health impact of sexual abuse may include unwanted pregnancy, miscarriage, sexually transmitted infections (STI) and other gynaecological problems. Similarly, FGM also results in heavy bleeding, infection and development of tetanus and other physiological problems (Black 2011).

British Muslim Women and DVA

Religion plays a vital role in the lives of many people and so also has an impact on how DVA is interpreted, experienced and addressed. There are contradictory views reported in the literature with regard to religion and DVA, and not limited to Islam. Evidence suggests that many religious communities give importance to family commitments, which is often interpreted as condoning DVA. Religion has also been used to impose adverse impacts on women and especially victims of DVA (Ghafournia 2017) by instructing them to cope with abuse, to stay in abusive relationships and to forgive the abuser (Fowler et al. 2011).

While there is no specific evidence to suggest that the prevalence of DVA in the British Muslim community is higher than in any other religious minority population (Chantler et al. 2019), given that Muslims are a minority in the country and the population is already affected by poverty and health inequalities, it is no surprise that British Muslim women experience additional barriers when seeking support. Muslim women make up one of the most disadvantaged groups in British society and often experience further inequalities due to expectations surrounding gender roles and behaviours rooted in concepts of honour culture (Milani et al. 2018). They experience an intense pressure to conform and suffer in silence. If they can find the courage to report their DVA experience to the appropriate services, they are taking a colossal step. If they then receive poor service, it can disempower and deter them (and others) from continuing with any reports made to the police or from making future reports, or they may choose not to pursue a case before it reaches court. Consequently, the women do not get justice and the perpetrators are not held accountable. This may also embolden perpetrators, leading to an increase in the DVA inflicted on the victim and an increase in the number of victims. The consequences of an inadequate service can sometimes be fatal.

It is important to recognise that Muslims in the UK (and worldwide) are a diverse group in order to understand the special issues concerning British Muslim women that affect their ability to recognise DVA, disclose that they are victims of DVA and seek appropriate help and support in a timely manner. These include the following:

Isolation

Abusers often impose isolation on their victims to enforce their dominating control. Isolation can also result from being an immigrant and the inability to speak English. The women may look and dress differently and may live far from familiar and potentially supportive friends and family members, impacting their ability to seek support. Isolation makes a woman vulnerable to DVA because she comes to depend on the perpetrator for all human contact, loses self-esteem and has no one to turn to when she needs support or an escape route (Mirza 2017). Islamophobia and prejudice of professionals may affect this further. For instance, women who wear the headscarf can feel isolated and misunderstood by professionals and those who do not are subjected to negative attitudes and reactions from within the community, making them feel isolated and stigmatised (Johnson 2017).

Stigma

DVA victims, regardless of their religion or any other affiliation, often feel ashamed of their victimisation. Acknowledging and disclosing their experiences of DVA can be especially difficult for Muslim women because they may believe that revealing abuse will disgrace their family (Ali et al. 2019). Additionally, Muslims as a group are already portrayed negatively in the media and so, like members of other stigmatised groups, Muslim victims of DVA may not want to disclose their experiences for fear of bringing increased negative attention to their family and community.

Discrimination

Confiding in others about DVA requires confidence, courage and a sense of trust. People who have experienced discrimination or who have been reviled by politicians are less likely to trust secular authorities with their intimate family matters and may find it difficult to talk about their experiences. Practitioners may not take them seriously and such experiences can further destroy trust and impact on the victim's ability to disclose their experiences and the practitioner's ability to support victims (Milani et al. 2018).

Staying in an abusive marriage

This may involve forcing someone to marry or to stay in an abusive marriage for the sake of the family and children. Divorce and remarriage, though acceptable from a religious point of view, are nonetheless frowned upon and so the victim may be reluctant to be open about her experience. However, from an Islamic perspective, divorce is completely acceptable especially if the marriage is not a happy one and the husband and wife want to separate. In fact, a woman does not have to 'come up' with a reason for divorce if she wants to end a marriage. When a couple divorce, the woman's property is not divided up and so whatever she owns or was given before and during the course of the marriage remains hers (Booley 2014). On the other hand, the man's property is divided if a divorce occurs according to the couple's marriage contract. A woman is also entitled to support and maintenance from her former husband if she requires (Jaafar-Mohammad and Lehmann 2011).

Lack of knowledge of rights within Islam

Although, as mentioned earlier, Islam does not condone beating or sexual assault of women perpetrators may seek and find religious justifications for their actions, and other people may encourage victims to stay in an abusive relationship and to obey the husband as a religious responsibility. However, it is important to remember that DVA is not acceptable in Islam and accepting and staying in abusive relationships should be discouraged.

Vulnerability with regard to immigration status

Many women come to the UK following marriage and their visa may be attached to their husband's immigration status. Some victims may not have access to their own passport and travel documents, making them highly vulnerable to threats and abuse. They may be very reluctant to get involved with authorities because of the risk of deportation. Women may also not want to go back to their country of origin due to the fear of stigma and bringing shame on themselves and their family.

Fear of losing custody of children or child abduction

DVA perpetrators often threaten to take away the children or, in the case of migrant couples, to take them back to the country of origin and make them 'disappear'. Victims are often unfamiliar with their rights and available services in their new country and therefore become trapped in the relationship and unable to seek help. They may also be fearful of children being taken away by social services and such fears may further limit their ability to seek appropriate support.

Support from religious figures

Muslim clerics are often ill-equipped to handle DVA in families, and yet they may be the first point of contact for Muslim families. These clerics are exclusively men, some of whom will interpret Islamic texts in ways that either condemn or support DVA, depending on their own interpretation and perspectives. If they do not know what to do or where to refer a victim for further support, they will often urge a woman to be patient, thus encouraging her to remain in a dangerous situation.

Unregistered Marriages and Coercive Control

Spouses are not protected by English law in unregistered religious marriages which have been conducted in the UK. Many women do not realise that that by only having an Islamic marriage (*nikah*) and not the civil registration alongside it, they have no legal status as a wife, and thus if the marriage breaks down, they cannot get any recourse from the legal system (Fairbairn 2020). When migrant Muslims initially settled in the UK, unregistered marriages from overseas were culturally recognised; migrant communities have not always been aware that such marriages are not legally recognised in Britain. Some men – or their family members – try to dissuade women from pursuing the legal civil registration of their marriage, telling them that the Islamic marriage is all that is needed. They do this deliberately to ensure that if the women does leave the marriage, she will not be entitled to anything. By law, this type of marriage is considered a 'non-marriage', with serious consequence in the case of death of a spouse or separation (Fairbairn 2020). There are issues with divorce too. Currently, where the marriage has been registered, Muslim women must go through a twofold divorce process, once through the civil court and then the Islamic divorce. A recently conducted review highlighted that the vast majority (over 90 per cent) of people using Sharia Councils (unofficial local religious bodies arbitrating in Muslim family disputes) are women seeking an Islamic divorce. The review also found that a significant number of Muslim couples do not register their religious marriage as a civil marriage and that some Muslim women therefore have no option of obtaining a civil divorce (Fairbairn 2020; Siddiqui 2018).

If the woman has a civil divorce then the Islamic divorce is issued automatically. Many Muslim women for whom faith is an important part of their identity say that they need to have an Islamic divorce alongside the civil divorce to ensure that they feel no longer spiritually connected to their husband and for their own families to recognise this too. Without the Islamic divorce many women would still be considered as the wife of their former husband even if the marriage has broken down completely. In addition, in the absence of civil marriage, 'some men had refused to give or agree to a divorce even though they had moved forward with their lives and remarried; refused or contested an Islamic divorce to extract a more favourable financial settlement from their wife' (Casey 2016).

Healthcare Professionals and DVA

Appropriate and effective help and support from HCPs and services can do much to prevent harm. However, accessing support from hospitals, primary care centres, GP surgeries and practitioners is often not straightforward for women (Briones-Vozmediano et al. 2014; Vives-Cases et al. 2014). The experiences of

Muslim women including migrants and those from BME backgrounds is even worse (Vives-Cases et al. 2014; Stockman et al. 2015).

Most British Muslims belong to South Asian communities that place a lot of emphasis on joint family systems (Rai et al. 2019). The combination of arranged marriage and the joint family system means that many DVA victims may also be experiencing DVA from other family members such as in-laws. Factors such as a lack of social networks and appropriate family support systems and lower personal income adds to their vulnerability to further abuse and coercive control by intimate partners and other family members (Stockman et al. 2015). If the victim is unable to communicate in English, social isolation can increase (Colucci et al. 2014). Likewise, access to health and social care services becomes increasingly difficult (Pearce and Sokoloff 2013; Reina et al. 2014). Victims find it difficult to disclose their experiences of abuse as in most situations they are accompanied by family members who function as interpreters, making it impossible to be open about their situation. Even when the interpreters are arranged, victims may not find it easy to be honest about their experiences to someone from the same community.

As HCPs regularly encounter DVA victims (Houry et al. 2008), they can play a crucial role in the identification, prevention and management of DVA (NICE 2014), although they need to be able to differentiate between injuries resulting from DVA and those with other causes, and provide person-centred, sensitive and empathetic care to all their service users. However, DVA victims often feel that HCPs blame them for abuse, do not show concern and do not address the issue (Yam 2000), even when DVA is obvious (Bradley et al. 2002). Many factors impact HCPs' ability to provide effective services to DVA victims, including a lack of time, lack of training (Gerbert et al. 2002; Gutmanis et al. 2007), and lack of confidence, knowledge and awareness about DVA and its impact (Ramsay et al. 2012; Sundborg et al. 2012). Evidence also suggests that practitioners often feel unprepared to meet the needs of DVA victims from a BME background and faith communities (Colucci et al. 2014; Kallivayalil 2007; Vives-Cases et al. 2014). To remove such barriers and ensure provision of appropriate care to Muslim victims of DVA, professionals need appropriate training and support.

Engagement with religious organisations such as mosques and other groups may help HCPs find useful ways to engage with the communities, not only to understand their needs better but also to plan and disseminate health promotion messages (Rai et al. 2019).

People who understand Islam need to be recruited and supported in the field of services for DVA as counsellors, advocates, police and lawyers. Muslim clergy and organisations should be educated about the real dynamics and risks of DVA and their individual roles and responsibilities in preventing it. Organisations need to have regular and meaningful cultural competence training to improve their ability to address the needs of cultural minority groups, including Muslims. Policies that support immigrant and refugee children, adults and families will decrease family stress, thus reducing violence and increasing options for DVA victims. People who view the police and other authorities as hostile forces will run from – rather than towards – services that might help them live free from violence and control.

Conclusion

This chapter has highlighted the issue of DVA, its forms and health impacts, and has explored factors affecting Muslim women's ability to access appropriate support. It is important for HCPs to understand that disclosing DVA and seeking help can be difficult and challenging. It is also important to recognise the special role HCPs can pay in detecting and intervening in DVA. To summarise, this chapter highlighted the following points:

- DVA is a major social and public health issue and millions of women, regardless of income, education, age or other characteristics, experience DVA in its various forms.
- DVA has dire consequences for victims, including short- and long-term physical, mental and emotional health problems.
- While men can also be victims of DVA, the intensity, frequency and severity of abuse experienced by women is much worse.
- Disclosing DVA experiences and seeking help from appropriate sources is not easy and the number of women seeking support from appropriate professionals and organisations including the police and HCPs remains extremely low.

References

Ahmed, H. M., Kareem, M. S., Shabila, N. P. and Mzori, B. Q. (2019). 'Religious leaders' position toward female genital cutting and their perspectives on the relationship between the Islamic religion and this practice'. *Women & Health*, 59(8), 854–66.

Al-Awa, M. S. (2019). *FGM in the Context of Islam*. Cairo: The National Council for Childhood and Motherhood.

Al Gharaibeh, F. M. (2016). 'Debating the role of custom, religion and law in "honour" crimes: implications for social work'. *Ethics and Social Welfare*, 10(2), 122–39.

Ali, P. and McGarry, J. (2020). 'Introduction to domestic violence and abuse within healthcare contexts', in P. Ali and J. McGarry (eds), *Domestic Violence in Health Contexts: A Guide for Healthcare Professions*. Cham: Springer, pp. 1–15.

Ali, P. A., Dhingra, K. and McGarry, J. (2016). 'A literature review of intimate partner violence and its classifications'. *Aggression and Violent Behavior*, 31, 16–25.

Ali, P. A., O'Cathain, A. and Croot, E. (2019). 'Not managing expectations: a grounded theory of intimate partner violence from the perspective of Pakistani people'. *Journal of Interpersonal Violence*, 34(19), 4085–113.

Bacchi, C. (2009). *Analysing Policy: What's the Problem Represented to Be?*. Melbourne: Pearson Higher Education Australia.

Baker, N. L., Buick, J. D., Kim, S. R., Moniz, S. and Nava, K. L. (2013). 'Lessons from examining same-sex intimate partner violence'. *Sex Roles*, 69(3–4), 182–92.

BBC (2011). '"Honour" attack numbers revealed by UK police forces', 3 December. Available at: www.bbc.co.uk/news/uk-16014368 (last accessed 11 May 2022).

Begikhani, N. and Gill, A. K. (2016). *Honour-based Violence: Experiences and Counter-strategies in Iraqi Kurdistan and the UK Kurdish Diaspora*. London: Routledge.

Bhanbhro, S., Cronin De Chavez, A. and Lusambili, A. (2016). 'Honour based violence as a global public health problem: a critical review of literature'. *International Journal of Human Rights in Healthcare*, 9(3), 198–215.

Black, M. C. (2011). 'Intimate partner violence and adverse health consequences: implications for clinicians'. *American Journal of Lifestyle Medicine*, 5(5), 428–39.

Booley, A. (2014). 'Divorce and the law of Khul: a type of no fault divorce found within an Islamic legal framework'. *Law, Democracy & Development*, 18(1), 37–57.

Bradley, F., Smith, M., Long, J. and O'Dowd, T. (2002). 'Reported frequency of domestic violence: cross sectional survey of women attending general practice'. *BMJ*, 324, 271.

Brandon, J. and Hafez, S. (2008). *Crimes of the Community: Honour-based Violence in the UK*. London: Civitas.

Briones-Vozmediano, E., Agudelo-Suarez, A. A., Goicolea, I. and Vives-Cases, C. (2014). 'Economic crisis, immigrant women and changing availability of intimate partner violence services: a qualitative study of professionals' perceptions in Spain'. *International journal for Equity in Health*, 13(1), 79.

Casey, L. (2016). 'The Casey Review: a review into opportunity and integration'. Available at: https://assets.publishing.service.gov.uk/government/uploads/system/uploads/attachment_data/file/575973/The_Casey_Review_Report.pdf (last accessed 11 May 2022).

Chantler, K., Gangoli, G. and Thiara, R. K. (2019). 'Muslim women and gender based violence in India and the UK'. *Critical Social Policy*, 39(2), 163–83.

Chesler, P. and Bloom, N. (2012). 'Hindu vs. Muslim honor killings'. *Middle East Quarterly* 19, 33, 43–52.

Colucci, E., O'Connor, M., Field, K., Baroni, A., Pryor, R. and Minas, H. (2014). 'Nature of domestic/family violence and barriers to using services among Indian immigrant women'. *Alterstice-Revue Internationale de la Recherche Interculturelle*, 3(2), 9–26.

Devries, K. M., Mak, J. Y., García-Moreno, C., Petzold, M., Child, J. C., Falder, G., Lim, S., Bacchus, L. J., Engell, R. E., Rosenfeld, L., Pallitto, C. and Vos, T. (2013). 'The global prevalence of intimate partner violence against women'. *Science*, 340(6140), 1527–8.

Dyer, E. (2015). *Honour Killings in the UK*. London: Henry Jackson Society.

Eisner, M. and Ghuneim, L. (2013). 'Honor killing attitudes amongst adolescents in Amman, Jordan'. *Aggressive Behavior*, 39(5), 405–17.

El-Damanhoury, I. (2013). 'The Jewish and Christian view on female genital mutilation'. *African Journal of Urology*, 19(3), 127–9.

Fairbairn, C. (2020). 'Islamic marriage and divorce in England and Wales'. Briefing Paper 08747. Available at: https://commonslibrary.parliament.uk/research-briefings/cbp-8747 (last accessed 11 May 2022).

Follingstad, D. R. and DeHart, D. D. (2000). 'Defining psychological abuse of husbands toward wives: contexts, behaviors, and typologies'. *Journal of Interpersonal Violence*, 15(9), 891–920.

Fowler, D. N., Faulkner, M., Learman, J. and Runnels, R. (2011). 'The influence of spirituality on service utilization and satisfaction for women residing in a domestic violence shelter'. *Violence Against Women*, 17(10), 1244–59.

García-Moreno, C., Jansen, H. A. F. M., Ellsberg, M., Heise, L. and Watts, C. (2005). *WHO Multi-country Study on Women's Health and Domestic Violence against Women: Initial Results on Prevalence, Health Outcomes and Women's Responses*. Geneva: World Health Organization.

García-Moreno, C., Pallitto, C., Devries, K., Stöckl, H., Watts, C. and Abrahams, N. (2013). *Global and Regional Estimates of Violence against Women: Prevalence and Health Effects of Intimate Partner Violence and Non-partner Sexual Violence*. Geneva: World Health Organization.

Gerbert, B., Gansky, S. A., Tang, J. W., McPhee, S. J., Carlton, R., Herzig, K., Danley, D. and Caspers, N. (2002). 'Domestic violence compared to other health risks: a survey of physicians' beliefs and behaviors'. *American Journal of Preventive Medicine*, 23(2), 82–90.

Ghafournia, N. (2017). 'Muslim women and domestic violence: developing a framework for social work practice'. *Journal of Religion & Spirituality in Social Work: Social Thought*, 36(1–2), 146–63.

Gill, A. and Mitra-Kahn, T. (2012). 'Modernising the other: assessing the ideological underpinnings of the policy discourse on forced marriage in the UK'. *Policy & Politics*, 40(1), 104–19.

Gutmanis, I., Beynon, C., Tutty, L. T., Wathen, C. N. and MacMillan, H. L. (2007). 'Factors influencing identification of and response to intimate partner violence: a survey of physicians and nurses'. *BMC Public Health*, 7, 12.

Hayford, S. R. and Trinitapoli, J. (2011). 'Religious differences in female genital cutting: a case study from Burkina Faso'. *Journal for the Scientific Study of Religion*, 50(2), 252–71.

Her Majesty's Inspectorate of Constabulary and Fire & Rescue Services (2015). 'The depths of dishonour: hidden voices and shameful crimes. An inspection of the police response to honour-based violence, forced marriage and female genital mutilation'. Report. Available at: www.justiceinspectorates.gov.uk/hmic/publications/the-depths-of-dishonour (last accessed 11 May 2022).

Home Office (2013). 'Forced marriage: how to protect, advise and support victims of forced marriage – information and practice guidelines for professionals'. Available at: www.gov.uk/guidance/forced-marriage (last accessed 11 May 2022).

Home Office (2018). 'Forced marriage unit statistics 2017'. Available at: https://assets.publishing.service.gov.uk/government/uploads/system/uploads/attachment_data/file/730155/2017_FMU_statistics_FINAL.pdf (last accessed 11 May 2022).

Houry, D., Kaslow, N. J., Kemball, R. S., McNutt, L. A., Cerulli, C., Straus, H., Rosenberg, E., Chengxing, L. and Rhodes, K. V. (2008). 'Does screening in the emergency department hurt or help victims of intimate partner violence?'. *Annals of Emergency Medicine*, 51(4), 433–42.

Ibrahim, N. and Abdalla, M. (2010). 'A critical examination of Qur'an 4:34 and its relevance to intimate partner violence in Muslim families'. *Journal of Muslim Mental Health*, 5(3), 327–49.

Iranian Kurdish Women's Rights Organisation (2014). 'Postcode lottery: police recording of reported "honour" based violence'. Available at: https://democracy.brent.gov.uk/documents/s22709/2-Appendix%208%20-%20IKWRO%20HBV%20FOI%20Report%20Postcode%20Lottery-04.02.2014-Final.pdf (last accessed 11 May 2022).

Jaafar-Mohammad, I. and Lehmann, C. (2011). 'Women's rights in Islam regarding marriage and divorce'. *Journal of Law and Practice*, 4(3).

Jewkes, R., Sen, P. and Garcia-Moreno, C. (2002). 'Sexual violence', in E. G. Krug, L. L. Dahlberg, J. A. Mercy, A. B. Zwi and R. Lozano (eds), *World Report on Violence and Health*. Geneva: World Health Organization, pp. 149–81.

Johnson, A. (2017). '"You're othered here and you're othered there": centring the clothing practices of Black Muslim women in Britain'. PhD thesis. University of Sheffield.

Kallivayalil, D. (2007). 'Feminist therapy: its use and implications for South Asian immigrant survivors of domestic violence'. *Women & Therapy*, 30(3–4), 109–27.

Kelleher, R. (2019). 'The cut in conflict: female genital mutilation and the concept of religious violence in the Western world'. *Journal of the Council for Research on Religion*, 1, 45–69.

Khan, R., Saleem, S. and Lowe, M. (2018). '"Honour"-based violence in a British South Asian community'. *Safer Communities*, 17(1), 11–21.

Khosla, R., Banerjee, J., Chou, D., Say, L. and Fried, S. T. (2017). 'Gender equality and human rights approaches to female genital mutilation: a review of international human rights norms and standards'. *Reproductive Health*, 14(1), 59.

Macfarlane, A. and Dorkenoo, E. (2015). 'Prevalence of female genital mutilation in England and Wales: National and local estimates'. Available at: https://www.trustforlondon.org.uk/publications/prevalence-female-genital-mutilation-england-and-wales-national-and-local-estimates (last accessed 11 May 2022).

Milani, A., Leschied, A. and Rodger, S. (2018). '"Beyond cultural sensitivity": service providers' perspectives on Muslim women experiences of intimate partner violence'. *Journal of Muslim Mental Health*, 12(1).

Mirza, N. (2017). 'South Asian women's experience of abuse by female affinal kin: a critique of mainstream conceptualisations of "domestic abuse"'. *Families, Relationships and Societies*, 6(3), 393–409.

Mulvihill, N., Gangoli, G., Gill, A. K. and Hester, M. (2019). 'The experience of interactional justice for victims of "honour"-based violence and abuse reporting to the police in England and Wales'. *Policing and Society*, 29(6), 640–56.

Munir, A. and Akhter, N. (2018). 'Marriage in Islam: an analytical study with a special focus on non-traditional marriages in Pakistan'. *FWU Journal of Social Sciences*, 12(2), 179–89.

Muslim Council of Britain (2015). 'British Muslims in numbers: a demographic, socio-economic and health profile of Muslims in Britain drawing on the 2011 census'. Available at: https://www.mcb.org.uk/wp-content/uploads/2015/02/MCBCensusReport_2015.pdf (last accessed 11 May 2022).

Muteshi, J. K., Miller, S. and Belizán, J. M. (2016). 'The ongoing violence against women: female genital mutilation/cutting'. *Reproductive Health*, 13, 44.

Myhill, A. (2017). 'Measuring domestic violence: context is everything'. *Journal of Gender-based Violence*, 1(1), 33–44.

NICE (2014). 'Domestic violence and abuse: multi-agency working'. Available at: www.nice.org.uk/guidance/ph50 (last accessed 11 May 2022).

NICE (2016). Domestic violence and abuse: Quality standard [QS116]. Available at: www.nice.org.uk/guidance/qs116 (last accessed 11 May 2022).

Office for National Statistics (2015). 'Intimate personal violence and partner abuse'. Available at: www.ons.gov.uk/peoplepopulationandcommunity/crimeandjustice/compendium/focusonviolentcrimeandsexualoffences/yearendingmarch2015/chapter4intimatepersonalviolenceandpartnerabuse (last accessed 14 July 2022).

Office for National Statistics (2020). 'Crime and justice'. Available at: www.ons.gov.uk/peoplepopulationandcommunity/crimeandjustice (last accessed 14 July 2022).

Pearce, S. C. and Sokoloff, N. J. (2013). '"This should not be happening in this country": private-life violence and immigration intersections in a US gateway city'. *Sociological Forum*, 28(4), 74–810.

Plugge, E., Adam, S., El Hindi, L., Gitau, J., Shodunke, N. and Mohamed-Ahmed, O. (2018). 'The prevention of female genital mutilation in England: what can be done?'. *Journal of Public Health*, 41(3), e261–e266.

Po-Yan Leung, T., Phillips, L., Bryant, C. and Hegarty, K. (2018). 'How family doctors perceived their "readiness" and "preparedness" to identify and respond to intimate partner abuse: a qualitative study'. *Family Practice*, 35(4): 517–23.

Rai, K. K., Dogra, S. A., Barber, S., Adab, P., Summerbell, C. and Childhood Obesity Prevention in Islamic Religious Settings' Programme Management Group (2019). 'A scoping review and systematic mapping of health promotion interventions associated with obesity in Islamic religious settings in the UK'. *Obesity Reviews*, 20(9), 1231–61.

Ramsay, J., Rutterford, C., Gregory, A., Dunne, D., Eldridge, S., Sharp, D. and Feder, G. (2012). 'Domestic violence: knowledge, attitudes, and clinical practice of selected UK primary healthcare clinicians'. *British Journal of General Practice*, 62(602), e647–e655.

Reina, A. S., Lohman, B. J. and Maldonado, M. M. (2014). '"He said they'd deport me": factors influencing domestic violence help-seeking practices among Latina immigrants'. *Journal of Interpersonal Violence*, 29(4), 593–615.

Renner, L. M., Wang, Q., Logeais, M. E. and Clark, C. J. (2019). 'Health care providers' readiness to identify and respond to intimate partner violence'. *Journal of Interpersonal Violence*, 36(19–20), 1907–34.

Saleem, F. and Martin, S. L. (2018). '"Seeking help is difficult"': considerations for providing mental health services to Muslim women clients'. *Canadian Journal of Counselling and Psychotherapy*, 52(2).

Schlytter, A. and Linell, H. (2010). 'Girls with honour-related problems in a comparative perspective'. *International Journal of Social Welfare*, 19(2), 152–61.

Shafak, E. (2012). '"Honour killings": Murder by any other name'. *The Guardian*, 30 April. Available at: www.theguardian.com/uk/2012/apr/30/honour-killings-spreading-alarming-rate (last accessed 11 May 2022).

Siddiqui, M. (2018). 'The independent review into the application of sharia law in England and Wales'. Cm 9560. Available at: https://assets.publishing.service.gov.uk/government/uploads/system/uploads/attachment_data/file/678478/6.4152_HO_CPFG_Report_into_Sharia_Law_in_the_UK_WEB.pdf (last accessed 11 May 2022).

Stockman, J. K., Hayashi, H. and Campbell, J. C. (2015). 'Intimate partner violence and its health impact on ethnic minority women'. *Journal of Women's Health*, 24(1), 62–79.

Sundborg, E., Saleh-Stattin, N., Wandell, P. and Tornkvist, L. (2012). 'Nurses' preparedness to care for women exposed to Intimate Partner Violence: a quantitative study in primary health care'. *BMC Nursing*, 11(1), 1.

The Asian Today (2019). 'Shafilea Ahmed – Honour Killing Documentary', 19 April. Available at: www.theasiantoday.com/index.php/2019/04/15/shafilea-ahmed-honour-killing-documentary/ (last accessed 8 July 2022).

United Nations (1993). 'Declaration on the elimination of violence against women'. Available at: www.un.org/documents/ga/res/48/a48r104.htm (last accessed 11 May 2022).

Vives-Cases, C., La Parra, D., Goicolea, I., Felt, E., Briones-Vozmediano, E., Ortiz-Barreda, G. and Gil-González, D. (2014). 'Preventing and addressing intimate partner violence against migrant and ethnic minority women: the role of the health sector'. Available at: www.euro.who.int/__data/assets/pdf_file/0018/270180/21256-WHO-Intimate-Partner-Violence_low_V7.pdf (last accessed 11 May 2022).

Waigwa, S., Doos, L., Bradbury-Jones, C. and Taylor, J. (2018). 'Effectiveness of health education as an intervention designed to prevent female genital mutilation/cutting (FGM/C): a systematic review'. *Reproductive Health*, 15(1), 62.

World Health Organization (2002). World report on violence and health: summary. Available at: https://apps.who.int/iris/bitstream/handle/10665/42512/9241545623_eng.pdf?sequence=1&isAllowed=y (last accessed 11 May 2022).

World Health Organization (2013). 'Global and regional estimates of violence against women: prevalence and health effects of intimate partner violence and non-partner sexual violence'. Available at: http://apps.who.int/iris/bitstream/10665/85239/1/9789241564625_eng.pdf?ua=1 (last accessed 11 May 2022).

World Health Organization (2014a). 'Violence against women'. Available at: www.who.int/publications/i/item/9789240022256 (last accessed 8 July 2022).

World Health Organization (2014b). 'Health care for women subjected to intimate partner violence or sexual violence: a clinical handbook'. Available at: https://apps.who.int/iris/bitstream/handle/10665/136101/WHO_RHR_14.26_eng.pdf (last accessed 11 May 2022).

Yam, M. (2000). 'Seen but not heard: battered women's perceptions of the ED experience'. *Journal of Emergency Nursing*, 26(5), 464–70.

Younis, T. and Jadhav, S. (2019). 'Islamophobia in the National Health Service: an ethnography of institutional racism in PREVENT's counter-radicalisation policy'. *Sociology of Health & Illness*, 42(3), 610–26.

Further reading

Muslin Women's Network: www.mwnuk.co.uk/history.php (last accessed 11 May 2022).

Muslim Marriage and Divorce: www.mwnhelpline.co.uk//go_files/issue/377623-MWNU%20M+D%20Booklet_WEB.pdf (last accessed 11 May 2022).

The Muslim Law (Sharia) Council UK: www.shariacouncil.org (last accessed 11 May 2022).

9

MEDICAL ENCOUNTERS BETWEEN OVERSEAS-TRAINED SOUTH ASIAN DOCTORS AND MARGINALISED PATIENTS IN THE UK: A RECIPROCAL DOCTOR– PATIENT RELATIONSHIP?

Yasmin Ghazala Farooq

Introduction

The doctor–patient relationship is considered a cornerstone of healthcare and the practice of medicine. It frequently appears in the literature of Western medicine and has a long history of being addressed from a sociological perspective (Bury and Monaghan 2013). There is a general consensus among scholars that Western scientific medicine is a product of social and cultural processes similar to the way medical knowledge and practices have developed in non-Western societies. In other words it means that sociocultural dimensions of medicine impact on the doctor–patient relationship (Lupton 2012).

Lupton (2012) argues that though 'culture' appears in the medical literature, it is usually used to refer to non-Western cultures. Concepts such as 'culturally competent' or culturally appropriate healthcare are used to draw attention of healthcare professionals such as doctors and nurses to the sensitivity of the disparity of health status and inequalities that is experienced due to the differences in social class, racial and ethnic groups.

Critics in medical sociology appear to agree that medicine acts as an important institution of social control and that powerful groups in possession of medical and scientific knowledge have been privileged over others. Their assertions, however, have centred on their tendency to focus on the micro-properties of interactions of doctors and patients rather than incorporating an analysis that includes the macro-level social and political context within which such encounters take place. It is argued that almost all existing studies focus on the powerful positions that the medical practitioners hold and portray patients as disadvantaged in one way or another (Lupton 2012).

In relation to the provision of culturally competent services, Lupton states that emphasis is placed on 'patient-centred communication' in which healthcare practitioners aim to make sense of the patients' culturally shaped understandings of their health through their raising awareness of ethnic and racial cultural differences in health practices.

Lupton emphasises a broadening of the above perspective as healthcare professionals also bring their own cultural beliefs into the medical encounter. The author refers to the concept of 'lifeworld', often used by sociologists and anthropologists, to depict the everyday sociocultural context within which meaning is generated. For lay people such as patients, lifeworld refers to a number of factors such as the concepts, perspectives and beliefs that they bring to the medical encounter which are shaped by their encounters with doctors and other healthcare professionals as well as their personal experiences. For example, how they interact with others, information they derive from the mass media and the internet, their social class, racial or ethnic group identity, gender or generational group all contribute towards formulating their lifeworld. Similarly, the healthcare professionals' own cultural beliefs that they bring into the medical encounter are shaped not only by their scientific training but also by other aspects of their own lifeworlds.

This chapter is an extract from my recent book (Farooq 2020), which is based on a doctoral study that investigated the identity and sociocultural integration experiences and perspectives of overseas-trained South Asian doctors in the UK. The study involved in-depth interviews with overseas-trained South Asian doctors who worked as general practitioners (GPs) in diverse geographical contexts in the UK. The chapter provides an overview of the doctors' perceptions of doctor–patient relationships from diverse backgrounds and geographical contexts. The insights into their experiences show that the overseas-trained South Asian doctors may have been able to form doctor–patient relationships that were more of a reciprocal nature than one of assumed medical dominance. By drawing on the empirical evidence, this chapter aims to shed light on various aspects of the lifeworlds of the doctors in the study which may have contributed to this reciprocity in the doctor–patient relationship.

The terms 'overseas-trained South Asian doctors' and 'South Asian migrant doctors' here refer to those doctors who obtained their basic medical degrees in India and Pakistan. These terms are used interchangeably at times. Only those doctors who practised as GPs were included in the analysis, as it was envisaged that GPs have a unique role in terms of their close relationships with patients and the local communities of their practice population.

Methodology

In order to investigate the process of sociocultural integration experiences and perspectives of overseas-trained South Asian doctors in the UK, which was the main objective of my doctoral study, a case study approach was applied with the expectation that localities are likely to have an impact on individuals' identity and community cohesion experiences (Holy and Stuchlik 1981; Equally Ours 2007). The study included twenty-seven in-depth interviews with overseas-trained South Asian doctors practising as GPs in the UK.

Areas with contrasting features were selected as case studies. For example, Manchester is a large urban area with high ethnic density, Sheffield an urban area with an ethnic density the same as the national average and Barnsley an ex-mining town with rural characteristics and very low ethnic density. The sample was selected using the snowballing method, and a thematic analysis was undertaken using Nvivo computer software. The themes developed included reasons for migration, experiences in the NHS, entrepreneurship, identity, experiences of racism and coping strategies, sense of belonging to Britain and the doctor–patient relationship. The interviewees were aged between 50 and 76, with the majority of doctors concentrated in the 60–75 age band. The characteristics of the doctors in the study and case study areas are illustrated in Table 9.1 and Table 9.2 respectively.

Table 9.1 Ethnic, gender and religious breakdown of GPs in the case study areas.

Ethnic origin	Sheffield		Barnsley		Manchester		Religion	
	Male	Female	Male	Female	Male	Female	Hindu	Muslim
Indian	7	1	2	1	6	1	14	4
Pakistani	3	0	4	1	1	0	0	9
Total	10	1	6	2	7	1	14	13

Table 9.2 Characteristics of geographical locales.

	Characteristics of place	Place
1	A major urban area with high ethnic density	Manchester
2	A large urban area with average ethnic density	Sheffield
3	A semi-rural area with low ethnic density	Barnsley

A cornerstone of the process in interpretive research is the researcher's own reflexivity (Paulus et al. 2008), as the researcher is always implicated in the research process of all qualitative methodologies in one way or another (Willig 1995). Personal reflexivity is related to the researcher's contribution to the research process. It is defined as follows by Willig (1995): 'Personal reflexivity involves reflecting upon the ways in which our own values, experiences, interests, beliefs, political commitments, wider aims in life and social identities have shaped the research'.

Bolognani (2007) refers to literature which places emphasis on interview matching' in the context of ethnic or linguistic similarity. I believe that the experiences of being a migrant, an Asian and a woman, of having had several professional roles in the UK and of being 'othered' while living in Britain served me well in enriching the quality of my research (Oguntokun 1998) and that my attributes enabled the participants to disclose information which may be regarded as of a highly sensitive nature (Song and Parker 1995). Moss (2002) takes the above a step further and questions the type of epistemology applied in research (such as Marxist, anti-racist or feminist), arguing that feminist scholars have had to fight not only for 'knowledge' to include 'women's voices' but also that the data might be affected by the gender of the researchers and the researched. The principles of anti-racist research are explained by Dei and Johal (2005) as follows: 'Anti-racist research does not just deal with "social facts", it is also about how people interpret those facts, how the researcher interprets those interpretations, contextualizes them, and assists the subject in developing theoretical understandings of their lived experiences.'

The epistemology of my research study was very much influenced by the above-mentioned perspectives.

From Migration to Settlement

In order to understand the subsequent relationships that the doctors in the study form with individuals and communities around them, it is important to understand the context of their migration. This section provides detailed descriptive accounts of the doctors that relate to their motivation to migrate and which sum up the economic, social, political and cultural practices involved in the migration process. It also provides a brief overview of how the doctors navigated the UK medical system upon arrival.

Migration Systems Theory comprises all dimensions of the migration experience incorporating the historical colonial link and has much to offer in analysing the complex sets of factors involved and how they interact with each other to facilitate migration. The approach adopted under this theory is based on a fundamental principle which assumes that a migratory movement is a consequence of the interaction of macro-micro-structures which are linked by a number of other intermediary agents known as meso-structures. The macro-structures are concerned with institutional factors, government policies etc., whereas micro-structures relate to the motivation of individuals/groups and their social networks. The meso-structures consist of intermediaries (such as recruitment agents) linking the macro- and micro-structures (Castles and Miller 2003).

The macro-structures include the laws, relationships and practices between sending and receiving countries that occurred in order to control migration settlement. They can act as lubricators in the migration process (Castles and Miller 2003). Esmail (2007) provides a detailed account of the historical back-ground of the migration of South Asian doctors in the UK.

In this section, I will focus on the micro-structures that relate to the moti-vation of individuals/groups and their social networks. Micro-approaches also relate to the processes underlying the decision to migrate and the influences that come to bear on the individual's decision to migrate and the choice of destination (Stillwell and Congdon 1991).

Almost all the doctors stated that their primary purpose for migration was to obtain a postgraduate medical qualification which linked with their career aspirations. Several interviewees of both Indian and Pakistani origin talked about the perceived superiority of UK qualifications in their countries of origin and the value that they add to one's human capital.

Migration to the UK was associated with academic opportunities. The ability to work with renowned professors and within prestigious hospitals in the UK, as well as to gain practical experience and clinical excellence, were things that cropped up in numerous accounts and were described as a tradition for those doctors migrating to the UK.

The historical colonial context may explain the urge of the doctors in the study to invest in their human capital by acquiring a Western education which would promise them social status in such a prestigious profession (Husband 1982). The majority of the interviewees in this study described how they had a preconceived image of the UK as a 'paradise'. Their accounts provide evidence of how an English-medium education, the school curriculum and the role of missionaries led to the mythologisation of England and impacted on their social lives as ex-colonised people. This impact is likely to be particularly strong for those towards the top of the status hierarchy which most of these doctors were. Two-thirds of the interviewees confirmed that family had played a significant part in planning to move.

Lahiri (2000) also contends that obtaining a British qualification was rarely an individual choice, and that parental aspirations lay behind this undertaking, for they perceived it as a window of opportunity for their children and an English hallmark that would be a ticket to success.

Van Manen (1990) refers to inter-related cultural, social and political complexities of migration which the interviewees in this study also identified as reasons for coming to Britain. Structural inequalities based on caste and class were cited as the most common reasons by interviewees of both Indian and Pakistani origin.

Apart from the influence of Western education, motivations for moving to the UK were also described in the cultural context. Culture can be defined in terms of language, religion and values (Castles and Miller 2003). The findings of this study lend support for Hagan and Ebaugh (2003) who argue that the role of religion and spirituality in the stages of migratory process has been neglected by scholars of both immigration and the sociology of religion, despite its prominence in immigrants' lives. The interviewees described how they were influenced by the revolutionary literary writings and Urdu poetry of their era. The following Muslim Pakistani origin interviewee explained by reciting the following poetic verse which he said had been inspirational for him in his decision to migrate; it also indicates how his faith shaped his way of thinking:

> When I was young, I used to read this Urdu poetry which I found very inspirational:
>> Mohabat mujhe un jwanu se hey,
>> Sitarun pa jo dalten hey Kamand.
> [Explains the meaning] The poet says, 'I love those kinds of people who have the ability to capture stars by throwing a noose at them'. What is meaningful here is that one must not make poverty or other problems as excuse. My own interpretation of this is that you try, God will then help. (GP2S)

For GP2S, reaching out to the stars equated with coming to the UK as it was considered a huge achievement in his era and he proved that with his determination he was able to do what may have been undoable for many. The majority of the doctors in the study referred to the strong cultural influences and values that they had been brought up with and which included the belief about *takdir* (destiny), that it is 'He who makes the plans and you are destined to it by your creator' (Sayeed 2006).

The migrants' creative use of religion was clearly evident in their accounts, not only in their decision-making processes, but also with regard to its provision as a spiritual resource.

Entry into General Practice

A very common experience among interviewees upon arrival to the UK was that of working at several temporary locum jobs, which generally lasted three to six months, followed by a longer job lasting a year, although in some situations it lasted only a few weeks. Specialties considered less prestigious were cited as their most common areas of work.

The push factors described for entry into general practice were listed as: harsh working conditions; mostly working as junior doctors despite having several years of experience in their country of origin; frequently moving to temporary jobs in areas of high demand; and being pigeonholed in the least desired specialties. Most stated that they were stagnating in jobs that did not relate to their career progression and there was no planned career path. A few interviewees stated that they had progressed to the post of a registrar, although they knew that they were going to be held back at some stage, as they had seen this happening frequently to their friends and colleagues. Many were unable to pass part of the postgraduate qualification exams, in part because their clinical experience did not relate to the desired qualification. Returning home was not an option as they were caught up in the migratory process, so for many the only viable option was that of general practice.

The role of institutional racism in the NHS was acknowledged by several of the doctors in the study:

> The bad thing here is that if you were competing with a local doctor, no matter how good you were, the English or the Scottish will always get the job. There is discrimination, and the thing is you could not even complain about it as it would be noted and then it will follow you wherever you go for the job and then you will have difficulty. (GP3B)

The above quote suggests that the interviewees were well aware of widespread discrimination and victimisation, but felt unable to complain given the existence of power inequalities and the likely implications for them if they were to speak up against more powerful people.

Ellis et al. (2007) argue that spatial accessibility to jobs may well be just as significant as social access to jobs. The majority of the interviewees stated that there was also a glass ceiling in GP jobs in sought-after practices which would be offered to 'local lads' (White British) first, whereas the overseas-trained South Asian doctors would only be successful if there was no competition.

The accounts of the doctors showed how, with determination and the use of their entrepreneurial skills, they were able to transform many deserted practices into something special, even outstanding. Other interviewees talked about utilising structure and agency for the transformations they undertook, which can be evidenced by the following:

> Yes someone was working there before, a White doctor; he moved to Spain, the practice was very deprived, debilitated. He was doing that Spanish practice for almost over a year, neglecting this altogether, so it was really neglected,

yes living in two places, hardly any . . . there wasn't even a list, only four or five patients. I did a lot, you see, that practice, you see, was in one of those terraced houses and hardly anything there, so then I think within three years more or less I built up a beautiful purpose-built practice in the area, and then it was like jungle mein mungal.[1] The result was in a few years' time I got the GP of the Year Award. (GP4M).

The following section provides evidence of how the doctors continued to integrate their cultural and/or religious values into their adaptation to Britain, importing innovation into their everyday experiences.

The Medical Encounters

The doctors' accounts show a variation in the experiences of the doctor–patient relationship. This relationship appeared to be stronger in Barnsley than in Sheffield and Manchester, even though the context of Barnsley was less reflective of the doctors' cultural identities. One interviewee described his patients as part of an extended family and others talked about having a strong bond with their patients. Emphasis was placed on respect by several of the interviewees:

My view is that you will only give me respect if I give you respect. (GP2B)

The following interviewee's account suggests that learning occurred on the part of both doctor and patient:

When I came I couldn't understand the dialect, because in the hospital surroundings it is different, whereas in general practice, they just, they use their own dialect, you see. I found it difficult . . . I couldn't understand, so I had to get my receptionist to come and tell me what they were on about [laughs], particularly 'tatoes', this gentleman would say that . . . 'tatoes' . . . potatoes . . . [laughs], he was going on saying . . . They could follow me but it is the bounce with dialect, you see. It is not too bad now, it used to be quite strong, the Barnsley accent, at that time in the 70s. (GP1B)

The above account suggests that such experiences contributed towards breaking the ice and the doctor and patient getting to know one another; these encounters were likely to have been instrumental in dismantling the power hierarchy which existed due to the dynamics of race, class and doctor–patient status. The fact that

---

[1] An Urdu expression meaning 'transforming a place from dry woodland into a wonderland'.

many interviewees experienced geographical isolation in rural areas where they had no immediate family or even community members may have created a need for the South Asian doctors to have a strong bond with their patients.

The integration of cultural values on a conscious and unconscious level was apparent in many of the interviewees' accounts, and helped build trust with White patients:

> When I see the patients on the streets, they always tell me how much they appreciate the service. When I stop and talk to them, I know most of them and I always ask how is your son, your daughter etc., I do this as an Indian because family values are ingrained in us, as you know, we are so used to asking about mama, chacha, baba [uncle, old man] you know, I didn't realise they would appreciate it so much, they feel good about it that I take an interest in them and their families, and that they appreciate it very much. Once I asked a patient, 'How is your dog with spots?' She said, 'Oh the dog died a while ago, but you have a good memory, doctor'. (GP1M)

He goes on to explain that through his interactions he learnt that White working-class family values were not so dissimilar to his own cultural values:

> I sometimes find similarities between White working-class family values and our culture, our experiences, they care and support for their families sometimes in the same way as we do. They appreciate it when I ask them about their extended family, there is class distinction here, and a vast majority of doctors in this country tend to be from the upper middle class, and I am not sure if a middle-class doctor from here would take an interest in what his/her [patient's] family are up to. These little things go a long way to build a trusting relationship between me and my patients and trust is so important in our doctor–patient relationship. (GP1M)

Evidence shows that the elite professionals incorporated their religious and spiritual beliefs into their practice. For example, the following interviewee states:

> I found myself often working with poor people for whom sometimes I could do little as a doctor to change their social circumstances. But I remember that one of our poets had once said '*Dard ke dawa na sehei, dard sun he liya hota*' [if you cannot cure pain, at least you could have just listened to it], so there was a lot of that. I could relate to some of the things, coming from Kashmir, where I had seen deprivation and poverty directly in the communities that I had worked with. (GP8S)

The doctor–patient relationship in Sheffield and Manchester was described as being more of a mixed nature. Working with marginalised communities, both White and Asian, as marginalised practitioners and the challenges that brought were mentioned by several of the interviewees:

> The English patients that we had, [they] were actually the ones no 'local' doctors wanted to keep as these patients were very demanding. (GP1M)

The accounts of the doctors in the study show that the nature of doctor–patient encounters had been shaped by the historical colonial context and this was more evident when working in deprived inner city practice areas.

> . . . some would show their arrogance by their body language that they were superior than us. You see they feel superior because they have ruled over you for hundreds of years or more, you know, they feel they are superior than all over the world not just us, they have colonised every part of the world. We did not think of the white working class as coming from lower strata because before us, they were English first. (GP10S)

Another interviewee's account points to the social hierarchies that exist within the UK social class system. He adds that being migrant doctors, their focus was on performing their duty well:

> We had no concept of demanding/non-demanding patients, we saw ourselves as the provider of the service and that we had to do our duty. These patients were very appreciative of our services and they had a lot of respect for us. In fact we often used to give their examples to our own community patients who were sometimes yelling for more help and we used to say, look at these patients who are so content with so little etc. These English patients were rejected by others but for us they were still better than our own in terms of their demands. (GP5M)

The above account refers to a number of issues such as the incorporation of cultural values which emphasise a sense of duty and the issues of working in deprived areas where patients are classified as demanding. The experiences of the marginalisation of overseas-trained South Asian doctors within the NHS may have better equipped them to empathise with patients from disadvantaged backgrounds, and their accounts provide evidence of insight into the symbiotic relationships that occur between marginalised practitioner and marginalised patients.

The account below would suggest that marginalised White working-class patients benefited from the perseverance of overseas-trained South Asian doctors:

At that time, if you were not happy with a patient, you simply wrote a letter for the patient stating that you were not happy to continue providing a service for them and then they had to find another one from the NHS list. I remember some patients used to say that they did not have a problem with me, why was I de-registering them, so I didn't in the end, and they were the ones who stayed in my surgery until I retired and were forever grateful for the service they received. (GP5M)

Interviewees talked about the diverse healthcare needs of their patients and the demands placed on the Asian doctors. In ethnically dense areas such as Manchester and Sheffield, the interviewees' accounts appeared less sympathetic to the issues confronting the South Asian patients, which may be linked to the complexity of the patients' healthcare needs.

The interviewees stated that being part of the same cultural group as the patient was both a benefit and a hindrance. Ahmad et al. (1991) also found a prevalence of less favourable attitudes among Asian doctors towards Asian patients. This may be due to a number of issues. Ethnic inequalities in health and healthcare is an area which has been well researched (Bhopal 2008; McAvoy and Donaldson 1990). Meeting the linguistic and cultural needs of such patients in deprived locales must place a disproportionate burden on overseas-trained South Asian doctors. Scaife et al. (2000) argued that South Asian patients are more likely to be frequent attendees at a GP practice. The Asian patients may regard Asian doctors as a member of their own community and make unrealistic demands on them. The Asian doctors, on the other hand, may not have wanted to be pigeonholed in the roles that were ascribed to them, that is to work with predominantly Asian patients, as some interviewees stated earlier. The difference in class identity of overseas-trained South Asian doctors and Asian patients may have acted as an additional barrier.

Interviewees in Manchester talked about the ever-changing demography of inner city practices, and meeting the needs and expectations of diverse communities such as Irish, Chinese, Polish and Nigerian. They described the transient nature of the population in an inner city practice.

Cutchin (1997) argues that the interaction between physician and the physical environment of a place presents challenges and responses and within such processes lies the act of integration. Cutchin adds that the physician becomes woven into the social fabric of the place through interacting, over time, with the evolving problems that exist in that place. The following account shows how specific contextual embedding was achieved by one of the doctors in the study:

There was a lot of community activities that I and other Asian doctors used to go to, there might be a dance, there might have been a pea and pie, whatever, small things, you know. I have a reasonably high profile in the community; I have served as a local councillor, well, this MBE was given to me by recommendation by my patients who are 99.9 per cent White . . . for my services in medicine. I am involved in charity work, there is the 'Lions club'.[2] (GP2B)

The above account shows the interaction of an overseas-trained South Asian doctor with lower- and higher-class strata that includes participation in community activities such as dancing, and pea and pie parties, which specifically relate to the culture of a working-class mining community. In rural areas, the interviewees talked about ways of embedding at both a social and professional level, for example through the membership of rotary clubs and golf clubs as well as getting involved in fundraising shows in the local area. Together with other innovative activities instigated by their practices, this projects an image of the doctors in the study as individuals who were genuinely interested in the wellbeing of local communities. The scarcity of resources in rural environments went hand in hand with the entrepreneurial spirit of the interviewees and such contexts provided them with perfect places in which to grow.

Bhabha (1994) refers to the Theory of Mimicry, whereby some of the Indians and Africans (colonised) imitated the language, dress, politics or cultural attitude of the British (colonisers). This is seen as opportunistic pattern of behaviour in which an individual copies the person in power so as to have access to that same power within the context of colonialism and immigration. In this case, membership of the Lions Club can be regarded as class membership which cannot be gained solely by one's job, but rather is a way of 'mimicking' a culture of that class which dictates its terms. Lahiri (2000) states that this theory can be reworked to apply to a specific historic moment and draws on a historical case in 1899 where an Indian student, Wagle, got an apprenticeship with a factory in Britain to study the British glass industry. In combating enormous hostility based on race and his middle-class status, Wagle learned that the greatest hostility he faced was due to his class and came from the factory workers rather than the factory owners, with one worker telling him, 'We hate all gents the same'. He therefore decided to integrate 'not in gentleman's clothes but as a fellow workman'. By adopting a cosmetic change and using phrases such as 'old chap' and 'chappie', shaking hands, acquainting himself with the workers' home lives and being aware of what was acceptable and unacceptable in that distinct working-class culture, Wagle eventually became accepted. Lahiri (2000) comments on this outward assimilation:

Wagle camouflaged his appropriation of imperial knowledge by adopting a mask of assimilation. But this time mimcry is relocated, away from the

---

[2] The Lions Club is a charitable organisation that serves the needs of local and global communities. Its ethos is that working together to initiate and carry out projects will make the community a better place. See www.lionsclubs.org/EN/our-work/index.php

colonial periphery to the metropolitan centre, Britain, and the new class dimension causes Wagle (the colonised) to mimic British working-class, metropolitan culture rather than middle-class, colonial culture.

It would appear from the interviewees' accounts that their interactions with the subsets of pluralist British society reflected both Bhaba's and Lahiri's approaches. The interviewees' accounts show that their own characteristics such as exposure to Western education in the countries of origin, professional status, and the specific characteristics of the place such as rural context and its need to sustain healthcare provision, may have facilitated the integration process.

The challenges of working in rural practices included dealing with complex chronic diseases as most of the patient population was described as ex-coalminers. The interviewees' accounts show sensitivity and empathy to the social context and the realities of most of the white working-class patients as they described how the occupation of mineworkers affected the life chances of those patients, and the ensuing demands placed on the doctors. It appears that the ethnicity of the doctors was also a resource here as many talked about the usefulness of their expertise gained in the country of origin:

> They [the miners] would invite us, just to get an idea of how people are working inside mines . . . sometimes they had to really, you know, crawl through small places [pause] people were getting more neck pain, sickness, chronic chest diseases, fortunately most of us [Asian doctors] had ample experiences of those illnesses from our own countries. (GP1S)

The empathy described in several of the interviewees' accounts towards the miners' circumstances shows that they engaged not only with the patients but also with the social contexts of those patients:

> I was aware that paperwork needed to be completed there and then. I mean like any compensation because people with mines . . . there were lots of people with pneumoconiosis [lung disease acquired in mines] and for pneumoconiosis, they had to give compensation, people were suffering a lot really. We had to write letters in a particular way and as quickly as possible. Sometimes you have to do more details . . . he [the patient] cannot breathe properly, he's out of breath like that he needs medication, and again these are those things because they were really working very hard, and in very adverse circumstances, you know they have to be inside long time, and they were getting this disease because of the . . . mine dust. (GP1S)

The ability and opportunity to achieve a vision and develop something of their own in the form of providing enhanced primary care services, and reducing the cost of secondary and tertiary care, was seen by many interviewees as offering the freedom to practise holistic medicine and continuity of care. Two of the female interviewees talked about focusing on offering enhanced primary care services for pregnant women and their newborn babies, services that did not previously exist. They were proud of their achievements, as previously female patients had had to travel long distances to attend hospital antenatal appointments whereas these services were brought to their doorsteps, as a result of the doctors' entrepreneurial activities that they undertook extensively to maximise opportunities.

Networking with local people on an individual level was instrumental and a reciprocal relationship appears to have existed in several of the interviewees' accounts. For example, one interviewee described how networking with a local woman, a retired tax officer, helped him become familiar with tax affairs; another mentioned how an ex-senior council manager, who subsequently worked for him, expanded his local links. Female interviewees talked about networking with local women for childcare arrangements. Such relationships appeared deeper and warmer than simply professional networking. Integration into the social fabric of the local community was evidenced in numerous accounts that showed that despite having multiple identities, human relationships often took precedence over any other social hierarchy:

> I had a patient [white male] who was always cleaning the outside area of my medical centre. I did not even know this until one day, he came in to see me, his hands had scratches all over and were bleeding. I said to him, 'What have you done to your hands?' He said, 'Oh nothing much.' It was then that I found out that it was him. He said I was just cleaning the bushes; actually I want to keep your place tidy. He died two weeks after. His wife was struggling a little after he died. I employed her as a cleaner. She became very friendly with my wife – it was like a mother–daughter relationship. I had many more positive relationships with local patients. I had 30 per cent our own patients and 70 per cent English patients. (GP4S)

Beider (2011) argues that in much of the literature, individuals belonging to White working-class communities are variously portrayed as perpetrators of racial harassment, antagonistic to immigration and with fixed views. However, the account above and others in the study show that there can be a bond between individuals that is not always shaped by racialised experiences. The interviewees mentioned such positive encounters with patients with some passion; these were memories they continued to treasure several years after their retirement. The interviewee below talks about how she 'bonded' with the families of patients:

So you go there and see all your patients and then they tell you what goes on in their family, so by going, by talking to them, yes . . . yes, by talking to them they will tell me everything, what goes on in their family, you see, so I would help as much as I could, whatever the system I needed to approach, so that's how I became well bonded to the community. Even now when I go there, the little ones . . . 'Doctor, do you remember me?' (GP1B)

Almost all the interviewees were able to recall occasions where they felt moved by having pleasant encounters with patients, and which strengthened their sense of belonging to Britain. The combination of place and person influences the integration process and leads to variation within the integration experiences (Cutchin 1997). The interviewees' accounts show that factors such as their exposure to Western education in their country of origin, their professional status and the specific characteristics of the place such as rural context and its need to sustain healthcare provision, may have facilitated the integration process.

With regard to identification with British identity, the interviewees frequently evaluated new situations through their old frame of reference, i.e. their own cultural/religious value system, and drew meanings from what they already knew. Below is a response from a doctor from a Pakistani Muslim background:

Adaptation . . . that question is very debatable, very hot question, if you take the religious point of view, there is a story that Umar Ibn Khattab [the second Caliph of Islam] was going from one city to another and was wearing silk that day. People objected and said to him, 'Hey, how come you are wearing silk when Islam forbids men to wear silk?' He said, 'The area that I am going to go, they wear silk there'. So, my learning from that is that *jaisa desh waisa bhais*' [when in London, do as the Londoners do]. (GP7S)

The study showed that the interviewees were not immune from racism, though there was spatial variation in the level of racial prejudice they experienced. Doctors were more likely to experience subtle racism in inner city areas.

Cox (1948) argues that racial prejudice is a social attitude that is propagated by the exploiting class against another group, stigmatising it as inferior in order to justify its own exploitation of its resources. Cox calls into play not only the economic relations that account for prejudice but also historical events such as colonisation which was justified by the Whites by stereotyping Blacks as inferiors who were seen as the 'white man's burden'. Cox, however, adds that the broader macro-level forces are mediated through a series of factors in which locality and personal circumstances at an individual level play a role. Such intersectionality was observed in the case study areas. For example, the interviewees referred to situations where their ethnicity created positive social capital for them, as the only non-White people in certain villages were the doctors. The intersectionality of race, the medical profession and their situations coupled with the remote areas' need for medical professionals mitigated against prejudice and enabled local people to use such cues not to exclude these migrant doctors. This can be evidenced by the following account:

> It's true that I also integrate my own religious values, e.g. I always say *Bismilaha* which means 'in the name of God' and aim to have good relations with patients. Sometimes, I do explain about my religion as well if someone is interested in knowing. I used to write *Bismilaha* on prescriptions. Once a White patient asked what it was. I said, 'This is my belief and I wish you good health'. The patient took it very well. In Qur'an it says '*Shifah unnas*', which means that it gives people physical as well as spiritual health, I say *dua* [prayer] when I see very ill patients. I hold their hand and recite *dua*. (GP7S)

He adds:

> The elderly people are neglected in this country, the sons and daughters don't like to know them, I mean British people. When I used to visit patients in hospital, I used to hold their hands and do dua because I believe dua has healing power, it certainly did good for patients spiritual health, they used to ask me when I was coming again. (GP7S)

The interviewees' accounts show that they negotiate belonging discursively and by the repositioning of self. Many of the interviewees talked about playing a role concerning the unmet needs of their own communities, but also contributing to enhancing community cohesion by connecting individuals with institutions:

> I used to teach Asian children the Qur'an because there was no proper system for religious teachings; they were children of Indian, Pakistani, Bengali Muslim families. I have been a chaplain for a long time and I visit patients in all of the hospitals in the city. Sometimes when someone dies and there is no relative for Muslim families around, I also organise for a Muslim burial. (GP7S)

Conclusion

This chapter set out to investigate the experiences of South Asian migrant doctors practising as GPs in different geographical locales of the UK. It focused on the evidence relating to how the doctors in the study build unique doctor–patient relationships in diverse contexts.

It was evident that these doctors had mixed experiences of being elite and marginalised simultaneously. The findings show that the standard theories concerning the sociocultural dimension of Western medicine do not fully reflect the experiences of overseas-trained South Asian GPs. The asymmetry in power relationships in the clinical discourse is reversed when this encounter is between a White patient and an overseas-trained South Asian migrant doctor, as both bring an imperial element into the encounter. The specific UK contexts serve as spaces where the identities of practitioners and patients are simultaneously negotiated against a backdrop of the legacy of the Empire. The insights into their doctor–patient relationships show that the South Asian migrant doctors may have been able to form relationships that were more of a reciprocal nature than one of medical dominance.

There were numerous examples that the interviewees were able to recall where there was an element of cohesiveness felt despite race and class differences. Just a few such examples are the adoption of a name given by an English nanny to an interviewee's daughter; a doctor describing how a white patient undertook gardening work at the back of his GP surgery without the interviewee's knowledge; another doctor saying how an encounter with a patient brought tears to her eyes because he waited for a considerable length of time outside a shop to be able to talk to her after she had been retired for several years; and another doctor repeatedly referring to his White patients as his 'extended family'.

The study showed how the interviewees had developed strategies to meet the needs of their diverse patient population and appear to have obtained the patients' trust. There was evidence that the interviewees had been able to dismantle the power relationships in their encounters with marginalised White patients. They believed that the experiences in their country of origin had prepared them to meet the needs of diverse communities, especially deprived rural communities. The doctors' ability to engage with not only with patients but also with the social contexts of those patients was evident throughout their accounts, which I believe helped build trust between them and the patients. The specific UK contexts served as spaces where the identities of doctors and patients were simultaneously negotiated. These contexts had a cooperative task at stake and shared common goals in environments.

This chapter has highlighted the need to have a diverse NHS workforce that understands the needs of marginalised communities. Examples of good practice can be developed from further exploration in this area.

Acknowledgements

I would like to acknowledge the doctors who were part of this study and without whom this chapter would not have been possible. I am grateful for their time, enthusiasm and for sharing their personal stories concerning their migration trajectories. I would like to extend my gratitude to the Economic and Social Research Council for providing the funding that enabled me to carry out this study and the case partner, British Association of Physicians of Indian Origin, for co-sponsoring. I am grateful for the support of my supervisory team that consisted of Dr Kingsley Purdam, Prof. Rob Ford, Prof. Aneez Esmail and Prof. Tarani Chandola at the University of Manchester.

References

Ahmad, W. U., Baker, M. R. and Kernohan, E. M. (1991). 'General practitioners' perceptions of Asian and non-Asian patients'. *Family Practice*, 8(1), 52–6.

Beider, H. (2011). 'Community cohesion: the views of white working-class communities. Joseph Rowntree Foundation. Available at: www.jrf.org.uk/sites/default/files/jrf/migrated/files/working-class-community-cohesion-full.pdf (last accessed 12 May 2022).

Bhabha, H. (1994). *The Location of Culture*. London: Routledge.

Bhopal, R. S. (2008). *Ethnicity, Race, and Health in Multicultural Societies: Foundations for Better Epidemiology, Public Health, and Health Care*. Oxford: Oxford University Press.

Bolognani, M. (2007). 'The myth of return: dismissal, survival or revival? A Bradford example of transnationalism as a political instrument'. *Journal of Ethnic and Migration Studies*, 33(1), 59–76.

Bury, M. and Monaghan, L. (2013). 'Practitioner-client relationships', in J. Gabe and L. Monaghan (eds), *Key Concepts in Medical Sociology*. London: SAGE Publications Ltd.

Castles, S. and Miller, M. J. (2003). *The Age of Migration: International Population Movements in the Modern World*. London: Macmillan Press Ltd.

Cox, O. C. (1948). *Caste, Class and Race*. New York: Doubleday.

Cutchin, M. P. (1997). 'Physician retention in rural communities: the perspective of experiential place integration'. *Health & Place*, 3(1), 25–41.

Dei, G. J. S. and Johal, G. S. (2005). *Critical Issues in Anti-racist Research Methodologies*. New York: Peter Lang.

Ellis, M., Wright, R. and Parks, V. (2007). 'Geography and the immigrant division of labor'. *Economic Geography*, 83(3), 255–81.

Equally Ours (2007). 'Commission on Integration and Cohesion final report'. Available at: https://www.equallyours.org.uk/commission-on-integration-and-cohesion-final-report (last accessed 14 July 2022).

Esmail, A. (2007). 'Asian doctors in the NHS: service and betrayal'. *British Journal of General Practice*, 57(543), 827–34.

Farooq, Y. G. (2020). *Elite Migrants: South Asian Doctors in the UK*. London: Transnational Press.

Hagan, J. and Ebaugh, H. R. (2003). 'Calling upon the sacred: migrants' use of religion in the migration process'. *International Migration Review*, 37(4), 1145–62.

Holy, L. and Stuchlik, M. (1981). *The Structure of Folk Models*. London: Academic Press.

Husband, C. (1982). 'Racial prejudice and the concept of social identity', *Ethnic Minorities and Community Relations, Part One*. Open University.

Lahiri, S. (2000). *Indians in Britain: Anglo-Indian Encounters, Race and Identity, 1880–1930*. London: Routledge.

Lupton, D. (2012). *Medicine as Culture: Illness, Disease and the Body*. London: SAGE Publications Ltd.

McAvoy, B. R. and Donaldson, L. J. (1990). *Health Care for Asians*. Oxford: Oxford University Press.

Moss, P. J. (2002). *Feminist Geography in Practice: Research and Methods*. Oxford: Blackwell.

Oguntokun, R. (1998). 'A lesson in the seductive power of sameness: representing Black African refugee women'. *Feminism & Psychology*, 8(4), 525–9.

Paulus, T. M., Woodside, M. and Ziegler, M. (2008). 'Extending the conversation: qualitative research as dialogic collaborative process'. *The Qualitative Report*, 13(2), 226–43.

Sayeed, A. A. (2006). *In the Shadow of My Taqdir*. Durham: Memoir Club.

Scaife, B., Gill, P., Heywood, P. and Neal, R. (2000). 'Socio-economic characteristics of adult frequent attenders in general practice: secondary analysis of data'. *Family Practice*, 17(4), 298–304.

Song, M. and Parker, D. (1995). 'Commonality, difference and the dynamics of disclosure in in-depth interviewing'. *Sociology*, 29(2), 241–56.

Stillwell, J. C. H. and Congdon, P. (1991). *Migrations Models: Macro and Micro Approaches*, London: Belhaven Press.

Van Manen, M. (1990). *Researching Lived Experience: Human Science for an Action Sensitive Pedagogy*. New York: Suny Press.

Willig, C. (1995). *Introducing Qualitative Research in Psychology*. Milton Keynes: Open University Press.

PART 3

THERAPEUTIC INTERVENTIONS

10

ISLAMOPHOBIA MAKES US SICK: THE HEALTH COSTS OF ISLAMOPHOBIA IN THE UK

Hina J. Shahid

Introduction

R acial inequities in social and health outcomes are well documented. How-ever, understanding the impact of Islamophobia, one of the most preva-lent discriminatory systems, is limited. In this chapter I look at Islamophobia as a global and intersectional system of oppression, exploitation and exclusion which produces discrimination, disadvantage and disparities. These shape Brit-ish institutions and society and impact the health of structurally pathologised populations and individuals. I draw on cross-disciplinary frameworks to anal-yse the multiple pathways through which Islamophobia directly, indirectly and intersectionally causes health inequities, mediating its effects through structural and social determinants, stigma and embodiment. I integrate public health and rights-based approaches with a unifying focus on ethics and justice to advocate the need to eliminate health inequities caused by Islamophobia.

A Brief History of Muslim Migration in the UK

Islam is the second largest religion in the UK with 2.8 million people, half of whom were born in the UK (ONS 2011; Elahi and Khan 2017). The presence of Islam in Europe spans centuries. Islamic culture influenced the arts, architecture, medicine, music, language, agriculture, law, education and technology in medieval Europe, laying the foundations of the European Renaissance (Essa and Ali 2012).

The majority of British Muslims have their origins in South Asia, reflecting British colonial legacy, but this demographic is shifting (MCB 2015). Muslim presence in the UK can be traced back to hundreds of years ago, when lascars and sailors arrived from the Indian subcontinent, South-East Asia and parts of the Middle East to work on docks (Ansari 2004). It was after the Second World War that destruction and labour shortages stimulated large-scale recruitment of British Commonwealth citizens, many of who were Muslim. Once the labour shortage was ameliorated, legislation was introduced by the British government to end large-scale migration, and after the 1970s migration shifted away from economic reasons to political and humanitarian emergencies, with refugees arriving from the the Middle East, Africa and Central Asia, and asylum seekers from the Muslim-majority European countries of Bosnia and Kosovo, creating an increasingly ethnically diverse community (Elahi and Khan 2017).

The first generation of Muslims felt strong ties to their home countries but from the early 1990s the prominence of an ethnic-centred identity has been gradually replaced with religious and faith-centred identification, particularly amongst second and third generations (Modood et al. 1997; Saeed et al. 1999). A 2001 Home Office Citizenship Survey found that for Muslims, religion was a more relevant marker of identity than ethnicity (O'Beirne 2004). Research also indicates that British Muslims feel a strong sense of religious identity, but that they are also more likely than the British public as a whole to say that their national identity as British is important to them (Kaur-Ballagan et al. 2018). Despite this, the concept of 'British Muslim' and 'British Islam' and what it means in relation to 'fundamental British values' has been the subject of fierce media and political debate and social tensions, opening the doors to discrimination.

Islamophobia in the UK: a System of Oppression

Islamophobia is a highly complex construct and the term has received much criticism as well as support. Islamophobia can be viewed as a system of oppression, exclusion and exploitation against Muslims within which discrimination takes place. This system is a product of historical and contemporary values and structures of power, privilege and dominance which 'hold down' a group, in this case Muslims. Islamophobia occurs on a spectrum, from values (principles), beliefs (ideas), attitudes (expressions) and behaviours (action).

In the UK, a consistent body of research shows that Muslims experience discrimination of a greater frequency and seriousness than other religious groups (Weller 2011). Discrimination is

> the process (or set of processes) by which people are allocated to particular social categories with an unequal distribution of rights, resources, opportunities and power, creating dominant and subordinate groups and enabling certain groups and individuals to be disadvantaged and oppressed. (Thompson 2017)

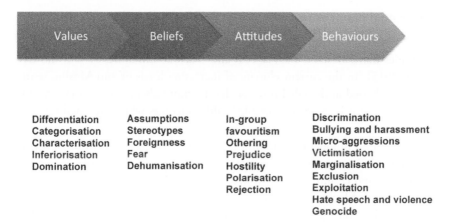

Values	Beliefs	Attitudes	Behaviours
Differentiation	Assumptions	In-group	Discrimination
Categorisation	Stereotypes	favouritism	Bullying and harassment
Characterisation	Foreignness	Othering	Micro-aggressions
Inferiorisation	Fear	Prejudice	Victimisation
Domination	Dehumanisation	Hostility	Marginalisation
		Polarisation	Exclusion
		Rejection	Exploitation
			Hate speech and violence
			Genocide

Figure 10.1 The spectrum of Islamophobia.

Linked to discrimination is the concept of stigma, defined as the 'co-occurrence of labelling, stereotyping, separation, status loss, and discrimination in a context in which power is exercised' (Hatzenbuehler et al. 2013).

The term Islamophobia was initially coined in the early 1900s (Allen 2016) but received widespread recognition in a 1997 Runnymede report (Elahi and Khan 2017). Islamophobia has been described as 'anti-Muslim racism' (ibid.) and as 'a type of racism that targets expressions of Muslimness or perceived Muslimness' (APPG 2018). The preference to view Islamophobia through the lens of racism is reflective of a secular liberal democracy like Britain. This secular awkwardness in acknowledging the contribution of religion-based discrimination is embedded in the Westphalian notion of the modern nation state being secular, a term which itself is frequently, and incorrectly, used interchangeably with atheist.

On the one hand, it is argued that while 'traditional' racist discourses based on biological differentiation have declined, those derived from perceptions of religious and cultural superiority now dominate expression of racism worldwide, creating a new type of 'racism without races' of which Islamophobia is a manifestation (Müller-Uri and Opratko 2016). However, while racism and religious discrimination may co-exist and are inter-related empirically, they are distinct analytically (Hussain and Bagguley 2012), as well as ideologically and legally. The Equalities legislation identifies race and religion as independent protected characteristics (UK Government 2010). Furthermore, 'religious discrimination may coexist with or supersede racial discrimination' (Laird et al. 2007a). Limiting the discriminatory experiences of Muslims centred on race alone underestimates the impact that Islamophobia has on individuals and societies.

Conceptual Framework

Health outcomes data on Muslim communities highlights the significant health disparities that Pakistani, Bangladeshi and Black communities face in the UK (MCB 2015). In the current climate of increasing levels of anti-Muslim sentiments and hatred in the UK I propose that Islamophobia is an important health determinant that leads to preventable health outcomes which are unethical and inequitable.

I integrate a number of frameworks to analyse the pathways through which Islamophobia impacts health outcomes. I argue that Islamophobia embedded in contexts and conditions contributes to multi-dimensional health inequities among British Muslims. These frameworks include the social determinants of health model (WHO 2008), theories of stigma (Hatzenbuehler et al. 2013) and concepts of embodiment (Krieger 2012). I conceptualise Islamophobia impacting health inequities through discrimination, disadvantage and disparities. Specifically, Islamophobia

1. is an intersectional system of oppression that affects multiple social and personal stratification axes experienced simultaneously and leads to discrimination, disadvantage and disparities
2. operates on multiple levels, from the global and societal to the individual, which are interacting and re-enforcing
3. is embedded in and an extension of spatiotemporal scales and sociocultural and historical contexts and in particular processes of oppression, exclusion and exploitation which shape current norms, values and structures
4. impacts health directly and indirectly through social determinants, stigma and embodiment
5. impacts multiple domains in a holistic model of health producing multi-dimensional disparities in health outcomes undermining capability, wellbeing and justice

Health outcomes are examined not only in terms of biological/physical health, but also psychosocial and spiritual wellbeing. The inclusion of the spiritual dimension, which is central to the identity of British Muslims, counters the epistemic religious discrimination inherent in the World Health Organization's (1995) secular description of health as a state of 'physical, mental and social well-being'.

Human rights, social justice and health are closely linked (Peñaranda 2015). Building further on the holistic view of health is the capability view which links wellbeing with social justice. A capability view of health assigns a special moral and ethical importance to health, arguing that health is a basic capability for human development (Nussbaum 2011) and that society has a moral obligation

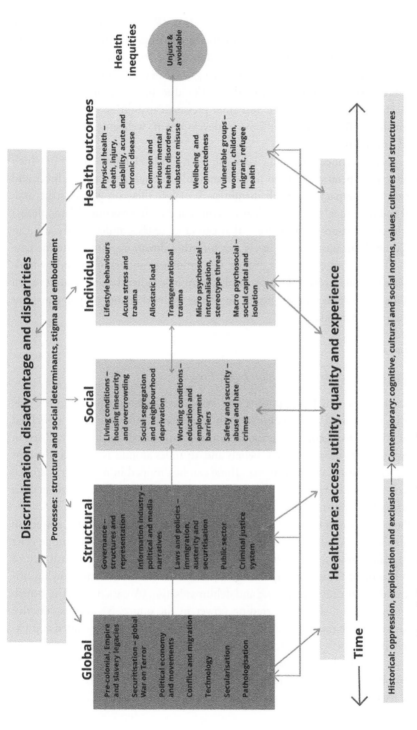

Figure 10.2 Islamophobia: an intersectional system of oppression.

to ensure freedom of wellbeing for every person (Ruger 2004). 'Functionings' are the 'beings and doings', and capabilities are the opportunities to be and do that which individuals and collectives value (Sen 1992). The role of capabilities and justice in global health is receiving increased attention (Khoo 2013). Discrimination, disadvantage and disparities due to Islamophobia operating and accumulating across space and time prevent capabilities and functionings of British Muslims and violate human development, wellbeing, and social and global health justice.

I apply this conceptual framework using a multi-level approach within which I analyse the operationalisation of Islamophobia through its direct, indirect and intersectional impact on health inequities. I analyse these on global, structural, social and individual levels, as well as junctures of their intersection. Islamophobia is an interactive and dynamic force that can cross levels simultaneously and can also 'jump' from upstream to levels much further down, bypassing intermediate levels. The healthcare system is unique as it influences and is influenced by multiple levels simultaneously. I choose health inequities rather than inequalities as an outcome measure because the health outcomes analysed are not only unequal but also unjust and avoidable.

Global Level

Internationalism: globalisation and glocalisation

The current wave of Islamophobia and associated health inequities in the UK must be understood in the context of an increasingly interdependent globalised world with convergent policies and cultures manifested locally, as well as an extension of pre-existing values, beliefs and attitudes around Islam and Muslims that span centuries and continents. These can be grouped into temporal, spatial and cognitive/cultural factors and will be mentioned here briefly as a full analysis is outside the scope of this chapter.

Pre-colonial events of the Crusades and the Spanish Reconquista centred on the ideology of Muslims as foreign invaders destroying a Christian Europe (Fitz 2009). This paved the way for brutal colonial rule through the construction of racial hierarchies based on superior genetics and culture and accompanying orientalist ideology causing othering and dehumanisation (Ansari 2003). The British Empire was also a dominant trading power in the oppressive and exploitative transatlantic slave trade (Jensen 2012). At its height, the Empire included approximately half of the world's Muslim population (Robinson 1999), and in the slave trade an estimated 30 per cent of slaves brought to America were Muslim, who then took on the name and religion of their Christian masters (Hill et al. 2005). These legacies of colonialism and slavery, which led to widespread and extensively documented illness, famine and deaths, continue to shape health outcomes and produce inequities.

Eleventh September 2001 ('9/11') was a watershed moment for relations between Islam and the West that resulted in the securitisation and criminalisation of the Muslim identity, and legitimisation of the War on Terror. This destabilised large parts of the Middle East and contributes to the ongoing wave of refugees and migrants to Europe, the majority of whom come from Muslim-majority countries (Pew Research Center 2017). This has deepened the divide between the West and Muslims, turning Muslims into a common enemy, defined predominantly by their religion rather than by ethnicity, nation of origin, sect, class or profession (Ahmed 2018). These events have also fuelled the rise of nationalistic and populist movements in the West and multiple Islamophobic policies across the world, intensifying stigma and social and structural discrimination.

Islamophobia is a transnational problem that spans borders; the Muslim Bosnian genocide (Mann et al. 1994), violence in Muslim-majority Kosovo (Wang et al. 2010), the public health crises in Indian-administered Muslim-majority Kashmir (Mirza 2019), persecution of the Rohingya community with poor healthcare access and outcomes (Mahmood et al. 2017), Chinese internment 're-education' camps for Muslim Uighurs (Stubley 2019) and barriers to healthcare services in Occupied Palestinian Territories (Giacaman et al. 2009) are all examples of Islamophobia's far-reaching and serious global health impact.

In a global world with increased political interactions between the West and Islam, the ideology of orientalism which promotes the 'West-and-Islam dualism' and the dehumanisation of 'the Other' has been reshaped, redistributed and accentuated, creating a new form of 'neo-orientalism' (Samiei 2010). Globalised Western imperialism produces norms and values centred on Eurocentric concepts of modernity and morality. These discourses converge on the pathologisation of Muslims and Islam globally in need of quarantine (the US Muslim travel ban, detention camps and torture cells), cleansing (integration policies in the West) and elimination (persecution and genocide in Kashmir, Palestine and Myanmar).

Globalisation produces an assemblage of local and global interlinkages of norms, values, cultures and structures which are co-produced and socialised by technological advances enabling rapid transfer of information. Orientalist and colonial discourses and the pathologisation of Muslims shape the institutional and everyday discrimination faced by non-White, non Judeo-Christian/atheist Others in modern European societies who bear a legacy of oppression that is responsible for economic marginalisation, political alienation, state and non-state violence, dehumanisation, and institutional and cultural barriers in healthcare delivery through discrimination and structural stigma. They impact the quality of care received from healthcare professionals who frame Muslim

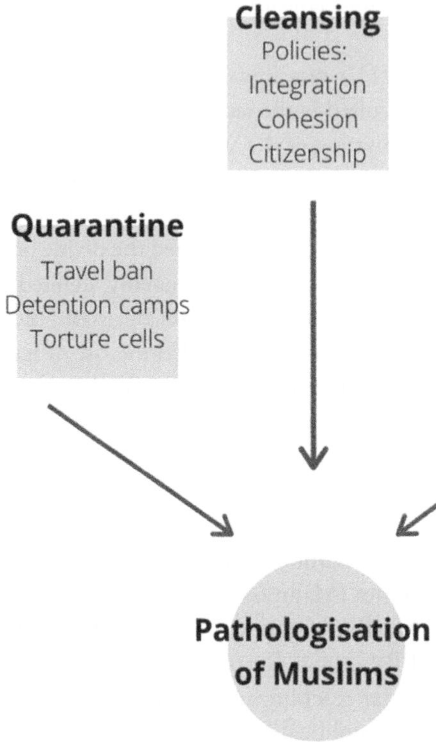

Cleansing
Policies:
Integration
Cohesion
Citizenship

Quarantine
Travel ban
Detention camps
Torture cells

Extermination
Hatred
Violence
Persecution
Genocide

**Pathologisation
of Muslims**

Figure 10.3 Pathologisation of Muslims.

patients as being problematic, subservient to backward traditions and posing health risks (Laird et al. 2007b). Transnational and national government authorities, media and social media align to form an 'Islamophobia information industry' that pathologises and stigmatises Muslims globally. These factors all have the combined effect of alienating Muslim communities, which can lead to a lack of trust in government authorities and healthcare services, impacting disease exposure, protection, and health-promoting and care-seeking behaviours.

Structural Level

Institutions: power and policies

Institutions target the fundamental causes of health inequities (Raphael and Bryant 2015) and play a critical role in the politics of health (Bambra 2016). Institutions are seats of power and privilege generating ideas and norms that structure society. They do this through arrangements which stratify multiple axes of power beyond the socioeconomic, such as race and religion, and inter-act with individual social positioning to produce potent downstream effects (Gklouleka et al. 2018). The concept of 'institutional imbrication' (Beckfield et al. 2015) is especially relevant as British Muslims are simultaneously affected by multiple institutional policies, determined by their intersectional social posi-tions, which entrenches stigma and social inequalities. Government policies, media, healthcare, education and criminal justice systems are key institutions where Islamophobia operates to produce health inequities.

Half of Muslim households live in poverty and just under half of Muslims are born in the UK (MCB 2015). Austerity and immigration policies therefore dis-proportionately impact Muslim communities. This institutional discrimination influences health through the 'social risk effect' of increasing socioeconomic risk factors and through a 'healthcare effect' from cuts to services, restrictions in access to care and reduced health coverage (Stuckler et al. 2017). In addition, welfare and austerity policies directly impact health and lead to mental health problems including depression, anxiety and suicide, as well as an increased incidence in communicable diseases (Barr et al. 2015; Quaglio et al. 2013). UK immigra-tion policies, epitomised by the Brexit vote and Windrush scandal, contribute to structural inequity and social segregation (Gee and Ford 2011). In the UK, immigrants are excluded from access to welfare benefits and types of healthcare (Legido-Quigley et al. 2019) which can lead to delays in accessing healthcare and presentation with more advanced disease, as well as increasing communicable dis-ease transmission and overall public health risk.

In addition to exclusionary policies, structural stigma impacts health out-comes through political and media rhetoric around integration, the underclass and welfarism. These generate Islamophobic prejudice and attitudes towards Muslims which can lead to a blame culture by health professionals who attribute the cause of illness and disability to the individual, ignoring the institutional structural and cultural barriers impacting healthcare access (Silva 2018). Struc-tural stigma is also independently associated with violence, homicide, suicide and cardiovascular disease (Hatzenbuehler et al. 2013; Lukachko et al. 2014) as well as social segregation and differential access to resources and determinants of health (Love 2009).

Surveillance policies which disproportionately impact Muslims are also asso-ciated with a range of adverse mental health outcomes (Medina Ariza 2014; Open Society for Justice Initiative 2016; O'Connor and Jahan 2014). The PRE-VENT and associated de-radicalisation Channel programmes, where public sec-tor workers have a statutory duty to report suspected extremists, are based on a 'problematic fusion' of terrorism rooted in psychological vulnerability and radi-calisation with child protection/safeguarding (Coppock and McGovern 2014). In the NHS, the PREVENT policy entrenches institutional Islamophobia through creating a climate of fear and suspicion (Younis and Jahav 2020) which can form a barrier for patients accessing healthcare. Research on the health impacts of PREVENT on children is very limited and is an area warranting further enquiry. What is known is that early exposure to discrimination has cumulative health impacts over the life course and also frames perceptions about the value and importance of diversity by society (Gee et al. 2012; Stevenson et al. 2017).

The criminal justice system is another key area in which Islamophobia is institutionalised. Muslims are a 'hyperincarcerated' group, making up 15 per cent of the total prison population (MCB 2015; Dumont et al. 2012). In the year ending June 2019, three-quarters of people in custody for terror offences were Muslim (Home Office 2019). Incarceration is associated with a range of acute and chronic physical health disorders such as tuberculosis and other communicable diseases, cancer and reproductive health problems, higher STI/HIV risk in children of those incarcerated and increased cardiovascular risk in female partners (Baussano et al. 2010; Binswanger et al. 2009; Khan et al. 2018; Geller et al. 2009; Gifford et al. 2019; Lee et al. 2014). Behavioural and mental health problems are well documented including drug and alcohol misuse, serious mental health disorders, self harm and death by suicide as well as violence and homicide (Fazel et al. 2016). This structural discrimination risks harming entire communities and contributes to health inequities among British Muslims.

Social Level

Inequalities: societies and stratification

Structural Islamophobia stratifies socioeconomic position and subsequent (unequal) distribution of power, resources and privilege that drive health inequities through discrimination, disadvantage and disparities across the life course, producing cumulative effects of increasing risk and poorer healthcare quality and access. Muslims in the UK have a more disadvantaged profile than any other minority faith group (Stevenson et al. 2017). The higher economic inactivity, lower incomes and large family sizes put Muslims at a higher risk of poverty which is more than double the national average (Heath and Li 2015). The impact of socioeconomic inequalities on health disparities in ethnic groups extends beyond genetic and cultural explanations (Nazroo 2003), embodied through increased expression of biomarkers of allostatic load, explained in more detail later (Sanders-Phillips et al. 2009).

Muslims are more likely than any other religious group to leave school at 16 with no qualifications (Hussain 2008). Religious discrimination, rather than racial, is strongly associated with school bullying (Weller et al. 2001). At school,

Muslim children are more likely to experience bullying, prejudiced attitudes, stereotypes and negative perceptions, exclusion, poorer grades and higher drop-out rates as well as a lack of role models and structures to challenge racism and Islamophobia (Stevenson et al. 2017). These cause stigma, low self-esteem and confidence, and an obstructed transition to the labour market (Stevenson et al. 2017). Education is key to one's position in the social stratification system, with a mediating effect on work and economic conditions, psychosocial resources and ability to cope with stressors, all of which impact health and lifestyle behaviours (Ross and Wu 1995). Poor educational attainment is linked with smoking, less physical activity and less engagement with preventative care, putting them at risk of developing serious illness with delayed presentation (Ross and Wu 1995).

Despite British Muslims being more likely to go on to higher education (Hussain 2008), they have unequitable access to high-status universities and courses (Stevenson 2017), have the highest rate of unemployment (Khattab and Modood 2015) and are less likely to progress to senior roles (Jivraj and Khan 2013). Unemployment is linked to suicide, higher mortality rates, acute and chronic physical health conditions, poor health behaviours, substance misuse, and poor wellbeing and mental health, with the greatest impacts seen in urban areas (Kasl and Jones 2000).

Muslims in the UK are also more likely to be in low-paid, high-risk jobs, which worsens health outcomes (Reynolds and Birdwell 2015). Income inequality affects health through perceptions of place in the social hierarchy, generating shame and distrust (Lynch et al. 2000) and worsening stigma. Job insecurity is associated with increased self-reported morbidity, premature mortality, mental health disorders, disability, poor obstetric outcomes, work absenteeism, increased GP and hospital outpatient consultations and increased medication use (Ferrie 2001; Burchell 2009; Caroli and Godard 2016; Mohren et al. 2003; Siegrist 1995). A range of poor health outcomes have been reported through embodied pathophysiological processes such as higher blood pressure, catecholamine secretion, cholesterol levels and arterial calcification (De Witte et al. 2015). The consequences of job insecurity are not limited to the individual; spill-over effects impact other dimensions of wellbeing such as family life, work-home interferences, life satisfaction and feelings of happiness (De Witte et al. 2015).

Islamophobia can lead to housing insecurity due to discrimination in the housing market, and data shows that Muslims in the UK are half as likely to own their homes and live in overcrowded houses (ONS 2011). Furthermore, residential segregation is a key determinant of racialised health inequalities and may originate from both discrimination and as a protective response to discrimination and disadvantage (Bailey et al. 2017). Social segregation is associated with increased mortality indirectly though poor-quality neighbourhood environment, socioeconomic disadvantage, access to quality healthcare and increased exposure to food insecurity and toxic air pollutants, and directly through increased prevalence of violent crime, cardiovascular disease, tuberculosis and adverse birth outcomes (Acevedo-Garcia and Lochner 2003; Bailey et al. 2017). Residential segregation through Islamophobic exclusionary policies systematically impacts healthcare access, acceptability, utilisation and quality, with a lack of adequate health promoting resources (Bailey et al. 2017) as well as a lack of high-quality and accessible primary and secondary care health services (Caldwell et al. 2017) and poorer uptake of screening programmes (Padela and Curlin 2013).

In social spaces, anti-Muslim hate crime maintains boundaries of 'them' and 'us', and creates fears about living in a particular locality because of feeling unwelcome, unsafe, vulnerable, insecure and excluded (Elahi and Khan 2017). These boundaries are not only geographical but include cyber spaces, becoming translated into 'emotional boundaries' which frame the way that safe spaces are perceived (Hopkins 2007). Furthermore, anti-Muslim hate crime is often experienced on multiple occasions, associated with cumulative psychological trauma and feelings of vulnerability, insecurity, fear and anxiety (Awan and Zempi 2015; Bowling 1999).

Individual Level

Intra- and inter-personal: humans and holism

We have seen in previous sections how Islamophobia acts primarily through pathways of structural and social stigma and determinants of health to leading to poorer health outcomes. In this section I further analyse the phenomenon of embodiment of Islamophobia and how this influences a range of biological and psychosocial processes at the individual level to produce adverse health outcomes in a range of dimensions: physical health, psychological health, social health and wellbeing, and spiritual health and wellbeing.

Research on discrimination and physical health outcomes is limited. Literature highlights how British Muslims experience poorer self-reported health and limiting long-term illness, especially in the over-50 age group, women and those living in certain areas (MCB 2015). Studies show the association between discrimination and financial strain, chronic stress, low levels of physical activity, poor nutrition and obesity, resulting in high blood pressure and cholesterol and worse self-rated health (Johnston and Lordan 2012). This is relevant to Muslim communities in the UK where data on Muslim majority ethnic groups shows they have lower physical activity and higher prevalence of cardio-metabolic disorders (Hayes et al. 2002; Bhopal et al. 1999; Sproston and Mindell 2006; Khunti et al. 2009), obesity (NHS Digital 2012), certain cancers (Fazil 2018) and poor self-reported health and disability (MCB 2015).

Islamophobia causes poorer health 'inside and 'outside' the body, which links individual and social pathology (Lynch et al. 2000). Internal biological effects are embodied through acute stress pathways generating psycho-neuro-endocrine, genetic, immunological and inflammatory pathological mechanisms mediated by cortisol, adrenaline, inflammatory markers and damage to genetic material, and stress-induced behaviours such as smoking and substance misuse as well as poor diet and physical activity. Additionally, direct trauma and violence can cause injury, disability and death. Externally, social effects are expressed as reduced civic participation, less cohesion and social capital within the community and individually, and antisocial abuse and violence, both online and offline.

In the UK, anti-Muslim hate crimes continue to increase year on year, accounting for almost half of all religiously motivated hate crime (Home Office 2018). About one in four people in the UK hold unfavourable views about Muslims (Carriere-Kretschmer 2008) and one in three believe that Islam threatens the British way of life (Carter and Lowles 2018). Verbal abuse which accompanies many anti-Muslim incidents shows several consistent stereotypes around terrorism, foreigners, competition, blame and paedophilia (Tell MAMA 2018). These stereotypes, prejudice and hate crimes create a socially devalued and stigmatised identity for British Muslims associated with population health disparities (Hatzenbuehler et al. 2013).

Of concern are the chronic daily microaggressions at work, in leisure settings and in public spaces, which have a stronger association with poor health outcomes including common mental disorders than acute experiences of harassment, threats and violence (Bailey et al. 2017). Additionally, parental stress can exacerbate the effects of similar experiences that may be faced by Muslim children in the school setting (Laird et al. 2007a). This sustained and cumulative exposure increases allostatic load, which leads to chronic activation of physiological and psychological stress pathways (McEwen and Stellar 1993). This is associated with high blood pressure and coronary artery calcification, high levels of C-reactive protein and oxidative stress, visceral fat, low birth weight infants, cognitive impairment, poor sleep, psychological distress, depression, anxiety, depressed pulmonary function, hippocampal atrophy, reduced telomere length and health damaging behaviours such as smoking (Paradies et al. 2015; Bailey et al. 2017; Berkman and Glass 2000). An emerging field of research is epigenetics, which analyses the impact that stress can have on development and gene expression and which may be associated with embodiment of racialised health disparities through transgenerational trauma (Kuzawa and Sweet 2009).

Islamophobia can have multiple and pervasive impacts on mental health by generating emotional distress, psychological burnout, and stressful circumstances and cognitive states, due to persistent deployment of defensive and adaptive strategies in the face of domination, oppression and victimisation, as demonstrated in racism studies (Pierce 1995; Comas-Diaz 2007). Islamophobia can also lead to internalised stereotypes, stigma, identity concealment and harmful coping mechanisms which can be detrimental to emotional and mental health (Pachankis 2007). 'Stereotype threat' is the activation of negative stereotypes among stigmatised groups which creates anxieties and expectations that negatively affect social and psychological functioning and physiological processes and contribute to stress and poor health (Aronson et al. 2013). A range of negative mental health outcomes have been observed with racism including cognitive impairment, insomnia, psychological distress, depression, anxiety and paranoia (Paradies et al. 2015; O'Connor and Jahan 2014).

Islamophobia disrupts social and community networks, engagement, cohesion, support and capital. This causes social isolation which is linked to a range of adverse physical and mental health outcomes including all-cause mortality, stroke, cardiovascular disease, infectious disease and substance misuse (Berkman and Glass 2000). While social cohesion refers to the the extent of solidarity and connectedness among groups in society, social capital refers to the resources available to individuals and communities, both tangible and intangible. A lack of social capital among British Muslims can lead to increased mortality, cardiometabolic disorders, cancer, infant mortality, poor self-rated health, poorer health behaviours, suicide, criminal behaviour and barriers accessing healthcare services (Kawachi and Berkman 2000).

Faith can moderate the impact of discrimination on health outcomes through the protective effects of faith beliefs and practices, social networks and identity affirmation. Research demonstrates the positive impact of faith on physical and mental health outcomes, including increased life expectancy, quality of life, coping skills, recovery from terminal illness and reduced anxiety, depression and suicide (Chattopadhyay 2007; Mueller et al. 2001). However, the current sociopolitical climate leads to stigma associated with belonging to a socially devalued group and consequent marginalisation and identity concealment of British Muslims, which can impact their sense of value, belonging, meaning, role, and a consistent and coherent sense of identity, which are all linked to wellbeing. Hostility and consequent stigma also makes it difficult for British Muslims to develop a community life, and faith identity becomes reconfigured as a stressor that is detrimental to health rather than protective as evidenced by anti-Muslim hate crime (Samari 2016). This may negatively impact spiritual wellbeing, meaning and connectedness.

Intersectional Identities and Inequities

An intersectional lens can be useful to understand experiences of discrimination and disadvantage towards multiple attributes of a person's identity where a number of stratifications and power axes are simultaneously embodied, compounding violent forms of social and health inequities (Gkiouleka et al. 2018). Situational intersectionality further looks at the social divisions most affecting people's lives which are specific to their context (Yuval-Davis 2015). Furthermore, deeper understanding of disadvantage, discrimination and disparties cannot be established without considering the various mechanisms producing and establishing privilege and that the impact on wellbeing may be more than the sum of these operating on individual social categories (Nash 2008).

Muslims in the UK are differentiated by intersectional combinations of race, ethnicity, gender, social class, national origin and immigration status. Any of these can be the target of social bias individually or simultaneously depending on context; thus experiences of Islamophobia are not homogeneous and universal. Islamophobia has a gendered component, as women who are visibly Muslim are the main targets of Islamophobic hate crime (Tell MAMA 2018) with health consequences such as panic attacks, anxiety, depression and social withdrawal (Awan and Zempi 2017). In the workplace, institutional Islamophobia results in Muslim women facing a triple penalty: being ethnic, female and Muslim, which impacts career progression (House of Commons Women and Equalities Committee 2016). This is also reflected in dress code policies in the NHS (Malik et al. 2019) and working environments for female NHS staff and disciplinary processes (Shahid and Abdulkareem 2018). Workplace-based discrimination is associated with a higher rate of common mental disorder such as anxiety and depression as well as psychosis-related disorders (Karlsen et al. 2005). This is particularly concerning due to the gendered nature of social and health inequities globally that already exist and are further exacerbated by Islamophobia (Bambra et al. 2009).

Gendered Islamophobia through stereotype threats is prevalent, such as views of Muslim female patients being excessively pious, traditional, oppressed or abused, which can lead to a breakdown in trust and rapport, stress, impaired health-promoting behaviours, delayed access to healthcare and discounting health professionals' advice (Laird et al. 2007a). In particular, women who wear the veil report more discrimination in healthcare settings, which is consistent with wider social trends, reporting increased discomfort, stereotypes, misunderstanding and fear of accessing healthcare, leading to delayed care and poor health outcomes (Hammoud et al. 2005; Vu et al. 2016). This also impacts access to preventative care and may account for lower cancer screening observed among Muslim women in the UK (Jack et al. 2014; Bansal et al. 2012; Szczepura 2005). Muslim women have reported negative experiences of maternity care which increases the risk to them and their babies through poor communication, stereotyping and inaccurate cultural assumptions, racism, and a lack of sensitivity and research around the linguistic and cultural needs of women from diverse populations (Reitmanova and Gustafson 2008; McFadden et al. 2013; Ali and Burchett 2004).

The impact of structural Islamophobia on mental health has been described previously. Mental health disorders are already known to be higher in ethnic minority groups and, in particular, among recent migrants and refugees with experiences of extreme physical and mental stress and trauma. The stigma associated with having a mental health problem in these communities combines with the structural stigma of belonging to a socially devalued group and can lead to a 'double stigma' (Gary 2005) of mistrust in mental health services and unmet need (Alang 2019). These also intersect with multiple barriers in accessing mental health services including communication difficulties, cultural differences and professionals' lack of understanding of the cultural and religious impact on beliefs and behaviours around mental health (Kirmayer et al. 2011). Asian women in particular have been identified as a special group at high risk of suicide (McKenzie et al. 2008). Studies also demonstrate that ethnic minorities are more likely to be hospitalised and treated with pharmacotherapy, and more likely to be given a diagnosis of a serious mental health disorder, perpetuating racist assumptions and a lack of attention to social and contextual issues (Corneau and Stergiopoulos 2012).

Research shows that Somalis form the largest refugee community in the UK and face the most social disadvantage with over a third experiencing a common mental disorder, high levels of stress, disrupted family life and child development, and poor wellbeing (Bhui et al. 2006; Warfa et al. 2006). Using a situational intersectional lens, this highlights the intersection of race, religion and immigration status with trauma and social disadvantage in contributing to poorer health outcomes in a highly vulnerable and marginalised group. Specifically, immigration status affects health outcomes through its influence on health-damaging conditions such as poverty, famine, persecution, conflict, movement causing physical and psychological trauma; on access to political, civil and human rights and health and social care services in host societies; and in shaping experiences of discrimination and everyday microaggressions within the current climate of increasing nationalism, populism, xenophobia and Islamophobia.

A life course or neo-material approach can be viewed as an extension of a situational intersectional lens. This focuses on the differential accumulation of exposures across the life course, lack of resources and systemic underinvestment across a range of infrastructure – human, physical, social and health – and is a result of historical, cultural and political-economic processes which affects the private resources available to individuals and shapes public infrastructure, thus acting as an index for broader social processes (Lynch 2000). These processes are embodied by British Muslim children who live with the worst forms of health inequities and which have the potential to accumulate and accentuate health inequities throughout the life course (Collings et al. 2020).

In this life course approach, Islamophobia may impact health outcomes by influencing processes and pathways at critical points in a person's (especially a child's) development and/or due to the cumulative effects of chronic psychosocial and physical stress and exhaustion. Racism can be internalised and in children has been linked to waist circumference, body fat distribution and insulin resistance (Mays et al. 2007). Health inequities are also exacerbated by interpersonal discrimination during encounters with healthcare providers (Smedley et al. 2002). In a study on African American women (Hilmert et al. 2014), a higher prevalence of low birth weight and pre-term infants was observed, attributed to high diastolic blood pressure specifically due to childhood racism operating across the life course, which may be relevant to Muslim women. Among Muslim girls, assumptions, prejudice and blaming families for poor healthcare access and engagement worsen health disparities (Laird et al. 2007a). Pakistanis have the highest infant mortality rate in England (Public Health England 2017) and research on Pakistani children has demonstrated higher death rates in children, disability and life-limiting conditions compared with other children (Corry 2014). Additionally, parents have reported that discrimination is a barrier to meet their children's mental health needs (Bradby et al. 2011).

Conclusions, Recommendations and Future Directions

We have seen how the conceptual framework outlined in this chapter highlights Islamophobia as an intersectional oppressive system that operates across society, globally and nationally, and at multiple levels, influenced by sociohistorical and cultural contexts to produce discrimination, disadvantage and disparities that impact multidimensional health outcomes directly and indirectly through the processes of stigma, social determinants and embodiment. These processes are dynamic and reciprocal, reinforcing what has been described as 'structural violence' embedded in and normalised by institutions and societies and which stops people from achieving their full potential (Galtung 1969). Additionally, reverse effects are also seen, for example someone who has developed a mental health disorder due to trauma from Islamophobia may be faced with decline in their social position or access to material resources such as housing, creating a positive feedback loop.

Oriental discourses, securitisation and secularisation on the global level create a stigmatised and socially devalued identity for British Muslims. Institutional policies, media narratives and political movements crystallise structural stigma and inequities which discriminate and disadvantage Muslims through social positioning and access to resources, power, privilege and social determinants of health. They also impact 'pathways to embodiment' (Krieger 2012) through access and quality of healthcare, health behaviours and psychosocial stressors. These generate multisystem psychological, cognitive, physiological and molecular responses linked to acute stress and trauma, long-term allostatic load and transgenerational epigenetic modification in response to legacies (of trauma and oppression).

Public health and human rights frameworks are rooted in a shared concern for equity, social justice and dignity, the very principles violated by Islamophobia which systematically dehumanises and oppresses Muslims by causing

> distinction, exclusion, or restriction towards, or preference against, Muslims (or those perceived to be Muslims) that has the purpose or effect of nullifying or impairing the recognition, enjoyment or exercise, on an equal footing, of human rights and fundamental freedoms in the political, economic, social, cultural or any other field of public life. (Elahi and Khan 2017)

Human rights can be considered, at their source, not only as moral rights ensuring that individuals live a life with dignity and aspirations, but also as a social practice which transcends their legal limitation by legitimising the struggle of excluded groups against dominant groups violating their recognition and development, as we see with Muslims currently and historically (Peñaranda 2015). Deprivation, state and non-state discrimination and violence prevent both capabilities and functionings of British Muslims through Islamophobia which violates human development, wellbeing, and social and health justice.

A rights-based approach (RBA) or human rights-based approach (HBRA) to health incorporates human rights into public health, encompassing both the delivery of health services and determinants of health to ensure that policies and programmes contribute to the fulfilment of human rights, particularly in relation to groups that are disadvantaged and excluded and affected by multiple unjust disparities (Gruskin et al. 2010). The PANEL framework can be used to operationalise a rights-based approach to develop policy and practice at structural and organisational levels that encourages participation, accountability, non-discrimination, empowerment and legality of rights of Muslim patients and the wider Muslim population (Mental Health Foundation 2015).

Drawing on a public health response to Islamophobia focused on addressing the 'causes of the causes'; interventions need to be targeted at multiple levels and require a multi-sectoral and multidisciplinary approach to eliminate multidimensional health inequities. A whole-system, whole-person humanitarian and public health approach is thus needed to reduce health disparities caused

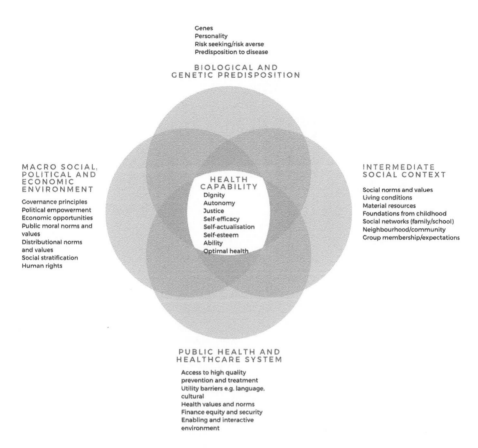

Figure 10.4 Achieving health capability for British Muslims using a human rights-based approach.

by Islamophobia with a particular focus on upstream factors and prevention. Inclusive and compassion-centred attitudes and practices that decolonise, re-humanise and replace the normative and exclusionary Eurocentric worldview in societies can improve individual and societal health through promoting an understanding of shared histories and humanity while simultaneously respecting diversity and individuality.

Globalisation has a critical role in shaping health, which relates to what has been called 'the inequality machine that is reshaping the planet', and governments have power to moderate its effect (Schrecker 2016). This begins with reviewing a number of policies to address the upstream factors which are likely to have the biggest impact on eliminating health inequities faced by British Muslims due to Islamophobia. There needs to be, as a priority, a clear government

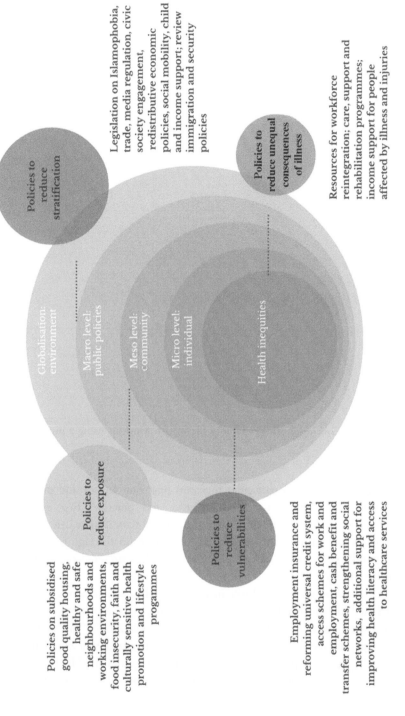

Figure 10.5 Public health response to reduce health inequities among British Muslims.

policy acknowledging and tackling Islamophobia and a need for the government to re-establish trust and credibility with the British Muslim community. There is a need for rigorous independent evaluation of any policies impacting Muslim communities and for the government to improve engagement with grassroots Muslim organisations that represent the insights and interests of the community. Adequate funding and resources for collaborative community action and co-production of knowledge and interventions is key to ensuring sustainable, equitable and impactful solutions.

There is a need for more effective and proactive media regulation in cases of alleged discriminatory reporting to reduce structural stigma. This needs to be coupled with improved support for victims of Islamophobia and appropriate resource allocation to tackle hate crime at local levels, as well as fair and proportionate criminal justice sanctions and rehabilitative interventions for hate crime offenders (Elahi and Khan 2017). Security policies need independent review and separation of the state's security apparatus from wider safeguarding or social policy strategies which can form a barrier for Muslims accessing health services. Workplace policies need to ensure that religious discrimination, as a protected characteristic in the Equality Act 2010, is monitored and effectively addressed within institutions, including the NHS.

Improved anti-poverty reduction strategies that are redistributive and empower Muslim communities are important to achieve health and social equity. Austerity policies which are regressive and worsen social disadvantage disproportionately experienced by British Muslims should be reversed and replaced with policies aimed at improving social mobility and access to healthcare and social determinants of health such as education, employment and income support, and higher-quality affordable housing. This requires strong and sustained intersectoral action, together with firm government commitment.

In key institutions and workplaces, policies and practices must be implemented which improve religious competency training and ensure appropriate interventions are in place to deal with discrimination, bullying and harassment against Muslims, provide access to faith and culturally congruent mentors and role models, and monitor and improve Muslim representation especially at senior levels where there is under-representation. Employers and employment support organisations should identify barriers to equal labour market participation, and implement policies addressing religious discrimination and lack of progression and senior representation in the workplace. For public-sector bodies, there needs to be monitoring and accountability of their compliance with the Public Sector Equality Duty (UK Government 2012).

In healthcare settings, improved religious competency and a faith impact assessment of policies such as dress codes needs to be considered, as well as a review of the Prevent policy. Improved data collection on the health of of Muslim and other faith groups will improve monitoring of health inequities. Information on religion as well as ethnicity should be routinely collected by local and national public health authorities, primary and secondary care, and death registration records to better assess needs and inform appropriate interventions, with information campaigns on the purpose of data collection to a community suspicious of any forms of surveillance. There is also a need for faith and culturally sensitive health interventions, especially in mental health services, to accommodate and support holistic and integrated health belief models.

Social participation and empowerment are key to ensure that British Muslims become active enablers and controllers of their own health, linking the human rights, capabilities and public health approaches. Governments hold primary responsibility for promoting health equity and human rights but participatory decision making with community and faith-based organisations within a pluralistic, transparent and accountable governance structure and policy environment is essential. Participation needs to move beyond performative acts of consulting and collaborating to sincerely and actively empowering communities. Empowerment too has different levels, progressing from satisfying basic needs and equality of access, to ensuring social and material resources, addressing structural and institutional discrimination, promoting shared decision making and finally control with autonomous decision making, recognition and reward (Longwe 1991). Empowerment initiatives must aim for autonomy, agency and accountability.

Further research and improved data collection is required on faith-based health outcomes for British Muslims as well as pathways to inequities, especially pathophysiological processes, moderating and mediating factors, domains and expressions of Islamophobia and direct health impacts, and subgroup and intersectional analyses. However, the dependence on evidence can be a double-edged sword, causing delays in implementing urgent and important policy changes. Rapid assessments and pragmatic approaches are essential to narrow the research–policy gap and save lives and livelihoods. Furthermore, increased importance must be given to qualitative data, especially narrative approaches that capture the diverse and dynamic lived experiences of Muslim communities to deepen understanding of Islamophobia and its social and health impact. Finally, there is a need for and legitimacy of research on Islamophobia as a determinant of health to eliminate preventable and avoidable health inequities among Muslims in the UK and beyond. It is only when the most marginalised and vulnerable in society are protected, and inequities and injustice eliminated, that harmonious and sustainable societies can flourish with health, wellbeing and dignity for all.

References

Acevedo-Garcia, D. and Lochner, K. A. (2003). 'Residential segregation and health', in I. Kawachi and L. F. Berkman (eds), *Neighborhoods and Health*. New York: Oxford University Press, pp. 265–87.

Ahmed, A. (2018). *Journey into Europe: Islam, Immigration, and Identity*. Washington, DC: Brookings Institution Press.

Alang, S. M. (2019). 'Mental health care among blacks in America: confronting racism and constructing solutions'. *Health Services Research*, 54(2), 346–55.

Ali, N. and Burchett, H. (2004). 'Experiences of maternity services: Muslim women's perspectives'. Available at: www.maternityaction.org.uk/wp-content/uploads/2013/09/muslimwomensexperiencesofmaternityservices.pdf (last accessed 19 May 2022).

Allen, C. (2016). *Islamophobia*. London: Routledge.

All Party Parliamentary Group on British Muslims (2018). 'Islamophobia defined: the inquiry into a working definition of Islamophobia'. Available at: https://static1.squarespace.com/static/599c3d2febbd1a90cffdd8a9/t/5bfd1ea3352f531a6170ceee/1543315109493/Islamophobia+Defined.pdf (last accessed 13 May 2022).

Ansari, H. (2004). *The 'Infidel' Within: The History of Muslims in Britain, 1800 to the Present*. London: C. Hurst & Co.

Aronson, J., Burgess, D., Phelan, S. M. and Juarez, L. (2013). 'Unhealthy interactions: the role of stereotype threat in health disparities'. *American Journal of Public Health*, 103(1), 50–6.

Awan, I. and Zempi, I. (2017). '"I will blow your face OFF"– VIRTUAL and physical world anti-Muslim hate crime'. *British Journal of Criminology*, 57(2), 362–80.

Bailey, Z. D., Krieger, N., Agénor, M., Graves, J., Linos, N. and Bassett, M. T. (2017). 'Structural racism and health inequities in the USA: evidence and interventions'. *The Lancet*, 389(10077), 1453–63.

Bambra, C. (2016). *Health Divides: Where You Live Can Kill You*. Bristol: Policy Press.

Bambra, C., Pope, D., Swami, V., Stanistreet, D., Roskam, A., Kunst, A. and Scott-Samuel, A. (2009). 'Gender, health inequalities and welfare state regimes: a cross-national study of 13 European countries'. *Journal of Epidemiology & Community Health*, 63(1), 38–44.

Bansal, N. Bhopal, R. S., Steiner, M. F. C., Brewster, D. H and Scottish Health and Ethnicity Linkage Study (2012). 'Major ethnic group differences in breast cancer screening uptake in Scotland are not extinguished by adjustment for indices of geographical residence, area deprivation, long-term illness and education'. *British Journal of Cancer*, 106(8), 1361–6.

Barr, B., Kinderman, P. and Whitehead, M. (2015). 'Trends in mental health inequalities in England during a period of recession, austerity and welfare reform 2004 to 2013'. *Social Science & Medicine*, 147: 324–31.

Baussano, I., Williams, B. G., Nunn, P., Beggiato, M., Fedeli, U. and Scano, F. (2010). 'Tuberculosis incidence in prisons: a systematic review'. *PLoS Medicine*, 7(12), e1000381.

Beckfield, J., Bambra, C., Eikemo, T. A., Huijts, T., McNamara, C. and Wendt, C. (2015). 'An institutional theory of welfare state effects on the distribution of population health'. *Social Theory & Health*, 13(3), 227–44.

Berkman, L. F. and Glass, T. (2000). 'Social integration, social networks, social support, and health'. *Social Epidemiology*, 1: 137–73.

Bhopal, R., Unwin, N., White, M., Yallop, J., Walker, L., Alberti, K. G., Harland, J., Patel, S., Ahmad, N., Turner, C., Watson, B., Kaur, D., Kulkarni, A., Laker, M. and Tavridou, A. (1999). 'Heterogeneity of coronary heart disease risk factors in Indian, Pakistani, Bangladeshi, and European origin populations: cross sectional study'. *BMJ*, 319(7204), 215–20.

Bhui, K., Craig, T., Mohamud, S., Warfa, N., Stansfeld, S. A., Thornicroft, G., Curtis, S. and McCrone, P. (2006). 'Mental disorders among Somali refugees'. *Social Psychiatry and Psychiatric Epidemiology*, 41(5), 400–8.

Binswanger, I. A., Krueger, P. M. and Steiner, J. F. (2009). 'Prevalence of chronic medical conditions among jail and prison inmates in the USA compared with the general population'. *Journal of Epidemiology & Community Health*, 63(11), 912–19.

Bowling, B. (1999). *Violent Racism: Victimization, Policing and Social Context*. Oxford: Clarendon Press.

Bradley, R. and Slade, P. (2011). 'A review of mental health problems in fathers following the birth of a child'. *Journal of Reproductive and Infant Psychology*, 29(1), 19–42.

Burchell, B. (2009). 'Flexicurity as a moderator of the relationship between job insecurity and psychological well-being'. *Cambridge Journal of Regions, Economy and Society*, 2(3), 365–78.

Caldwell, J. T., Ford, C. L., Wallace, S. P., Wang, M. C. and Takahashi, L. M. (2017). 'Racial and ethnic residential segregation and access to health care in rural areas'. *Health & Place*, 43, 104–12.

Caroli, E. and Godard, M. (2016). 'Does job insecurity deteriorate health?'. *Health Economics*, 25(2), 131–47.

Carriere-Kretschmer, E. (2008). 'Unfavorable views of Jews and Muslims on the increase in Europe'. The Pew Global Attitudes Project. Available at: www.pewresearch.org/global/2008/09/17/unfavorable-views-of-jews-and-muslims-on-the-increase-in-europe (last accessed 16 May 2022).

Carter, R. and Lowles, N. (2018). 'Britain divided? Rivers of blood 50 years on'. Hope Not Hate. Available at: https://hopenothate.org.uk/wp-content/uploads/2018/04/Britain-Divided-50-years-on.pdf (last accessed 16 May 2022).

Chattopadhyay, S. (2007). 'Religion, spirituality, health and medicine: Why should Indian physicians care?'. *Journal of Postgraduate Medicine*, 53(4), 262–6.

Collings, P. J., Dogra, S. A., Costa, S., Bingham, D. D. and Barber, S. E. (2020). 'Objectively-measured sedentary time and physical activity in a bi-ethnic sample of young children: variation by socio-demographic, temporal and perinatal factors'. *BMC Public Health*, 20(1), 109.

Comas-Diaz, L. (2007). 'Ethnopolitical psychology: healing and transformation'. Available at: https://api.semanticscholar.org/CorpusID:21368106 (last accessed 16 May 2022).

Coppock, V. and McGovern, M. (2014). '"Dangerous minds"? Deconstructing counter-terrorism discourse, radicalisation and the "psychological vulnerability" of Muslim children and young people in Britain'. *Children & Society*, 28(3), 242–56.

Corneau, S. and Stergiopoulos, V. (2012). 'More than being against it: anti-racism and anti-oppression in mental health services'. *Transcultural Psychiatry*, 49(2), 261–82.

Corry, P. C. (2014). 'Consanguinity and prevalence patterns of inherited disease in the UK Pakistani community'. *Human Heredity*, 77(1–4), 207–16.

De Witte, H., Vander Elst, T. and De Cuiyper, N. (2015). 'Job insecurity, health and well-being', in J. Vuori, R. Blonk and R. H. Price (eds), *Sustainable Working Lives*. Dordrecht: Springer, pp. 109–28.

Dumont, D. M., Brockmann, B., Dickman, S., Alexander, N. and Rich, J. D. (2012). 'Public health and the epidemic of incarceration'. *Annual Review of Public Health*, 33: 325–39.

Elahi, F. and Khan, O. (2017). 'Islamophobia: still a challenge for us all. A 20th-anniversary report'. The Runnymede Trust. Available at: www.runnymedetrust. org/publications/islamophobia-still-a-challenge-for-us-all (last accessed 16 May 2022).

Essa, A. and Ali, O. (2012). *Studies in Islamic Civilisations: The Muslim Contribution to the Renaissance*. London: International Institute of Islamic Thought.

Fazel, S., Hayes, A. J., Bartellas, K., Clerici, M. and Trestman, R. (2016). 'Mental health of prisoners: prevalence, adverse outcomes, and interventions'. *The Lancet Psychiatry*, 3(9), 871–81.

Fazil, Q. (2018). 'Cancer and black and minority ethnic communities'. Better Health Briefing 47. Available at: http://raceequalityfoundation.org.uk/wp-content/uploads/2018/07/REF-Better-Health-471-1.pdf (last accessed 16 May 2022).

Ferrie, J. E. (2001). 'Is job insecurity harmful to health?'. *Journal of the Royal Society of Medicine*, 94(2): 71–6.

Fitz, F. G. (2009). 'La Reconquista: un estado de la cuestión'. *Clío & Crimen*, 6: 142–215.

Galtung, J. (1969). 'Violence, peace and peace research'. *Journal of Peace Research*, 6(3), 167–91.

Gary, F. A. (2005). 'Stigma: barrier to mental health care among ethnic minorities'. *Issues in Mental Health Nursing*, 26(10), 979–99.

Gee, G. C. and Ford, C. L. (2011). 'Structural racism and health inequities: old issues, new directions'. *Du Bois Review: Social Science Research on Race*, 8(1), 115–32.

Gee, G. C., Walsemann, K. L. and Brondolo, E. (2012). 'A life course perspective on how racism may be related to health inequities'. *American Journal of Public Health*, 102(5), 967–74.

Geller, A., Garfinkel, I., Cooper, C. E. and Mincy, R. B. (2009). 'Parental incarceration and child well-being: implications for urban families'. *Social Science Quarterly*, 90(5), 1186–202.

Giacaman, R., Khatib, R., Shabaneh, L., Ramlawi, A., Sabri, B., Sabatinelli, G., Khawaja, M. and Laurance, T. (2009). 'Health status and health services in the occupied Palestinian territory'. *The Lancet*, 373(9666), 837–49.

Gifford, E. J., Kozecke, L. E., Golonka, M., Hill, S. N., Costello, E. J., Shanahan, L. and Copeland, W. E. (2019). 'Association of parental incarceration with psychiatric and functional outcomes of young adults'. *JAMA Network Open*, 2(8), e1910005.

Gkiouleka, A., Huijts, T., Beckfield, J. and Bambra, C. (2018). 'Understanding the micro and macro politics of health: inequalities, intersectionality and institutions – a research agenda'. *Social Science & Medicine*, 200, 92–8.

Gruskin, S., Bogecho, D. and Ferguson, L. (2010). '"Rights-based approaches" to health policies and programs: articulations, ambiguities, and assessment'. *Journal of Public Health Policy*, 31(2), 129–45.

Hammoud, M. M., White, C. B. and Fetters, M. D. (2005). 'Opening cultural doors: providing culturally sensitive healthcare to Arab American and American Muslim patients'. *American Journal of Obstetrics and Gynecology*, 193(4), 1307–11.

Hatzenbuehler, M. L., Phelan, J. C. and Link, B. G. (2013). 'Stigma as a fundamental cause of population health inequalities'. *American Journal of Public Health*, 103(5), 813–21.

Hayes, L., White, M., Unwin, N., Bhopal, R., Fischbacher, C., Harland, J. and Alberti, K. G. M. M. (2002). 'Patterns of physical activity and relationship with risk markers for cardiovascular disease and diabetes in Indian, Pakistani, Bangladeshi and European adults in a UK population'. *Journal of Public Health*, 24(3), 170–8.

Heath, A. and Li, Y. (2015). 'Review of the relationship between religion and poverty; an analysis for the Joseph Rowntree Foundation. CSI Working paper 2015-01'. Available at: http://csi.nuff.ox.ac.uk/wp-content/uploads/2015/03/religion-and-poverty-working-paper.pdf (last accessed 17 May 2022).

Hill, S. S. and Lippy, C. H. (eds) (2005). *Encyclopaedia of Religion in the South*. Macon, GA: Mercer University Press.

Hilmert, C. J., Dominguez, T. P., Schetter, C. D., Srinivas, S. K., Glynn, L. M., Hobel, C. J. and Sandman, C. A. (2014). 'Lifetime racism and blood pressure changes during pregnancy: implications for fetal growth'. *Health Psychology*, 33(1), 43–51.

Home Office (2018). 'Individuals referred to and supported by the Prevent Programme, April 2017 to March 2018'. Home Office Statistical Bulletin. Available at: www. gov.uk/government/statistics/individuals-referred-to-and-supported-through-the-prevent-programme-april-2017-to-march-2018 (last accessed 17 May 2022).

Home Office (2019). 'Operation of police powers under the Terrorism Act 2000 and subsequent legislation: arrests, outcomes, and stop and search: year ending June 2019'. Available at: www.gov.uk/government/statistics/operation-of-police-powers-under-the-terrorism-act-2000-quarterly-update-to-june-2019 (last accessed 11 July 2022).

Hopkins, P. (2007). 'Young Muslim men's experiences of local landscapes after 11 September 2001'. *Geographies of Muslim Identities: Diaspora, Gender and Belonging*, 189–200.

House of Commons Women and Equalities Committee (2016). 'Employment opportunities for Muslims in the UK'. Second Report of Session 2016–17. Available at: www.publications. parliament.uk/pa/cm201617/cmselect/cmwomeq/89/89. pdf (last accessed 16 May 2022).

Hussain, S. (2008). *Muslims on the Map: A National Survey of Social Trends in Britain*. London: Tauris Academic Studies.

Hussain, Y. and Bagguley, P. (2012). 'Securitized citizens: Islamophobia, racism and the 7/7 London bombings'. *The Sociological Review*, 60(4), 715–34.

Jack, R. H., Møller, H., Robson, T. and Davies, E. A. (2014). 'Breast cancer screening uptake among women from different ethnic groups in London: a population-based cohort study'. *BMJ Open*, 4(10), e005586.

Jensen, N. T. (2012). *For the Health of the Enslaved: Slaves, Medicine and Power in the Danish West Indies, 1803–1848*. Copenhagen: Museum Tusculanum Press.

Jivraj, S. and Khan, O. (2013). 'Ethnicity and deprivation in England: how likely are ethnic minorities to live in deprived neighbourhoods'. Dynamics of Diversity: Evidence from the 2011 Census. Available at: https://hummedia.manchester. ac.uk/institutes/code/briefingsupdated/ethnicity-and-deprivation-in-england-how-likely-are-ethnic-minorities-to-live-in-deprived-neighbourhoods%20(1). pdf (last accessed 18 May 2022).

Johnston, D.W. and Lordan, G. (2012). 'Discrimination makes me sick! An examination of the discrimination–health relationship'. *Journal of Health Economics*, 31(1), 99–111.

Karlsen, S., Nazroo, J. Y., McKenzie, K., Bhui, K. and Weich, S. (2005). 'Racism, psychosis and common mental disorder among ethnic minority groups in England'. *Psychological Medicine*, 35(12), 1795–1803.

Kasl, S. V. and Jones, B. A. (2000). 'The impact of job loss and retirement on health', in L. F. Berkman and I. Kawachi, *Social Epidemiology.* New York: Oxford University Press, pp. 118–36.

Kaur-Ballagan, K., Gottfried, G. and Mortimore, R. (2018). *A Review of Survey Research on Muslims in Britain.* London: Ipsos Mori Social Research Institute.

Kawachi, I. and Berkman, L. (2000). 'Social cohesion, social capital, and health', in L. F. Berkman and I. Kawachi, *Social Epidemiology.* New York: Oxford University Press, pp. 174–90.

Khan, M. R., Scheidell, J. D., Rosen, D. L., Geller, A. and Brotman, L. M. (2018). 'Early age at childhood parental incarceration and STI/HIV-related drug use and sex risk across the young adult lifecourse in the US: heightened vulnerability of black and Hispanic youth'. *Drug and Alcohol Dependence*, 183, 231–9.

Khattab, N. and Modood, T. (2015). 'Both ethnic and religious: explaining employment penalties across 14 ethno-religious groups in the United Kingdom'. *Journal for the Scientific Study of Religion*, 54(3), 501–22.

Khoo, S.-M. (2013). *Health Justice and Capabilities: A Turning Point for Global Health?* London: Sage Publications Ltd.

Khunti, K., Kumar, S. and Brodie, J. (2009). 'Diabetes UK and South Asian Health Foundation recommendations on diabetes research priorities for British South Asians'. Available at: www.diabetes.org.uk/resources-s3/2017-11/south_asian_report.pdf (last accessed 18 May 2022).

Kirmayer, L. J., Narasiah, L., Munoz, M., Rashid, M., Ryder, A. G., Guzder, J., Hassan, G., Rousseau, C., Pottie, K and the Canadian Collaboration for Immigrant and Refugee Health (2011). 'Common mental health problems in immigrants and refugees: general approach in primary care'. *CMAJ*, 183(12), e959–e967.

Krieger, N. (2012). 'Methods for the scientific study of discrimination and health: an ecosocial approach'. *American Journal of Public Health*, 102(5), 936–44.

Kuzawa, C. W. and Sweet, E. (2009). 'Epigenetics and the embodiment of race: developmental origins of US racial disparities in cardiovascular health'. *American Journal of Human Biology*, 21(1), 2–15.

Laird, L. D., Amer, M. M., Barnett, E. D. and Barnes, L. L. (2007a). 'Muslim patients and health disparities in the UK and the US'. *Archives of Disease in Childhood*, 92(10), 922–6.

Laird, L. D., de Marrais, J. and Barnes, L. L. (2007b). 'Portraying Islam and Muslims in MEDLINE: a content analysis'. *Social Science & Medicine*, 65(12), 2425–39.

Lee, H., Wildeman, C., Wang, E. A., Matusko, N. and Jackson, J. S. (2014). 'A heavy burden: the cardiovascular health consequences of having a family member incarcerated'. American Journal of Public Health, 104(3), 421–7.

Legido-Quigley, H., Pocock, N., Tan, S. T., Pajin, L., Suphanchaimat, R., Wick-ramage, K., McKee, M. and Pottie, K. (2019). 'Healthcare is not universal if undocumented migrants are excluded'. *BMJ*, 366: l4160.

Longwe, S.H. (1991). 'Gender awareness: the missing element in the Third World development project'. OXFAM Publications.

Love, E. (2009). 'Confronting Islamophobia in the United States: framing civil rights activism among Middle Eastern Americans'. *Patterns of Prejudice*, 43(3–4), 401–25.

Lukachko, A., Hatzenbuehler, M. L. and Keyes, K. (2014). 'Structural racism and myocardial infarction in the United States'. *Social Science & Medicine*, 103, 42–50.

Lynch, J. W., Smith, G. D., Kaplan, G. A. and House, J. S. (2000). 'Income inequality and mortality: importance to health of individual income, psychosocial environment, or material conditions'. *BMJ*, 320(7243), 1200–4.

Mahmood, S. S., Wroe, E., Fuller, A. and Leaning, J. (2017). 'The Rohingya people of Myanmar: health, human rights, and identity'. *The Lancet*, 389(10081), 1841–50.

Malik, A., Qureshi, H., Abdul-Razakq, H., Yaqoob, Z., Javaid, F. Z., Esmail, F., Wiley, E. and Latif, A. (2019). '"I decided not to go into surgery due to dress code": a cross-sectional study within the UK investigating experiences of female Muslim medical health professionals on bare below the elbows (BBE) policy and wearing headscarves (hijabs) in theatre'. *BMJ Open*, 9(3), e019954.

Mann, J., Drucker, E., Tarantola, D. and McCabe, M. P. (1994). 'Bosnia: the war against public health'. *Medicine and Global Survival*, 1(3), 130–46.

Mays, V. M., Cochran, S. D. and Barnes, S. W. (2007). 'Race, race-based discrimination, and health outcomes among African Americans'. *Annual Review of Psychology*, 58, 201–25.

McEwen, B. S. and Stellar, E. (1993). 'Stress and the individual: mechanisms leading to disease'. *Archives of Internal Medicine*, 153(18), 2093–101.

McFadden, A., Renfrew, M. J. and Atkin, K. (2013). 'Does cultural context make a difference to women's experiences of maternity care? A qualitative study comparing the perspectives of breast-feeding women of Bangladeshi origin and health practitioners'. *Health Expectations*, 16(4), e124–e135.

McKenzie, K., Bhui, K., Nanchahal, K. and Blizard, B. (2008). 'Suicide rates in people of South Asian origin in England and Wales: 1993–2003'. *British Journal of Psychiatry*, 193(5), 406–9.

Medina Ariza, J. J. (2014). 'Police-initiated contacts: young people, ethnicity, and the "usual suspects"'. *Policing and Society*, 24(2), 208–23.

Mental Health Foundation (2015). 'Dementia, rights and the social model of disability'. Policy Discussion Paper. Available at: www.mentalhealth.org.uk/sites/default/files/dementia-rights-policy-discussion.pdf (last accessed 18 May 2022).

Mirza, Z. (2019). 'Humanitarian crisis in Kashmir: don't shoot the messenger'. *The Lancet*, 396(10255), e45.

Modood, T., Berthoud, R., Lakey, J., Nazroo, J., Smith, P., Virdee, S. and Beishon, S. (eds) (1997), *Ethnic Minorities in Britain: Diversity and Disadvantage*. London: Policy Studies Institute.

Mohren, D. C., Swaen, G. M., van Amelsvoort, L. G., Borm, P. J. and Galama, J. M. (2003). 'Job insecurity as a risk factor for common infections and health complaints'. *Journal of Occupational and Environmental Medicine*, 45(2), 123–9.

Mueller, P. S., Plevak, D. J. and Rummans, T. A. (2001). 'Religious involvement, spirituality, and medicine: implications for clinical practice'. *Mayo Clinic Proceedings*, 76(12), 1225–35.

Müller-Uri, F. and Opratko, B. (2016). 'Islamophobia as anti-Muslim racism: racism without "races", racism without racists'. *Islamophobia Studies Journal*, 3(2), 116–29.

Muslim Council of Britain (2015). 'British Muslims in numbers: a demographic, socio-economic and health profile of Muslims in Britain drawing on the 2011 census'. Available at: https://www.mcb.org.uk/wp-content/uploads/2015/02/MCBCensusReport_2015.pdf (last accessed 13 May 2022).

Nash, J. C. (2008). 'Re-thinking intersectionality'. *Feminist Review*, 89(1), 1–15.

NHS Digital (2012). 'National Child Measurement Programme – England, 2011–2012 school year'. Available at: https://digital.nhs.uk/data-and-information/publications/statistical/national-child-measurement-programme/2011-12-school-year (last accessed 15 July 2022).

Nazroo, J. Y. (2003). 'The structuring of ethnic inequalities in health: economic position, racial discrimination, and racism'. *American Journal of Public Health*, 93(2), 277–84.

Nussbaum, M. C. (2011). *Creating Capabilities*. Cambridge, MA: Harvard University Press.

O'Beirne, M. (2004). 'Religion in England and Wales: findings from the 2001 Home Office citizenship survey'. Available at: www.semanticscholar.org/paper/Religion-in-England-and-Wales%3A-findings-from-the-O%E2%80%99Beirne/6588afbdbb53e13a9b9b5ce5c1ce06b75af7c534#paper-header (last accessed 11 July 2022).

O'Connor, A. J. and Jahan, F. (2014). 'Under surveillance and overwrought: American Muslims' emotional and behavioral responses to government surveillance'. *Journal of Muslim Mental Health*, 8(1), 95–106.

Office for National Statistics (2011). 'Religion in England and Wales 2011'. Available at: www.ons.gov.uk/peoplepopulationandcommunity/culturalidentity/religion/articles/religioninenglandandwales2011/2012-12-11 (last accessed 19 May 2022).

Open Society for Justice Initiative (2016). 'Eroding trust: the UK's PREVENT counter-terrorism strategy in health and education'. Available at: www.justiceinitiative.org/

publications/eroding-trust-uk-s-prevent-counter-extremism-strategy-health-and-education (last accessed 19 May 2022).

Pachankis, J. E. (2007). 'The psychological implications of concealing a stigma: a cognitive-affective-behavioral model'. *Psychological Bulletin*, 133(2), 328–45.

Padela, A. I. and Curlin, F. A. (2013). 'Religion and disparities: considering the influences of Islam on the health of American Muslims'. *Journal of Religion and Health*, 52(4), 1333–45.

Paradies, Y., Ben, J.,Denson, N.,Elias, A., Priest, N., Pieterse, A., Gupta, A., Kelaher, M. and Gee, G. (2015). 'Racism as a determinant of health: a systematic review and meta-analysis'. *PloS ONE*, 10(9), e0138511.

Peñaranda, F. (2015). 'The individual, social justice and public health'. *Ciencia & Saude Coletiva*, 20, 987–96.

Pew Research Center (2017). 'Europe's growing Muslim population'. Available at: www.pewresearch.org/religion/2017/11/29/europes-growing-muslim-population (last accessed 19 May 2022).

Pierce, C. (1995). 'Stress analogs of racism and sexism: terrorism, torture, and disaster'. *Mental Health, Racism, and Sexism*, 33: 277–93.

Public Health England (2017). 'Focus on ethnicity'. Public Health Outcomes Framework: Health Equity Report. Available at: https://assets.publishing.service.gov.uk/government/uploads/system/uploads/attachment_data/file/733093/PHOF_Health_Equity_Report.pdf (last accessed 15 July 2022).

Quaglio, G., Karapiperis, T., Van Woensel, E., Arnold, E. and McDaid, D. (2013). 'Austerity and health in Europe'. *Health Policy*, 113(1–2), 13–19.

Raphael, D. and Bryant, T. (2015). 'Power, intersectionality and the life-course: identifying the political and economic structures of welfare states that support or threaten health'. *Social Theory & Health*, 13(3–4), 245–66.

Reitmanova, S. and Gustafson, D. L. (2008). '"They can't understand it": maternity health and care needs of immigrant Muslim women in St. John's, Newfoundland'. *Maternal and Child Health Journal*, 12(1), 101–11.

Reynolds, L. and Birdwell, J. (2015). 'Rising to the top'. DEMOS. Available at: https://demos.co.uk/project/rising-to-the-top (last accessed 19 May 2022).

Robinson, F. (1999). 'The British empire and the Muslim worlds', in J. Brown and W. R. Louis (eds), *Oxford History of the British Empire*, vol. 4. Oxford: Oxford University Press, pp. 398–420.

Ross, C. E. and Wu, C.-I. (1995). 'The links between education and health'. *American Sociological Review*, 60(5), 719–45.

Ruger, J. P. (2004). 'Health and social justice'. *The Lancet*, 364(9439), 1075–80.

Saeed, A., Blain, N. and Forbes, D. (1999). 'New ethnic and national questions in Scotland: post-British identities among Glasgow Pakistani teenagers'. *Ethnic and Racial Studies*, 22(5), 821–44.

Samari, G. (2016). 'Islamophobia and public health in the United States'. *American Journal of Public Health*, 106(11), 1920–5.

Samiei, M. (2010). 'Neo-Orientalism? The relationship between the West and Islam in our globalised world'. *Third World Quarterly*, 31(7), 1145–60.

Sanders-Phillips, K., Settles-Reaves, B., Walker, D. and Brownlow, J. (2009). 'Social inequality and racial discrimination: risk factors for health disparities in children of color'. *Pediatrics*, 124(Supplement 3), S176–S186.

Schrecker, T. (2016). 'Globalization, austerity and health equity politics: taming the inequality machine, and why it matters'. *Critical Public Health*, 26(1), 4–13.

Sen, A. K. (1992). *Inequality Reexamined*. Oxford: Oxford University Press.

Shahid, H. and Abdulkareem, B. (2018). 'The triple penalty: Muslim doctors in the NHS'. Muslim Doctors Association. Available at: https://muslimdoctors.org/wp-content/uploads/2021/02/The-Triple-Penalty-Muslim-Doctors-in-the-NHS-.pdf (last accessed 19 May 2022).

Siegrist, J. (1995). 'Emotions and health in occupational life: new scientific findings and policy implications'. *Patient Education and Counseling*, 25(3), 227–36.

Silva, S. (2018). 'Cultures: how different are they? A nursing perspective'. *Senior Honors Theses and Projects*, 577. Available at: https://commons.emich.edu/honors/577 (last accessed 19 May 2022).

Smedley, B., Stith, A. and Nelson, A. (2002). 'Unequal treatment: What healthcare providers need to know about racial and ethnic disparities in health-care'. Washington, DC: National Academy Press. Available at: https://nap.nationalacademies.org/resource/10260/disparities_providers.pdf (last accessed 19 May 2022).

Sproston, K. and Mindell, J. (2006). *Health Survey for England 2004: Health Survey for England 2004: The Health of Minority Ethnic Groups*. Leeds: The Information Centre.

Stevenson, J., Demack, S., Stiell, B., Abdi. M., Clarkson, L., Ghaffar, F. and Hassan, S. (2017). 'The social mobility challenges faced by young Muslims'. Social Mobility Commission. Available at: https://assets.publishing.service.gov.uk/government/uploads/system/uploads/attachment_data/file/642220/Young_Muslims_SMC.pdf (last accessed 19 May 2022).

Stubley, P. (2019). 'Muslim women "sterilised" in China detention camps, say former detainees'. *The Independent*, 12 August. Available at: www.independent.co.uk/news/world/asia/uighur-muslim-china-sterilisation-women-internment-camps-xinjiang-a9054641.html (last accessed 19 May 2022).

Stuckler, D., Reeves, A., Loopstra, R., Karanikolos, M. and McKee, M. (2017). 'Austerity and health: the impact in the UK and Europe'. *European Journal of Public Health*, 27 (suppl 4), 18–21.

Szczepura, A. (2005). 'Access to health care for ethnic minority populations'. *Postgraduate Medical Journal*, 81(953), 141–7.

Tell MAMA (2018). 'Beyond the incident: outcomes for victims of anti-Muslim prejudice'. Executive Summary. Available at: https://tellmamauk.org/wp-content/uploads/2018/07/EXECUTIVE-SUMMARY.pdf (last accessed 19 May 2022).

Tell MAMA (2019). 'Tell MAMA Annual Report 2018: normalising hatred'. Available at: https://tellmamauk.org/tell-mama-annual-report-2018-_-normalising-hate (last accessed 19 May 2022).

Thompson, N. (2017). *Promoting Equality*. 4th edn. London: Macmillan International Higher Education.

UK Government (2010). 'Equality Act 2010'. Available at: www.legislation.gov.uk/ukpga/2010/15/contents (last accessed 19 May 2022).

UK Government (2012). 'Public sector equality duty'. Available at: www.gov.uk/government/publications/public-sector-equality-duty (last accessed 15 July 2022).

Vu, M., Azmat, A., Radejko, T. and Padela, A. I. (2016). 'Predictors of delayed healthcare seeking among American Muslim women'. *Journal of Women's Health*, 25(6), 586–593.

Wang, S.-J., Salihu, M., Rushiti, F., Bala, L. and Modvig, J. (2010). 'Survivors of the war in the Northern Kosovo: violence exposure, risk factors and public health effects of an ethnic conflict'. *Conflict and Health*, 4(1), 11.

Warfa, N., Bhui, K., Craig, T., Curtis, S., Mohamud, S., Stansfeld, S., McCrone, P. and Thornicroft, G. (2006). 'Post-migration geographical mobility, mental health and health service utilisation among Somali refugees in the UK: a qualitative study'. *Health & Place*, 12(4), 503–15.

Weller, P. (2011). Religious discrimination in Britain: A review of research evidence, 2000–10'. Equality and Human Rights Commission, Research Report 73. Available at: www.equalityhumanrights.com/sites/default/files/research_report_73_religious_discrimination.pdf (last accessed 19 May 2022).

Weller, P., Feldman, A. and Purdam, K. (2001). *Religious Discrimination in England and Wales*. London. Home Office.

World Health Organization (1995). 'Constitution of the World Health Oganization'. Available at: https://apps.who.int/iris/handle/10665/121457 (last accessed 19 May 2022).

World Health Organization (2008). 'Closing the gap in a generation: health equity through action on the social determinants of health'. Commission on Social Determinants of Health final report. Available at: https://apps.who.int/iris/bitstream/handle/10665/43943/9789241563703_eng.pdf (last accessed 18 May 2022).

Younis, T. and Jadhav, S. (2019). 'Keeping our mouths shut: the fear and racialized self-censorship of British healthcare professionals in PREVENT training'. *Culture, Medicine and Psychiatry*, 43(3), 404–24.

Younis, T. and Jadhav, S. (2020). 'Islamophobia in the National Health Service: an ethnography of institutional racism in PREVENT's counter-radicalisation policy'. *Sociology of Health & Illness*, 42(3), 610–26.

Yuval-Davis, N. (2015). 'Situated intersectionality and social inequality'. *Raisons politiques*, 58(2), 91–100.

11

'WELL DONE FOR COMING BECAUSE YOUR KIND DON'T NORMALLY COME TO THINGS LIKE THIS' – IDENTITY STRUGGLES FOR SECOND- AND THIRD-GENERATION BRITISH MUSLIMS AND ENGAGEMENT WITH HEALTH INFORMATION: A REFLECTIVE PERSPECTIVE

Rukhsana Rashid

Introduction

The way in which a subject is first broached can often determine what message is received. The intention of the messenger and the message itself may become clouded if the choice of words was poor. Healthcare professionals, like everyone else, can sometimes hold pre-judged ideas about certain groups of people. It is very difficult to be completely unbiased despite one's best intentions. Even in blind randomised controlled trials, there is always an element of bias. You may be able to blind individual participants; however if you are recruiting in a certain hospital in a particular town, for example, you will know certain demographics about local residents which can lead to bias. It is therefore important that bias is managed and does not disproportionately and negatively affect certain communities. The current social and political climate highlights that bias and prejudice can disadvantage people in certain groups from healthcare services all the way through to access to the judicial system. If anything, it creates further disharmony in an already fractured society.

Identities are a complex thing. In a rapidly changing world, it is becoming harder to characterise people with a somewhat outdated set of characteristics. In this chapter, I will draw on some of my own experiences as someone who has a hybrid identity and doesn't fit in a neat and concise identity box that we often use to characterise people in order to show how this can be problematic when delivering health information or services. The problems are deep-rooted and in a world built around systems, challenges can be presented from both sides of the equation.

The Importance of Narratives in Delivering Effective Health Information and How they Have Been Used

First and foremost, it is important to understand how people use narratives. A number of narratives can be generated which are a function of linguistic form. Not only do they provide a view on what people do and how they do it, but also how they feel about what it is they do. As much as the person telling their story selectively chooses certain dynamics or experiences to emphasise, this is further complicated by the fact that the narrator makes their own decisions as to what is regarded as important or significant. Further, through this process a certain interpretation emerges which tells a particular story. How this is rationalised and internalised by other readers then also becomes important in the context of determining whether what is found is a specific objective truth or a view on the world in general.

In particular, the narrative approach appears to suggest meaningful and purposive opportunities for engagement and effective delivery. One model uses the notion of 'culture-centricity' as a way to suggest culturally specific interventions that target communities through an engagement with narratives and metaphors. The process includes understanding the community through a kind of ethnographic methodology that means listening, understanding and conceptualising a particular set of cultural norms and values for various ethnic groups without necessarily placing any pre-existing paradigms at the fore (Campbell and Quintiliani 2006). Larkey and Hecht (2010) state that:

> Many remarkable programmes of health promotion have done just that, both nationally and internationally, taking an ethnographic inventory regarding health behaviours and developing educational interventions that take into account cultural factors that function as barriers and facilitators, or incorporating cultural content to make messages more relevant.

Moreover, the 'model acknowledges the value of going beyond conventional theory and adopting a culturally grounded view of how behaviour is shaped and normed within sociocultural contexts' (ibid).

These cultural scripts are, however, contextual in that they relate to specific cultural, social and psychological norms and values of different communities across the world. Research carried out on the understanding of dying in the USA and Japan found that there were different characterisations of the experience and how people prepared themselves for the inevitable outcome. Much of this was maintained through a cultural lens such that 'the process of creating and maintaining cultural scripts requires the active participation of ordinary people as they in turn respond to the constraints of post-industrial technology, institutions, demographics and notions of self' (Long 2004). Here, the roles of culture, religion, identity and practice are omnipotent in the understanding of how different people across the world appreciate dying and how they prepare for it. Different health service fraternities across the world need to remain aware of the variations in cultural expectations and narratives that ensue from them, particularly for those with hybrid identities. This chapter highlights that there are significant gaps between the expectations of individual patients and the preconceptions of medical and health services.

All of these issues become important in the context of the ways in which individuals and communities appreciate and understand the nature of the healthcare that they receive. While culturally sensitive health education is a way in which to target certain groups, it is important to understand that individuals (especially those that have hybrid identities) engaging with such matters have their own 'logic of choice', which affects their attitudes and behaviour in relation to healthcare programmes. Therefore, within the constraints of trying to ensure an effective policy and cultural approach in managing the health needs of minority groups, there are existing concerns that exist within the groups themselves that are mediated at an individual level based on issues of psychology, physiology and social context (Henwood et al. 2001).

When there are issues relating to questions of health, a number of other factors come into play. Doctors and nurses can play a crucial role in constructing, shaping and re-affirming certain health narratives that can aid the process of healing and recovery. These professionals can (and that is a key word here) employ empathetic methods of listening and learning, ensuring that they can fully appreciate the nature of the patient's problems without coming to predetermined conclusions which may well be damaging to the individual in the short term. This process establishes a rapport that sustains reflection on problems, perceived and actual, and encourages a fuller and franker interaction. This process also reflects on the general nature of medical professional practices, which maintain the need to determine an explicitly scientific conclusion for diagnosis and treatment. While this is a necessary element of any aspect of treatment, without a clearer and more nuanced analysis of the qualitative dimensions of the illness, there is the potential for certain limits to understanding and application.

The essential element is interpretation. Oral traditions have been lost in the recent experiences of Western medicine, but they continue to provide valuable approaches to treatment, which are potentially being overlooked in the current period. It can be argued that there is a need to move away from a more structured and disciplined method of analysis to one that is based more on qualitative interpretation and individual case study analysis. The upshot of this is that for a research project looking at the medical treatment experiences and particular forms of health education, such a method has a certain purchase that is informative, evaluative and cost-effective in the long run. In the context of the particular challenges facing ethnic minorities (or the majority within minorities, which is what the focus is on here), such a method potentially provides considerable opportunities (Greenhalgh and Hurwitz 1999).

The Research Problem

Health services, interventions and policies are no doubt influenced and determined by research findings, meaning the role of research and research conduct is the first vital step to appropriateness and efficiency in practice.

How we record and use information is also important in shaping our understanding. In the UK (and indeed around the world), there are many large cohort studies that follow the lives, health and wellbeing of participants over many years. However, it is often the case that demographic information that was first collected on participants at baseline is not regularly updated. There is no doubt that some demographics will not change but there are other features that may, and not updating such information can lead to mistargeted interventions or understanding. The language question is one such example. If a cohort that started fifteen years ago recruited participants where 50 per cent of them were non-English speakers, is it acceptable to assume that fifteen years later that balance would not have changed? Because information like this is not regularly updated, the assumption is always that the sample consists of 50 per cent non-English-speaking participants and therefore resources will continue to be directed into translated documents and results will be presented that are based on baseline demographic data. A lack of consideration is given to the fact that this kind of demographic information can change. This in turn can lead to misleading and misdirected outcomes. For example, if a survey on the uptake of prenatal education classes was conducted with a cohort in 2020 based on demographic information collected in 2005, when 50 per cent of participants were non-English speaking, one might conclude from this study that language barriers were an issue that reflected the uptake numbers. It would assume that in fifteen years language skills had not improved and resources should focus on making education more accessible when in actual fact the low uptake may be a result of other issues which are not being given as much attention. Factors such as systematic racism, social isolation and deprivation can contribute to low uptake and poor access to services. Indeed, these factors are much more difficult to address than a language barrier. We need to move on from this idea of basing things on what can be referenced from historical literature.

There are a number of important issues in the appreciation of the context of second- and third-generation (South Asian) Muslim minority identities in the UK. Apart from the socioeconomic issues that impact on groups there are also a whole host of sociocultural concerns. It is important that the changing identity dynamics are recognised and understood among health professionals in order to engage and cater for a group that is largely ignored in the literature because the literature has not moved beyond describing British Muslims (who are largely from a South Asian background) as non-English speaking, curry-eating, introverted individuals. Far too often, health professionals presume that in order to engage people from minority ethnic backgrounds the focus should be on translating literature and seeking out 'gatekeepers' from the community. Fifteen years ago, when I started out in this field, it was common and robotic practice to auto-translate information if you had minority participants. Although we now have a new generation of British (Asian) Muslims who are likely to be British-born and some to British-born parents, the practices for 'reaching out' have not changed. Who are the gatekeepers or community leaders anyway? What qualifies someone to be one? Why do only minority groups have community leaders? Why isn't there an attempt to understand individual groups through their own lens rather than be represented by someone who is more often than not of a first generation, an older person, male and generally not very 'representative' of the majority of the active population who tend to be more closely aligned to the British culture that they were born into. I can fully appreciate that for some research or engagement activities, there is a need for 'gatekeepers'. For example, if a Western researcher wanted to meet locals in a remote part of Timbuktu, using a local 'gatekeeper' who can help with access and local knowledge would be very helpful. Do we really have communities in the UK that are so inaccessible that we need 'community leaders' to engage with them?

I am somewhat relieved to see that in most instances we have now moved away from using terms such as 'hard-to-reach communities'. Although a prominent feature in literature that referred to minority communities around ten years ago, it is now slightly more widely accepted that minority communities are not 'hard to reach' but in fact the approaches that were used to engage them were perhaps problematic (Symons 2017). Not everyone will engage with traditional methods of research, and there is a need for more novel approaches:

> Ethnography has much to offer health informatics research, but its contribution may remain in the shadows until the field acknowledges the need not merely for new methodologies but also new ontologies, new epistemologies and new definitions of what is of value. (Greenhalgh 2001)

Making Sense of Hybrid Identities

When it comes to people with hybrid identities in the UK, this can add a further layer of complication to characterising people and therefore understanding them. It is however very important because British-born ethnic minorities is a large and distinct group. The approach that healthcare professionals take is a vital tool in how messages about health and wellbeing are received (Bibi et al. 2014). This section will now explore how second- and third-generation British South Asian Muslims who identify with a more hybrid identity are missing from the debate and how they can be key to promoting better health within this wider minority group if properly engaged.

For many UK nationals descended from second-, third- or fourth-generation migrants, their identity can sometimes become an issue of confusion as self-identification may not match how others may choose to identify them. This is something that I regularly experience and struggle to make sense of because I am often described as or seen through a lens of an identity that I do not necessarily identify with. Here is an example from a personal account: 'Well done for coming because your kind don't normally come to things like this'. These were the 'encouraging words' uttered to me by a nurse when I attended my GP surgery for a routine cervical screening test. For a short moment I contemplated what she meant by '[my] kind'. Was it a reference to women? Was it a reference to women in their mid-thirties? Or was it a reference to a wider definition: short women in their mid-thirties with long dark hair who wear glasses? Cynicism aside, I do not believe that any of those identities were visible in her observation of '[my] kind'. The reality is that the reference was clearly about my perceived ethnicity and/or race, which was evident from the colour of my skin. This unfortunate choice of words took my attention away from the very valid and correct point that she was making. The attendance for cervical screening in the UK among women of a South Asian background is disappointingly low (Anderson de Cuevas et al. 2018). Many reasons for this have been identified in the literature and, sure enough, some of these point to cultural taboos and barriers. There is clearly a need for improvement in uptake; however, if this was an attempt at motivation, I'm afraid it failed to encourage me at least. In fact, it probably had the opposite effect from the desired impact. First, how I self-identify did not match the box that she was perhaps placing me in, which is quite common among British-born minorities. However, this identity argument is almost completely absent from the mainstream. Race/ethnicity categories used for data collection are still defined as they were in the 1960s. I am unable to reference this claim because it is ignored in research; however from my lived experiences, I know that there are significant differences between, for example, people of South Asian origin born in the UK and their migrant parents in how they access health services. British-born 'South Asians' are a significantly large minority group; nevertheless, in the literature, 'Asian or British Asian' is often a homogeneous category.

Clearly we cannot have separate categories to define every different group in a multicultural society; it wouldn't be feasible to do so. However it is unfortunate that the stereotypes associated with 'South Asians' have not evolved in the way the actual community has. This stereotyping and preconceived labelling is at best unhelpful.

One may hope that instances such as the example above are isolated; however, they are actually more common than we would like to think. It is important to remember that NHS staff are ordinary members of society outside their professional capacity. So a nurse politely telling me 'my kind don't come' in reality is no different from a woman in a queue at the theme park maliciously telling a young girl that '[her] kind are not welcome here'. Nevertheless, it is important to point out that there is clearly a difference of intent here even though the narrative is the same. We cannot decode a person's intentions; however, the point is that semantics are important. For those who are more accustomed to being on the receiving end of such comments, the feeling of being 'profiled' or discriminated against based on a single characteristic such as race or ethnicity is demoralising and it does not help facilitate engagement. In post-Brexit Britain, this sense of constantly being reminded that you are an 'Other' to the mainstream is more prevalent in society generally but it should not be an experience reinforced within a public body such as the NHS and other healthcare services. Effectively engaging people may help with uptake of some services where this is lacking.

My list of lived experiences of this kind could, unsurprisingly, go on and on. As mentioned previously, the intent is not always malicious. It may well be and probably is considerate. However, it cannot be stressed enough how important semantics and the execution of a message is. Perhaps it is an oversensitivity but it is the case for a large proportion of 'minority communities'. Shaping discourse based on preconceived ideas that are often outdated (regardless of how subtly it is done) is not helpful. I recall these narratives from my experiences often and remember them in detail because of the effects they had. Here is another example. When my child was a newborn, the midwife came to speak to me about childhood immunisations and asked if I wanted the tuberculosis (TB) injection for him. 'I think you should go for it because you are a high-risk group and when you go to India or Pakistan [clearly unsure about which one would apply] that are high-risk countries, then at least you are protected'. Just like the first example, this was a perfectly valid and correct point but unfortunately it was mixed up with confusing and disengaging narratives. She was absolutely correct that people of South Asian origin are at higher risk of contracting TB (Offer et al. 2016) but to then follow up with a presumption about 'when' we take our child to Pakistan is unfortunate. As someone who has not yet visited any part of South Asia themselves, it wasn't a given that my child would be visiting. The presumption from the midwife, however, was that we would because our parents/grandparents (who were early migrants) did and therefore that's what all we brown folks do. Would similar implications be made to a Caucasian person? Benidorm in Spain is a popular holiday destination for many working-class White British families. Would anyone imply to a White person that they 'will' visit Benidorm? It could be considered pre-judgemental, confusing and even offensive. So why is there an assumption that everyone from a South Asian background identifies and lives in a particular assumed way? That the dominant practices of the early migrant population of the 1950s and 1960s still define subsequent generations? From an engagement point of view, these narratives are not reflective of second- or third-generation British Asians and are outdated and disengaging.

The need to intervene in improving awareness of health issues among ethnically diverse communities has been researched in the recent past with the general result that community-orientated projects provide additional space for impact, combined with the importance of a change in behaviour patterns to help fight obesity, for example. While much of this research is scientifically methodological, there are also studies that are community-orientated action research projects focusing on changing attitudes as well as outcomes. One of the findings often repeated is that if there is a communication strategy in relation to health awareness that involves a number of health interventions, namely diet, exercise and counselling, multi-purpose outcomes can be achieved (Resnicow et al. 2006). Although a receptive audience can be found in this way, it is important that the information given is also relevant. For example, second- and third-generation British (Asian) Muslims don't eat curry and chapatti every day of the week (like their parents). Instead, they are more likely to eat a low-nutrition fast-food takeaway if they live in a deprived neighbourhood where such food outlets are many. It is therefore important that health information takes into account a generationally relevant and holistic approach. Unlike their parents, second- and third-generation British (Asian) Muslims (although well below the national average) tend to be better educated and so it is important to acknowledge how knowledge of positive health choices is utilised and actualised between generations (Landman and Cruickshank 2001).

Emergence of the British Muslim Identity

For many Muslims, their religious identity holds far more relevance than their ethnic identity in defining their characteristics and lifestyle. In many ways there has been a strategic shift away from ethnic and cultural identification because much of it is embedded in traditional Indo-Hindu practices that are largely deemed as contradictory to Islamic values. It is therefore important to elaborate on the questions that impact on the study of British (Asian) Muslims in relation to their health needs and in the raising of awareness of certain treatment programmes that specifically target minority 'ethnic' communities.

It seems that community-driven literature has outpaced academic literature and acknowledged that communities in the UK adopt more hybrid identities. Take, for example, Ilm2Amal, an educational resource developed by imams and madrassahs in the UK (ilm2amal.org) that looks at society and identity. It has correctly identified that British Muslims' cultural heritage is less significant to them than their faith-based and British identity. It is important for mainstream literature to acknowledge this as an identity in itself otherwise we risk alienating a whole generation of people who have carved a clear identity in the present which is not dictated by the past but looks towards the future.

In order to properly construe this argument, it is important that we first explore some of the historical context and understand why there is sensitivity around identity politics among some groups. The religion question appeared in the 2001 Census for the first time since 1850, and 92 per cent of the population gave a response to the voluntary question. Muslims of a South Asian background (particularly Pakistani) are the single largest ethnic religious group in Britain, with approximately 1.5 million in the UK today based on current estimates from the 2011 UK census (ONS 2011).

During the 1950s and 1960s, as a result of the push-pull forces of emigration and migration, many of the first migrants from Pakistan, especially from the Azad Kashmir region of the country, settled in the poorer older towns and cities where the jobs were at the time, with places such as Bradford becoming one of the most attractive due to its textile industry, metal manufacturing and engineering sectors. But because of de-industrialisation and globalisation, there had been a concentration of migrant Pakistanis who experienced deskilling and underemployment, which prevented social mobility and impacted on a process of cultural and religious maintenance in response to racism and discrimination that has seen this group locked out of the local economy and society (Abbas 2010a). Unfortunately, several generations on and this limited social, economic and educational mobility, with its associated poor health outcomes, is still quite evident and as a result perceptions of British South Asians by the host population have not changed much even though the community has evolved through the generations, particularly in terms of how they self-identify.

The regional concentrations in the UK vary, with South Asians in the north of England more likely to be monocultural, monoethnic, monolingual Mirpuris compared with those in the south of England who are more likely to be the opposite, that is multicultural, multiethnic and multilingual. The terms 'Azad Kashmiri' and 'Mirpuri' have not achieved recognition in the academic literature in the same way as 'Pakistani', but often when discussions of inequality and disadvantage are mentioned, there is an indirect reference to the Mirpuris. Moreover, politically speaking, it is important to mention that some would not regard the region of Azad Kashmir as part of Kashmir and nor would some regard Azad Kashmir as part of Pakistan. There are ongoing challenges of identity construction and formalisation that have often found greater space for discussion in the context of diaspora communities in Britain (Shaw 2001).

In the post 9/11 climate, where issues of terrorism are in the media domain, British Muslims have been at the sharp end of negative discourses in relation to the othering, where ideas of failed multiculturalism have been intertwined with a debate on securitisation (Abbas 2011). When it comes to matters of religion, there tends to be a wish for many second and third generations of British South Asian Muslims to identify with any form of 'Islamisation', particularly in the post-9/11 period (Abbas 2007). Young Muslims are increasingly shaping their identities by focusing on religion rather than ethnicity. This is determined by forces that may be external to the community or, indeed, internal, creating a local-global nexus of Islamicised identity politics. Part of the reason is intergenerational change, that is that younger Muslims are having another look at religion's original sources for themselves, re-interpreting it and making it relevant for their needs today, without it in any way seemingly going against doctrine (Ijaz and Abbas 2010). This is shaping their perceptions of identity far more than their ethnic origins as, having spent their lives in the UK, their association with a British lifestyle and language is more relevant to them within the realms of Islamic boundaries. The systematic discrimination and disadvantages faced by their parents have brought about a new form of identity for British Muslims in an attempt to shake off the negative experiences of their predecessors.

In order to improve the health behaviour of patients and those at risk of certain illnesses, it remains crucial to understand the factors that drive various social norms and values in specific ethnic and religious minority communities (Patel et al. 2012). Before this can be done, it is important to understand the hybrid and evolved identity with which some identify, as without proper understanding we can neither understand nor deliver. Scholars have questioned how existing research has tended to misunderstand the factors associated with ways in which South Asian groups perceived the cause of their illnesses, and greater researcher sensitivity is presented as a way in which to alleviate the problems of research design bias and misconceptualisation (Lawton et al. 2007). This sensitivity is also important on the part of the clinicians, who have been known to show a lack of awareness at some level, but crucially to misinterpret cultural sensitivity as a lack of knowledge per se, or that the wider communities in which these South Asians find themselves did not show the support or awareness that would otherwise be seen as purposive for the patient concerned (Grace et al. 2008).

While there are considerable 'theoretical benefits' for marginalised ethnic minority groups in accessing effective healthcare (Greenhalgh 2001), it remains inconclusive whether their engagement through a series of ethnic minority sensitive gateways actually led to the changed outcomes. One of the key reasons is that studies carried out to determine this process have not always been able to capture the entire period of the programme and thus have not been able to measure the course of action over a dedicated period of time. Greenhalgh et al. (2011) argued that more enhanced research techniques are potentially required in order to fully ascertain how the individual ethnic minority storyteller is able to determine a set of healthcare solutions by 'linking membership of a story-sharing group with individual clinical care planning and regular review of goals' (ibid.).

There are far too many leaflets out there that are translated into Urdu when in fact the majority of even the first generation of South Asians from the Mirpur region do not read or speak the language to any great extent. Although such practices may tick the boxes for inclusivity, they are often useless. On the other hand, that is not to say that the British population as a whole should be viewed homogeneously. Of course there are differences based on ethnic origin, however the point is that other forms of self-identification and lived experiences of communities in the UK should not be ignored. Unfortunately, South Asian Muslims are among the most marginalised and alienated in British society (Abbas 2010b), not just in terms of health promotion but also with regard to social mobility.

Conclusion

How people remember social facts and recall memories are a function of the ways in which the brain differentiates between different types of memory (Squire 1992). Schank and Abelson (1995) have argued that

> if the core of social knowledge and the essence of social communication both consist of a bank of stories and a set of story processing structures, then it should be the case that the understanding of other people's utterances is story-based, too.

That is, what people understand as knowledge is effectively the sum of the recollection of stories, invariably in response to other stories, which act as stimuli. Once the stories are told and retold, they eventually begin to allow memories to be formed. Therefore, stories can be suppressed and affect what is recalled, or not as the case may be. What we choose to remember is a function of what we choose to forget and vice versa. Determining comprehension in relation to a story requires finding degrees of similarity between the various narratives of the storyteller and the listener. Therefore, what we choose to remember, and how we choose to tell the story about that particular memory, affects what we understand from it and therefore what we communicate to others as our recollection and understanding of the event (Schank and Abelson 1995).

While these psychological processes within the brain are determined through experience, there is also the effect it has on the ways in which individuals can challenge the systems they face, that is to assess modes of education and understanding from a more critical perspective, ultimately improving understanding and their engagement with the social world. Therefore, storytelling and narrative building is not just a way of improving learning and understanding among adults, it is also a way in which to actively change their behaviour and actions (Carter 1993).

There is clearly a link between the academic literature and health information that is produced based on that literature. However, with evolving communities and hybrid identities, there is a need for more work to be done with communities in a present and future tense rather than historical contexts. Before attempts are made to develop interventions, it is vital that researchers conceptualise who the target audience is and what their lived experiences are rather than nuanced ethnicities.

The need and the solution here are simple. Currently contemporary understandings of second- and third-generation minority communities are sometimes missing. It is important to see them through a lens that is representative of their lives and experiences and not just their ethnicity or cultural background. Identity can be a complex phenomenon. Putting people in predefined boxes is not always the best approach and nor can we not apply characteristics. As individual as everyone is, it is important on a macro level that there is some definition of different groups. My argument in this chapter is a simple one. Second- and third-generation British Muslims are a significant group in the UK and we need to recognise that their identities and their experiences differ significantly from those of their predecessors if services are to be targeted effectively.

Many studies comparing health outcomes for South Asian communities with those of the Caucasian population tend to imply that South Asians are at higher risk or are more susceptible to certain illnesses. The problem, however, is that such studies paint a somewhat distorted picture. Although there is acknowledgment that in some cases the fact that British South Asian families live in deprived neighbourhoods feeds into the health inequalities they face, the right level of importance is not placed on this. Would the Caucasian population in these circumstances still have better health outcomes? Would they still have better educational and social mobility outcomes? I would say probably not. The suggestion here is not that all Caucasians are better off. Of course this is not the case. There are many, particularly in towns in the north of England, who live in deprived neighbourhoods with low educational attainment and overall poverty. I suggest the difference is racial discrimination. They probably never hear the words 'well done for coming because your kind don't come to things like this'. Maybe if that phrase stopped at 'well done for coming' the impact would be vastly different. A sensitive, unbiased and identifiable approach may improve the accessibility to and uptake of health information and services among an invisible group within a marginalised community.

References

Abbas, T. (2007). 'Muslim minorities in Britain: integration, multiculturalism and radicalism in the post-7/7 period'. *Journal of Intercultural Studies*, 28(3), 287–300.

Abbas, T. (2010a). 'The British Pakistani diaspora: migration, integration and the intersection of race, ethnicity and religion'. *Orient*, 2, 49–55.

Abbas, T. (2010b). 'Islam and Muslims in the UK'. Available at: www.thebritishacademy.ac.uk/sites/default/files/08-Abbas.pdf (last accessed 16 May 2022).

Abbas, T. (2011). *Islamic Radicalism and Multicultural Politics*. London: Routledge.

Anderson de Cuevas, R., Saini, P., Roberts, D., Beaver, K., Chandrashekar, M., Jain, A., Kotas, E., Tahir, N., Ahmed, S. and Brown, S. (2018). 'A systematic review of barriers and enablers to South Asian women's attendance for asymptomatic screening of breast and cervical cancers in emigrant countries'. *BMJ Open*, 8, e020892.

Bibi, R., Redwood, S. and Taheri, S. (2014). 'Raising the issue of overweight and obesity with the South Asian community'. *British Journal of General Practice*, 64(625): 417–19.

Campbell, M. K. and Quintiliani, L. (2006). 'Tailored interventions in public health: where does tailoring fit in interventions to reduce health disparities?'. *American Behavioral Scientist*, 49(6): 775–93.

Carter, K. (1993). 'The place of story in the study of teaching and teacher education'. *Educational Researcher*, 22(1), 5–18.

Grace, C., Begum, R., Subhani, S., Kopelman, P. and Greenhalgh, T. (2008). 'Prevention of type 2 diabetes in British Bangladeshis: qualitative study of community, religious, and professional perspectives'. *BMJ*, 337, a1931.

Greenhalgh, T. (2001). 'Storytelling should be targeted where it is known to have greatest added value'. *Medical Education*, 35(9), 818–19.

Greenhalgh, T., Campbell-Richards, D., Vijayaraghavan, S., Collard, A., Malik, F., Griffin, M., Morris, J., Claydon, A. and Macfarlane, F. (2011). 'New models of self-management education for minority ethnic groups: pilot randomized trial of a story-sharing intervention'. *Journal of Health Services Research & Policy*, 16(1), 28–36.

Greenhalgh, T. and Hurwitz, B. (1999). 'Narrative based medicine: Why study narrative?'. *BMJ*, 318, 48–50.

Henwood, F., Harris, R. and Spoel, P. (2011). 'Informing health? Negotiating the logics of choice and care in everyday practices of "healthy living"', *Social Science & Medicine*, 72(12), 2026–32.

Ijaz, A. and Abbas, T. (2010). 'The impact of inter-generational change on the attitudes of working class South Asian Muslim parents on the education of their daughters'. *Gender and Education*, 22(3), 313–26.

Ilm to Amal (2022). Available at: http://ilm2amal.org/faq_category/resources (last accessed 16 May 2022).

Landman, J. and Cruickshank, J. K. (2001). 'A review of ethnicity, health and nutrition-related diseases in relation to migration in the United Kingdom'. *Public Health Nutrition*, 4(2B), 647–57.

Larkey, L. and Hecht, M. (2010). 'A model of effects of narrative as culture-centric health promotion'. *Journal of Health Communication: International Perspectives*, 15(2), 114–35.

Lawton, J., Ahmad, N., Peel, E. and Hallowell, N. (2007). 'Contextualising accounts of illness: notions of responsibility and blame in white and South Asian respondents' accounts of diabetes causation'. *Sociology of Health & Illness*, 29(6), 891–906.

Long, S. O. (2004). 'Cultural scripts for a good death in Japan and the United States: similarities and differences'. *Social Science & Medicine*, 58, 913–28.

Offer, C., Lee, A. and Humphreys, C. (2016). 'Tuberculosis in South Asian communities in the UK: a systematic review of the literature'. *Journal of Public Health*, 38(2), 250–7.

Office for National Statistics (2018). Population of England and Wales. Available at: www.ethnicity-facts-figures.service.gov.uk/uk-population-by-ethnicity/national-and-regional-populations/population-of-england-and-wales/latest (last accessed 16 May 2022).

Patel, M., Phillips-Caesar, E. and Boutin-Foster, C. (2012). 'Barriers to lifestyle behavioral change in migrant South Asian populations'. *Journal of Immigrant and Minority Health*, 14(5), 774–85.

Resnicow, K., Davis, R. and Rollnick, S. (2006). 'Motivational interviewing for pediatric obesity: conceptual issues and evidence review'. *Journal of the American Dietetic Association*, 106(12), 2024–33.

Schank, R. C. and Abelson, R. P. (1995). 'Knowledge and memory: the real story', in R. S. Wyer, Jr (ed.), *Knowledge and Memory: The Real Story*. Hillsdale, NJ: Lawrence Erlbaum Associates, pp. 1–85.

Shaw, A. (2001). *A Pakistani Community in Oxford*. Oxford: Basil Blackwell.

Squire, L. R. (1992). 'Declarative and nondeclarative memory: multiple brain systems supporting learning and memory'. *Journal of Cognitive Neuroscience*, 4(3), 232–43.

Symons, J. (2017). '"We're not hard to reach, they are!" Integrating local priorities in urban research in Northern England: an experimental method'. *The Sociological Review*, 66(1), 207–23.

12

ADDRESSING MENTAL HEALTH THROUGH ISLAMIC COUNSELLING: A FAITH-BASED THERAPEUTIC INTERVENTION

Stephen Abdullah Maynard

Understanding the Relationships of Faith, Experience and Mental Health in UK Muslim Communities

Little emphasis is placed on mental health in comparison with physical health, concerning health provision in general and specifically regarding the wellbeing of Muslim communities. For this reason, there is a need to highlight concerns about Muslim mental health for Muslim communities themselves, as well as for policy makers, commissioners and service providers. Globally, 1.8 billion people are Muslim and so share the belief system that is Islam through which they interpret their experience of self and reality. This chapter presents some of the key issues around common mental health conditions and the experience of them by Muslims. In doing so there is a need to draw attention to the inequalities experienced by Muslims in the context of the present lack of equality of appropriate provision in mental healthcare.

Faith or religion is not a common point to start from in considering mental wellbeing or the impact of variables that concern it. In itself, faith or religion is not necessarily considered as a critical factor in understanding mental health as our social, as opposed to biological, conceptions are generally based in cultural contexts (WHO and Calouste Gulbenkian Foundation 2014). As the social determinants of mental health are primarily understood within cultural paradigms which are often reduced to ethnicity, much of the thinking in the UK about social policy and service provision is implicitly secular. For this reason, let us start by understanding religion as 'a social identity that is grounded in a system of guiding beliefs, and may serve as a powerful tool to shape psychological and social processes' (Ysseldyk et al. 2010).

Research has shown that in and of itself, religion contributes to the experience of greater positive and fewer negative emotions for the people who believe in it (Kim-Prieto and Diener 2009). However, despite a significant amount of data gathered generally about the relationship between faith and mental health, much of this concerns Christianity (Cornah 2006). Christianity has a long historical impact on Western thinking and is fundamentally linked to Aristotelian epistemology in the development of the sciences. Islam being not classically 'European', however, creates in the UK a different perspective on reality. Though it is often considered as a religion in Western contexts, within its own context it is the *deen*. The word *deen* does not accurately translate as 'religion' (*madhhab* is the Arabic word for religion). The *deen* can be seen to have multiple meanings in a variety of contexts. These include 'the way', 'governance' and 'judgement', all of which relate to the life transaction between humans and the Creator (Esposito 2014). Islam is, then, a way of being that grounds experience identity and conception within a frame of reality defined by this transaction. It is both absolute and relative, adaptive and contextual and at the same time universal and true.

In light of the above Islam can be understood as a fundamental 'cognitive schema'. Here reality is held in a way that allows for experience and knowledge – including scientific empirical knowledge – to be held in a greater context of *ilm* ('knowledge' as understood in Islam). Here there is no duality between scientific knowledge and divine knowledge, simply different degrees and ways of things being known. This allows flexibility in experiencing life phenomenologically and through rational observation, allowing for the coexistence of realities that some may find contradictory.

Muslims have many interpretations of Islam. Shia-ism, Sufism, Sunnism, liberal Islam, conservative Islam, practising and not practising Islam each impact on how individuals and groups construct value and meaning within lived experience. These understandings of reality interact and come to bear on the construction of self-worth and emotional resilience, and the interpretation of experience, enabling many Muslims to maintain their psychological integrity in adverse conditions as is the case in other communities defined by spirituality or religion (Koenig 2012).

Muslim communities are faith communities existing as coherent bodies based on shared networks of belief. As part of the Abrahamic tradition, they relate to Christian and post-Christian rational empiricism though in some respects their relationships with empiricism may be distinct. This is not to say that there is a conflict with the main body of Western thought, nor that they are better or worse, simply different. Similarly, as Western thought has its nuances, so too does Islamic thought.

The cumulative history of Western thinking has shaped the thoughts, beliefs and core concepts of its mental health professionals and therapeutic models alike. The cumulative history of Islamic thinking has shaped the psychological reality of Muslims. An example of the way these distinctions impact on mental wellbeing and therapeutic interventions is the greater Western emphasis on thought and action, as seen in the emphasis in cognitive *behavioural* therapy, compared with the Islamic emphasis on being, as seen in the way the state of the heart[1] is emphasised within Islamic counselling and psychology (Frager 1999). In addition, identity in Muslim culture and Islam in general, as with many Eastern religions and philosophies, is defined more in terms of relationships and is less individualistic than many northern European conceptions (Oyserman and Lee 2008). Northern European individualism can be a factor Muslims living in the UK grapple with, as it impacts differently across generations. Competing understandings of self and family mean that well-intended therapeutic interventions may undermine and challenge self-concepts that are core to the client's identity.

Western and Islamic thought create different narratives of reality requiring Muslims living in the UK, as well as the mental health practitioners who work with them, to understand both. Muslims must be cultural navigators regarding their faith and British modernity (Considine 2018).

Current health practice regarding Muslim mental wellbeing – decision making, data and ethno-religious identification

The life transaction of 'being Muslim' impacts Muslim conceptions and experiences of reality; it is important, therefore, to consider how such faith-based inner worlds are met within the field of mental health.

---

[1] The significance of the heart and intentionality does not contradict the generally understood importance of Islamic law but is an a priori. The following hadith indicate the significance of the condition of the heart and intention. 'Beware, in the body there is a flesh; if it is sound, the whole body is sound, and if it is corrupt, the whole body is corrupt, and behold, it is the heart' (Faith in Allah (n. d.), Al-Bukhari and Muslim hadith no. 6). 'All actions are judged by motives, and each person will be rewarded according to their intention. Thus, he whose migration was to God and His Messenger, his migration is to God and His Messenger; but he whose migration was for some worldly thing he might gain, or for a wife he might marry, his migration is to that for which he migrated' (Faith in Allah (n. d.), Saheeh Al-Bukhari, Saheeh Muslim hadith no. 1).

The Department of Health and Social Care has statutory duties under the Equality Act 2010 which require it when making decisions to take into account the need to

- eliminate discrimination, harassment and victimisation
- advance equality of opportunity
- foster good relations between different parts of the community

These requirements are across the protected characteristics of age, disability, gender reassignment, marital or civil partnership status, pregnancy and motherhood, race (including ethnic or national origin, colour and nationality), religion or belief (including lack of belief), sex and sexual orientation.

The needs of faith communities generally have remained invisible in planning and service provision. Religion and belief is one of the eight protected characteristics to be addressed in directing the development, provision, resourcing and monitoring of health service provision. However, to date there has been a lack of recorded focus on this protected characteristic compared to gender, age or race. This has been the case in health-related planning, policy and service development, and service delivery in general[2]. In the absence of clear direction from the Department of Health and Social Care, inaction concerning statutory duty regarding religion and belief is all too often evident in the decision making of bodies such as NHS England, specifically about Muslim mental health

---

[2] This problem is indicated in the following, though the Department of Health and Social Care's 'No Health Without Mental Health: Cross-Government Mental Health Strategy for People of All Ages' (2012) identifies its commitment to the 2010 Equalities Act including religion and belief, and commits to reducing mental health inequalities in line with this, the actual 'No Health Without Mental Health' implementation framework only acknowledges religious belief with respect to the department's responsibilities under the Act, giving no guidance for strategy regarding how government departments will plan around religion and belief. Following on from this, the current NHS England strategy for mental health, the 'Five Year Forward View for Mental Health', does not refer to faith, belief or religion, while it does address ethnicity, sex, age, sexual orientation, pregnancy and motherhood. Further, neither the current NHS Scotland mental health strategy, 'Mental Health Strategy 2017–2027' (Scottish Government Population Health Directorate 2017) nor the current NHS Wales mental health strategy, 'Together for Mental Health Delivery Plan 2019–2022' (Welsh Government 2019) refers to faith, religion or religious belief. The Health Northern Ireland Service Framework for Mental Health and Wellbeing 2018–2021 (Department of Health 2018) does, however. commit to providing services to all irrespective of religious belief, perhaps because of the historical and political context.

and related services. Much of mental illness is social in origin, not genetic, and often a response to life events and/or negative conceptions of self-worth. By not considering faith, understanding mental health provision has adopted a bio-psychosocial model of understanding mental ill health without recognising the significance of faith.

Therapeutic recovery, however, is a personal process relating to the restoration of the ability to function within the contextual environment and the establishment of value and autonomy for the individual through a process that is valid for them. Much of this comes back to identity and belief.

Muslims are self-defining communities that see their critical point of referencing identity as their faith (Maynard 2007). Muslim communities in the UK are ethnically diverse and include members originating from across at least four continents. However, in the context of such diversity ethno-religious assumptions and identifications often subsume the faith identity of Muslims in health policy and service provision. Approximately 60 per cent of British Muslims are of Pakistani, Bangladeshi or Indian origin. This proportion is decreasing over time as ethnic diversity has been increasing with more Muslims originating from 'Black African', 'Black other' and 'Asian other' origins (ONS 2011 Table DC2201EW; ONS 2012). However, with the history of thinking about ethnicity in health planning and the lack of data collected on faith, Muslim identity is not seen as specific in most mental health provision and is considered as addressed in 'working with' the Asian or the Pakistani community. This process not only renders significant proportions of the Muslim community invisible regarding mental health, but it also bypasses aspects of the lived reality and identity of the individual service user and prevents the active consideration of how Islam can help to structure experience.

Mir (2005) examined the impact of the two predominant European conceptual frameworks regarding Muslim identity on health and healthcare, namely (1) the Enlightenment notion that religion is a private matter to be disassociated from public life, and particularly from scientific enterprise; and (2) the orientalist tradition of portraying Islam as inferior to Western culture and Muslims as people to be feared and controlled.

Mir identified

that dominant conceptualisations of religion and of Islam corrupt the communication process between Pakistani people and health practitioners; discussion of religious influences on self-care is avoided by patients and practitioners alike and Pakistani people are exposed to stereotypical ideas about their beliefs and practices. Consequently, they receive inadequate support in decision-making about chronic illness management and are more likely to develop complications. This disadvantage is exacerbated by ethnicity and gender . . .

The disadvantage to which Muslim identity appears to expose individuals and groups suggests a possible explanation for higher levels of mortality and morbidity within this community compared to other minority ethnic communities. (Mir 2005)

With regard to clinical practice, policy research and engagement with Muslim communities concerning health, Mir goes on to state that

developing shared understanding and common ground with Muslim perspectives is highlighted as a necessary focus for policy and practice development. Policy support for Muslims to organise on the basis of faith identity is also indicated if health inequalities within the Pakistani Muslim community are to be effectively addressed. (ibid.)

In the presence of the two assumptions identified by Mir and the absence of an understanding of Muslim faith-based identity in statutory mental health provision, ethno-religious assumptions also prevent the collection of data relevant to developing an understanding of mental health within specifically Muslim communities. The assumption is that ethnic data collected on the Pakistani community provides the same information. However, this lack of focus has implications. Data that is collected and examined about ethnicity is interrogated from within that frame of reference. Ethnicity or race is seen as the one significant factor concerning findings from the data with regard to assessment, treatment and service delivery. This means that practitioners focus on ethnically defined cultural competence as the most significant way to deliver appropriate services to diverse communities. Culture and ethnicity are relevant factors in consideration of the wellbeing of a distinct community. But where is the evidence that the dyad ethnicity and culture defined by place of origin are the most significant driving factors that need to be taken into consideration to account for health inequalities in ethnically diverse communities such as Muslims? Here also such identification can be irrelevant through its lack of precision. Consider, for example, the ethnic identifiers 'Asian' or 'Black African', which refer to diverse peoples in the UK who originate from continents in which 1,500 to 2,300 different languages are spoken.

There appears to be recognition that Pakistanis (and implicitly Muslims), like other minority communities, experience mental health inequalities. But even when data is collected concerning faith rather than ethnicity the data is limited. There also is a lack of analysis as to what may be the significant factors within mental health needs, appropriate treatments or health outcomes that correlate with this difference. The Improving Access to Psychological Therapies (IAPT) programme (NHS England 2013), a central core of current mental health strategy in England, does monitor the faith of patients receiving treatment. In this context, the 2016 Increasing Access to Psychological Therapies Report (on the national programme of talking therapies used to address patients in primary care) (UK Government 2016) identified Muslims, the UK's second-largest faith group, as one of the two faith groups least well served.

IAPT provides a central aspect of the Five Year Forward View for Mental Health, the national strategy for mental health within NHS England. As mentioned above (see footnote 2), this strategy does not refer to faith, religion or belief, indicating a lack of consideration of religion or belief in the strategic planning of mental health provision for England. This omission may have practice implications related to Muslim identity and mental health, such as

- unidentified external stressors contributing to mental illness within Muslim communities such as Islamophobia (Amer and Hovey 2012)
- preventing engaging in more effective treatments through working with faith-based internal resilience to mental illness such as that evidenced in research relating to faith and mental health (Cornah 2006)
- biased consideration of faith beliefs and client-related interpretations of experience creating obstacles to the effective application of standard treatments (Mir 2005)
- missed opportunities for the development of personalised appropriate treatments (for example, the incorporation of Islamic counselling into treatment regimens and/or research trials).

As significant proportions of Muslim communities are from Black, Asian or minority ethnic communities, the situation within the NHS is further exacerbated by Black and South Asian patients being less likely to have mental health problems recognised by their GP (Gillam et al. 1989; Odell et al. 1997; Bhui et al. 2001). GPs may also experience South Asian patients as somaticising their condition, making the presentation of some mental health problems unclear. In a small study carried out in a GP surgery with a majority of Muslim patients (70 per cent), research found that frequent attenders at this practice from Muslim Pakistani and Pashtun (on the Afghanistan/Pakistan border) backgrounds had high rates of psychological distress (Fazil et al. 2004).

In addition to the identified absence of religion and belief in the NHS England mental health strategy, it is also important to consider the role of the National Institute for Health and Care Excellence (NICE). Through its guidance, NICE sets standards of practice for health provision nationally.

Such guidance includes Quality Standard QS167 (NICE 2018b), 'Promoting health and preventing premature mortality in black, Asian and other minority ethnic groups'. Again, emphasis is placed here on ethnicity, not religion or belief. There is no separate NICE Quality Standard that considers religion and belief in this way. Further, at the time of writing this chapter, NICE is revising its guidance on adult depression following consultation. The circulated draft guidelines (NICE 2018a) referred to DSM-5[3] in its recommendations regarding assessment. However, no mention was made of the supplements to DSM-5 regarding the (new) Cultural Formulation Interview (CFI). The CFI assesses both the cultural and ethnic groups to which the patient belongs and how such groups' understanding and experiences may impact the patient's experience of wellbeing. In the absence of such a reference in NICE guidelines, it is unlikely that the CFI would be widely used by mental health practitioners here. Confusion around the NICE position on race and ethnicity is further demonstrated by unclear and inconsistent requirements. NICE (2005) states the following (emphasis added):

> Healthcare professionals in primary care, schools and other relevant community settings should be trained to detect symptoms of depression and to assess children and young people who may be at risk of depression. Training should include the evaluation of . . . *ethnic and cultural factors* . . .
>
> Child and Adolescent Mental Health Services (CAMHS) tier 2 or 3 should work with health and social care professionals in primary care, schools and other relevant community settings to provide training and *develop ethnically and culturally sensitive systems for detecting*, assessing, supporting and referring children and young people who are either depressed or at significant risk of becoming depressed.
>
> Healthcare professionals in primary, secondary and relevant community settings *should be trained in cultural competence to aid in the diagnosis and treatment of depression in children and young people* from black and minority ethnic groups.

This indicates the importance of an awareness of cultural factors in the assessment and treatment of depression in children that is not evident in the assessment of adults (as would be indicated by the use of the CFI in adults). Further regarding

---

[3] The *Diagnostic and Statistical Manual of Mental Disorders*, 5th edn, is the 2013 update to the *Diagnostic and Statistical Manual of Mental Disorders*, the taxonomic and diagnostic tool published by the American Psychiatric Association in the USA.

children, no guidance is given as to what such awareness would entail, to what standard it should be expected or how it should be gained. In this NICE guidance concerning race and ethnicity across ages appears confused and that regarding religion and belief absent.

Detailed consideration of the way in which statutory services interact with Muslim clients is essential in understanding Muslim mental health. The most effective means of addressing many mental health problems is through talking therapies which require the counsellor or therapist and the client or patient to develop a working alliance based on rapport. Muslim clients, in addition to being of a specific faith that is most often different from that of the counsellor, may also be of a different class from their counsellor. The majority of Muslims being BME and the majority of counsellors being White European also means that clients are often of a different ethnicity from their counsellor. These differences imply that neither these nor the core faith identity of the client are easily engaged with. The outcome of this is the degree to which the Muslim client is generally disabled or enabled in the therapeutic relationship. Over the last forty years, whilst much has been written about ways of actively engaging people of colour in therapy regarding mental health, at the same time this parallel problem of the relationship between Muslim clients and mental health interventions remains largely unconsidered. It is also important to recognise in this context the cultural significance of wider geopolitical factors (for example forced migration) regarding Muslim identity in the UK, and how these impact on the wellbeing and mental health of the individuals and Muslim communities. Being Muslim in the UK for many includes the reality of being a refugee. It also includes the significance of living in a post 9/11 context and the questioning this engenders for a person living in the West following the faith of Islam.

These are critical contexts in which counsellors and therapists need to be able to empathetically navigate the development of rapport to work effectively – this is not assisted by obfuscating people's faith-based self-conceptions and understandings of reality by ethnic identities which may externally impose inaccurate or less significant identifiers to the client through ethno-religious identification.

This is significant in the context of the Department of Health and Social Care's contribution to the UK Government's Prevent strategy, particularly its guidance for healthcare workers. The UK is the only country worldwide to embed counter-terrorism into health and social care. This development is in the context of recent experiences of 'Islamic' terrorism originating from organisations such as Daesh, as opposed to previous experiences of terrorism in the context of Northern Ireland. Warwick University's research (Heath-Kelly and Strausz 2018) on the use of Prevent in the NHS found that mental health professionals were unclear regarding what their role was or how to assess the risk of radicalisation. The research found some cases of mental health professionals referring people to Prevent for watching TV in Arabic or going to Mecca for the Islamic pilgrimage.

Ethno-religious identification in the provision of mental healthcare to the Muslim communities in statutory health structures reduces the possibility for faith to be explored as a positive factor concerning Muslim mental health. It also creates barriers to researching and evidencing any relationship between faith and condition, or faith and treatment. This lack of information gathering regarding faith and condition is of specific importance in the UK at a time of heightened religious hatred, evidenced by the increase in hate-based crime recorded by the police concerning Muslim communities (BBC 2018). In this context, with the focus in statutory health remaining on ethnicity, there is no strategic consideration of key questions such as: What is the psychological impact of increased violence on Muslims? How is it internally/psychologically represented? Does that impact on the incidence of anxiety?

How well will a therapeutic model (which at its core rationally interrogates the belief and understandings of its clients to dismiss myths) practised by mental health professionals without understanding of faith-based beliefs within Muslim communities facilitate long- term mental health improvement?

Islamic Counselling, an Evaluation

In this context sits the following evaluation of a faith-based therapeutic intervention used in an NHS setting with Muslims experiencing common mental health problems. Islamic counselling is a developing modality of therapeutic counselling practised in the UK since 2000.[4] This is work that has been developed by

---

[4] Islamic counselling and Islamic psychotherapy as interrelated fields have been developing since the early 1990s. The term 'Islamic counselling' was coined by Aliya Haeri who, with Shaykh Fadhlalla Haeri, developed the initial model based on Islamic teachings in the science of Tasawwuf into a contemporary therapeutic approach. This work was then taken on by Sabnum Dharamsi and the author who since 1996 have developed the model, and since 1998 have established Counselling and Psychotherapy Central Awarding Body accredited training programmes to level 5 and developed Islamic counselling services. Dharamsi and the author have published regarding this work and there are trained professional Islamic counsellors competent in this model in practice. This chapter presents evidence of the efficacy of this model. Numerous conference presentations and papers by Dharamsi and the author have presented the methodology as well as the aetiology of mental health problems and human development from the Islamic counselling perspective.

Sabnum Dharamsi and the author of this chapter. It has a clear theoretical base derived from Islamic teachings as opposed to models that are hybrids or adaptations of contemporary therapeutic models and Islam. This differentiates this work from a number of other therapeutic practices from the last twenty years that have also adopted the same name. For this reason, all further references to Islamic counselling will be to this model, i.e. the one developed by Stephen Maynard & Associates. The aim of Islamic counselling is to enable people to develop and grow by finding a path of balance through their reflections on their experiences and themselves. Islamic counselling is derived from Qur'anic verses, hadith and the teachings of Tasawwuf (the Islamic science of the self). In this, it is distinct from culturally appropriate models of counselling Muslims based on cultural similarity between counsellor and client, or the integration of Islamic teachings or quotes into alternate contemporary therapeutic models, or the 'cultural competence' of counsellor or therapist.[5]

Islamic counselling has been taught through accredited training to the level of a professional qualification since 2000. It has been provided as a therapeutic intervention in partnership with the NHS to Muslim communities in London or Birmingham since 2002 and by a small pool of Islamic counsellors working in other contexts. The following evaluation relates the work of Islamic counsellors at the Lateef Project and its partnership from 2011 with the Pearl Medical Centre in Birmingham.

The Lateef Project is an Islamic counselling service developed to work with Muslim communities in Birmingham following on from the Department of Health and Social Care Muslim Mental Health Scoping Report (Maynard 2007). After its first year, during which it provided a telephone-based service in Birmingham in partnership with the local mental health trust, the Lateef Project entered into the provision of an embedded counselling service at Pearl Medical Centre, a surgery with 10,000 patients, 7,000 of whom are Muslim. This work was independently externally evaluated for the first year.

Pearl Medical Centre is located in Washwood, Heath. It serves a diverse community many of whom live in relative deprivation originating from either

---

[5] Though all approaches to Islamic counselling start from the Qur'an and hadith, in the 2007 Department of Health Muslim Mental Health Scoping Report the author identified the two broad approaches to Islamic counselling intrinsically rooted in Islamic teachings, those being Islamic counselling models that are derived from Tibb medicine (the medicine of the last prophet) and those derived from Tasawwuf. The model discussed in this chapter is based on Tasawwuf. Further information on this model of Islamic counselling can be found in Maynard (1998), Maynard (2007), and Dharamsi and Maynard (2012).

Pakistan or Afghanistan. In this context the presentation of common mental health conditions frequently related to at least one of the following factors:

- Islamophobia and racism
- histories of trauma related to domestic violence
- histories of child sexual abuse or neglect
- post-traumatic stress disorder (PTSD) from these or other forms of violence including the experience of war among refugees and asylum seekers as well as within established communities that have experienced war
- forced marriage
- substance misuse related to depression

A common theme that presented was a mental health problem (most often anxiety with depression) co-morbid with a long term condition (LTC) such as cardiovascular disease, diabetes or chronic obstructive pulmonary disease (COPD). Alternatively, there were also presentations of a common mental health problem co-morbid with medically unexplained symptoms (MUS) or somatic symptoms. These themes of co-morbidity coincided with these patients presenting most frequently to the surgery each year.

This cohort of patients with complex co-morbid presentations were identified as a target group to enable the evaluation of the impact of Islamic counselling. MUS research evidence indicates that it accounts for up to 20 per cent of GP consultations and is associated with 20–50 per cent more outpatient costs as well as 30 per cent more hospitalisation (Simon et al. 2005; Simon and Von Korff 1991; Reid et al. 2001; Fink 1992). Relative costs to healthcare are also significant as co-morbid mental health problems exacerbate physical illness and complicate its treatment. This raises the total healthcare cost by at least 45 per cent per person with co-morbid mental health and long-term physical health conditions (Naylor et al. 2012). This demonstrates the importance of appropriate psychological interventions with such patients in reducing the frequency of attendance at secondary care as well as in improving healthcare.

The Methodology

The evaluation of Islamic counselling was carried out by an independent consultant over a one-year period starting from December 2011. The evaluation was completed by a consultant. Secondary care appointment/attendance/admission data by quarter for the period of the evaluation was collected and anonymised by staff of the Birmingham East and North Primary Care Trust. The consultant, as a mental health professional, developed and evaluated several mental health services. As an evaluation of service, this study did not require ethical approval.

For the evaluation, the participants consisted of all adult Muslim patients of the surgery referred on to the Lateef Project who presented with a common mental health problem and either a long-term physical health condition or symptoms classified as MUS and who had attended the surgery more than thirty times in the previous year before the Islamic counselling intervention. In selecting patients with high rates of primary care attendance it was found that these correlated to high rates of secondary care attendance. This presented eighty-three adult participants in the service evaluation. Patients diagnosed with long-term conditions were identified through primary care and tracked with regard to their secondary care usage over the research period. Patients within the study reflected the gender distribution, social class, age, family formation and networks common within the wider Muslim patient community of the surgery referred on to mental health support at the time. A decision was made not to include a control group in the context of the long-term service evaluation to increase the depth of analysis of Islamic counselling.

The hypotheses that were tested were (1) the consultation rate in primary care would slightly increase/be more contained for those patients within the Lateef cohort and (2) the use of secondary care (planned and unplanned) would significantly reduce for those patients within the Lateef cohort. It was the belief that engaging with the lived reality of the patients in a way that enabled acceptance of their experience in the context of their beliefs would enable a deep therapeutic relationship through which with time resilience could be developed. This would enable patients to reframe their experience of their symptoms, resulting in greater psychological wellbeing, and an increased capacity to facilitate their physical wellbeing resulting in a reduced reliance on secondary care. In this context, there was a possibility that counselling would increase patient attendance at the surgery whilst at the same time reducing attendance at secondary care.

The counselling interventions were between eight and sixteen sessions long, equivalent to a high-intensity IAPT intervention. These took place within the normal conditions of the surgery. The cohort consisted of both men and women. Following the data collection, there was an analysis of the acute activity before and after the date of intervention for a year for each NHS number by codification, speciality and diagnostic code.

This evaluation was designed as a simple efficacy study concerning Islamic counselling. Patient secondary care activity was seen as an inverse measure of generalised patient wellbeing as well as an indication of the level of patient reliance on secondary care considering the impact of their psychological wellbeing on their physical health.

Outcomes of the evaluation concerning working hypothesis 1 (consultation rate within primary care would increase/be contained)

The attendance/consultation rates for the cohort at the surgery in 2011 (i.e. before referral) were analysed and compared to years 2012 and 2013 (i.e. after referral) using the data sources identified. Despite the small overall sample size, a small number of individuals showed a dramatic reduction in their attendance rate. The overall trend, however, showed an increase in patient attendance at the surgery (Table 12.1, Figure 12.1).

Table 12.1 Total cohort attendances at surgery, 2011–13.

Year	2011	2012	2013
Attendance	2,582	3,028	3,127

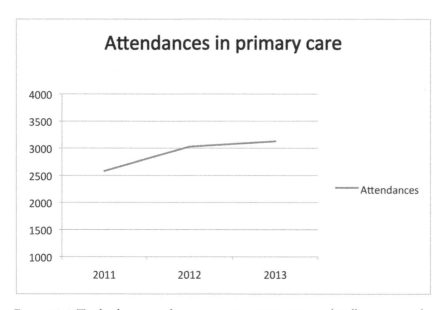

Figure 12.1 Total cohort attendances at surgery, 2011–13, graphically represented.

Outcomes of the evaluation concerning working hypothesis 2 (attendance rate within secondary care would significantly reduce)

Using NHS numbers the evaluation analysed the appointment/attendance/admission rate for the cohort of patients by quarter (three months) in 2011 before referral to Islamic counselling and compared this by quarter for four quarters post Islamic counselling intervention (Table 12.2, Figure 12.2).

Table 12.2 Total cohort secondary care attendance before and after Islamic counselling intervention in figures and percentages.

	Before	**After**	
			Percentage change
Elective admissions	21	6	71% reduction
Non-elective admissions	50	16	68% reduction
Outpatients	299	22	92% reduction
Accident and emergency	73	33	55% reduction
All activity	**443**	77	**82% reduction**

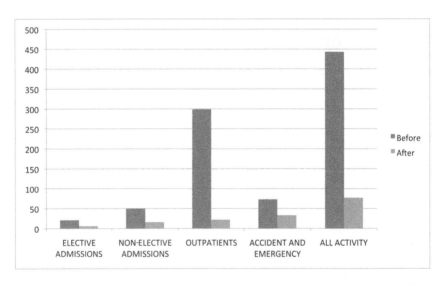

Figure 12.2 Total cohort secondary care attendance before and after Islamic counselling intervention in figures, graphically represented.

Using standard t testing at a p-value of 0.05, these results are statistically significant. The p-value for the total evaluation across all four conditions was 3.87698E-10. The p-value for elective admissions was 0.001672. The p-value for non-elective admissions was 0.012363. The p-value for A&E was 1.002E-7 and outpatients 0.000212.

When a smaller group of patients who had attended secondary care five or more times within the year before receiving Islamic counselling were considered (sub-cohort 2, comprising thirty-two patients) the figures demonstrated a greater reduction in secondary care usage (Table 12.3, Figure 12.3).

Table 12.3 Sub-cohort 2: secondary care attendance before and after Islamic counselling intervention in figures and percentages for patients who in the prior year had attended secondary care five or more times.

Before		After	
			Percentage change
Elective admissions	11	1	91% reduction
Non-elective admissions	44	7	84% reduction
Outpatients	234	11	95% reduction
Accident and emergency	44	11	75% reduction
All activity	**331**	**30**	**91% reduction**

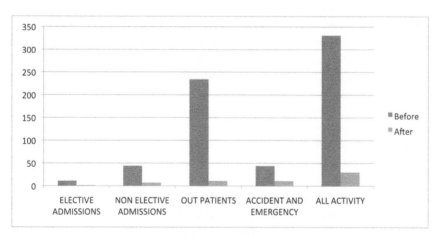

Figure 12.3 Sub-cohort 2: secondary care attendance before and after Islamic counselling intervention in figures, graphically represented.

The data shown in the preceding three figures clearly illustrate the reduction in patient use of secondary care across all areas following Islamic counselling. As illustrated in Figures 12.2 and 12.3 the greatest reductions in patient attendance in secondary care occurred in outpatient appointments. The evaluation demonstrates changed behaviour following the therapeutic intervention. This warrants further research work towards achieving appropriate and effective shifts of Muslim patient activity from secondary to primary care on a sustainable basis. This in itself would also require greater knowledge of Muslim physical and mental health co-morbidity and understanding of the impact of current medical practice on such co-morbidity as well as Muslim health-related decision making and behaviour (Mir and Sheikh 2010).

It is accepted that there could be confounding variables affecting the data, but the significance of the shift and the consistency of shift suggests a strong causal link. It is also acknowledged that appropriate targeting of patients with a particular profile/pattern of healthcare usage and presentations needs to be central to any 'scaling up' of such work.

Following the initial one-year post evaluation of this first cohort of Muslim patients receiving Islamic counselling in primary care, there has also been a three-years prior three-years post analysis (Maynard forthcoming) which also indicated significant reductions in inpatient use of secondary care.

The evidence from this work shows that Muslims co-morbid with common mental health problems and LTC/MUS who receive Islamic counselling present patterns of reduced use of secondary care, including A&E, following counselling and that these patterns are present one year after the intervention. It should be noted that De Lusignan et al. (2014) in their IAPT LTC/MUS Pathfinder Evaluation were overall unable to find changes in clinical or economic outcomes across several therapeutic interventions after three months.

Previous research on the impact of faith on the therapeutic relationship can assist in understanding the outcome of this evaluation. There is a considerable body of evidence that indicates that spirituality and religious identity have a direct impact on the quality of therapeutic work when working with mental health. Clients believe religious issues are generally appropriate in the counselling session and even display a preference for discussing spiritual and/or religious concerns (Rose et al. 2001). In another study (Kelly 1995), 81 per cent of respondents wanted counsellors to integrate beliefs and values into therapy. Where clients had spiritual or religious discussions in counselling, most report that they were responsible for initiating these conversations (Morrison et al. 2009). Because of this lack of addressing religion and spirituality on the part of counsellors, clients were less willing and less likely to find it appropriate to discuss religion and spirituality in counselling sessions (Richards and Bergin 1997). Christians and members of other religions prefer counsellors' beliefs to be similar to their own (Guinee and Tracey 1997), believing that counsellors with similar beliefs are more likely to support their beliefs rather than challenge them. Challenging produces fear because clients are worried psychotherapists will try to alter beliefs and convert the client to their religion (Quackenbos et al. 1985). Belaire and Young (2000) studied the influences of spirituality on counsellor selection and found that while client spirituality may have less influence over counsellor selection, the counsellor's ability to effectively implement religion and spirituality into counselling affects client preference of counsellors.

Considering the evidence above, enabling Muslim clients to be in therapeutic relationships that hold their reality both experientially and spiritually would appear to have a direct positive impact on the outcome of the therapeutic relationship in the complex and difficult settings evaluated in the above work.

The ability for Muslims to be engaged holistically therapeutically without the forms of judgement that were identified in the work of Mir (2005) or judgements from 'others' within the community appears to provide a space in which they can reflect on the reality of their experience and engage it depth in a process of change.

In this context, it can be argued that a therapeutic model that enables the spiritual reality of the client to be part of the framework of their understanding of the self, situation and wellbeing enables them to bring to the therapeutic relationship their spiritual resilience and understanding of reality as powerful tools supporting resilience in addressing wellbeing in complex contexts. At this time the author is aware of no other evidence of the efficacy of Islamic counselling or Islamic psychotherapy models. Verification of the therapeutic impact of this and other interventions is important to the mental wellbeing of Muslims in the UK and globally.

Research Indications of Muslim Mental Health Inequalities

To understand the implications of this evaluation it is necessary to develop a wider understanding of Muslim mental health. As previously explained, this is difficult as much of the information regarding Muslim mental health has to be extrapolated due to ethnic identification. Some work specifically focuses on Muslim mental health; there is also data collected in Muslim majority countries or among Muslim minorities elsewhere. Altalib et al. (2019) mapped global Muslim mental health research trends from 2000 to 2015 and found that 'the common theme of the MMH [Muslim mental health] literature is that Islam as a religion often informs how emotional distress is conceptualized and expressed, shapes interpersonal roles and relationships, and impacts health-seeking behavior in Muslim subcultures'. This supports engaging with faith and spirituality in the provision of mental health treatments. However, they also found that:

> The volume of MMH research is grossly disproportionate to the global Muslim population. For instance, the total number of MMH articles globally is less than

the number of mental health publications of many individual academic institutions in the USA and UK during the same period (and not related to MMH).

Original research on the role of Islam and Muslim culture on the expression of and coping with emotional distress constitutes <5% of the MMH literature and is primarily published by researchers based in medium- and high-income Muslim-majority countries such as Turkey, Iran, and Malaysia.

They also report:

MMH research themes topics related to 'trauma', 'violence', 'war', and post-traumatic stress were the most prominent. Other common psychiatric topics such as generalised anxiety disorders, substance use, and psychotic disorders were not prominently represented across regions. By contrast, in the more general mental health literature, substance abuse, depression, anxiety, psychotic disorders, and dementia are prominently featured across countries' mental health research.

Here, as with the clients in the evaluation above, acute, complex, traumatic mental health presentations appear to be more common. They conclude that 'further research in basic mental health needs, access to services, and effectiveness of MHS [mental health service] delivery to the nearly two billion Muslims globally is greatly needed'.

Accepting the limitations of the research, the following papers present themes indicative of the complexities of Muslim mental health, describing a distinct profile of mental health service needs that remain unaddressed in generic provision.

According to figures from the UN Refugee Agency (UNHCR 2017), globally 68 per cent of the world's refugees originated from Syria, Afghanistan, South Sudan, Myanmar or Somalia; three of these countries have significant Muslim majority populations, and 1.2 million Muslims left Myanmar due to religious persecution. In the UK a significant proportion of refugees are Muslim. People of refugee background experience multiple forms of disadvantage, including rates of long-term physical and psychological problems that are more significant than for other immigrants (Kulkens 2009; Department of Human Services 2008). People from a refugee background are also known to be at higher risk of suicide (Baron 2002; Vijayakumar and Jotheeswaran 2010).

Where prevalence studies exist reviews of these (e.g. Davidson et al. 2008; Fazel et al. 2005; Gerritsen et al. 2004) show a huge range in reported mental health disorder prevalence rates among people of refugee background, due to the heterogeneity (especially sample size) of the study population, and the measurement instruments and process (e.g. interviewer non-native to the refugee's ethnic group as opposed to native). The prevalence rates for depression range from 2 per cent to 88 per cent and from 3 per cent to 86 per cent for PTSD. Similar percentages are reported for the prevalence of anxiety (2 per cent to 80 per cent).

With a significant proportion of Muslim refugees having escaped from regions of conflict, the Gupta et al. (2014) paper on the relationship between armed conflict, domestic violence and probable PTSD among women in the Ivory Coast (a country where the largest religious group is Muslim – 39 per cent) is of note. Their study indicated that domestic violence is more strongly associated with past-week probable PTSD than remote domestic violence directly related to the crisis. Not only did the authors identify a relationship between probable PTSD, conflict and domestic violence, they also argue that 'domestic violence in such contexts must be considered within humanitarian mental health and psychosocial programming'.

Here there is a frightening sense that traumatised people who have been brutalised will commonly perpetrate and/or be victims of domestic violence.

Concerns regarding Muslim women and mental health have been under discussion in UK healthcare since 1990. These include the high prevalence of suicidal behaviour and ideation among Asian adolescent females (Bhugra 2002). Recent concerns also include the relationship between domestic violence and mental health problems, and the relationship between Muslim women's mental health and the wider family context as mediated by factors such as forced or arranged marriage.

Continuing to focus on Muslim women and domestic violence, also pertinent to Muslim women of the UK is the research of Kanwal Aslam et al. (2015). Their study on 'vertically transmitted' domestic violence through victims identified the continuation of spousal violence in the lives of women in Pakistan, and its transmission as a 'learned behavior' from mothers to daughters. Such trans-generation patterns of abuse were also identified in Morocco in the earlier work of Mernissi (1975). Here Mernissi argued that such behaviour, often initiated by the mother-in-law, becomes learned behaviour and is perpetrated inter-generationally.

Forced marriage statistics for 2017 indicate that 1,196 new cases were known to and engaged with by the Home Office in 2017 (Home Office 2018). Here again, though not all of these relate to Muslim women, over 60 per cent of cases relate to countries with over 90 per cent Muslim populations. These figures, however, relate only to those that come to the attention of the Home Office and do not provide any information on the psychological impact of forced marriage on the individual or the family. The prevalence of forced marriage in Muslim communities is not known. The psychological implications are currently only evident through casework.

With regard to research that focuses on Muslim children and young people, there is a lack of UK data specifically on mental health. Some lessons can be learned from the data that exists on this subject concerning ethnicity. The 2014 report by the Afiya Trust highlights how specialist child and adolescent mental health services (CAMHS), as well as the various programmes and initiatives aimed at prevention and early intervention, are falling short regarding the provision of services to BME children and young people. This is significant with respect to Muslim communities, as approximately a third of all Muslims in the UK are under the age of 16.

The Department of Health's publication 'No health without mental health' (HM Government 2011) indicated that 10 per cent of children and young people aged between 5 and 16 are believed to have a mental health problem. Though figures are available for mental health disorders for adults regarding ethnicity, none appear to be available for BME children and young people or specifically for Muslims considering the disproportionate weighting of Muslim communities towards the under-16s. In addition, identified risk factors for children and young people regarding mental health rarely include Islamophobia, racism or racial harassment.

There is a correlation between relative deprivation and mental illness (WHO and Calouste Gulbenkian Foundation 2014). In this context, three out of four Bangladeshi children aged 7 living in England were found to be living in deprivation. Pakistani and Bangladeshi families were over three times more likely than White British people to live in the most deprived 10 per cent of neighbourhoods in England[6] (Platt et al. 2014; UK Government 2018). This is further complicated by the overall poor assessment and treatment of Black and minority ethnic parents and children's mental health problems and the ongoing effect in this context that poor parental mental health can have on the wellbeing of BME children (Greene et al. 2008).

The above information forms the context for the concerns relating to the mental health of Muslim children and young people that remain unaddressed. These include:

- anxiety in third-generation Muslim young people who through their interactions across communities must form multiple or hybrid identities to interact effectively across cultures
- mismatch or discontinuity of values and practices between the school and home environment placing psychological strains on Muslim children and young people,

---

[6] Over 90 per cent of people in Bangladesh and Pakistan are Muslim.

specifically girls, over and above those experienced by White counterparts, causing tension and anxiety

- in this mismatch of values, the misinterpretation of Muslim values where, for example, respectfulness is seen as submissiveness and modesty construed as traditionalism, leading to a minority of Muslim girls and young people not learning to cope with this but instead suffering from psychosomatic illnesses, depression or anxiety
- institutional neglect impacting young people, particularly men, in emergent Muslim communities and established communities in areas of relative poverty where apparent social problems including poor educational performance and street crime may be related to psychological problems such as ADHD. (ADHD is a psychological problem which may develop from emotional trauma, presenting in such experiences as being an unaccompanied minor asylum seeker, wider issues of migration and forced migration or poverty.)
- difficulties experienced by young women regarding relationships and/or abuse and the related emotional distress and suffering of the individual as it is valued relative to the honour of the family.

Muslim men remain a difficult group to identify in mental health research data beyond current concerns regarding radicalisation, which in reality relate to very small numbers of Muslim men. It is concerning that there is a lack of research on the mental health of half the community.

Muslim communities as a whole do however experience Islamophobia. Though much has been noted in crime figures, as mentioned above, particularly the spikes in anti-Muslim hate crime in the wake of terrorist incidents, the anxiety this creates in Muslim communities is generally not addressed in mental health work. Data on the effect of Islamophobia on Muslim mental health is absent in the UK and relatively scarce elsewhere. Amer and Hovey (2012), in their study of anxiety and depression in Arabs in the US post-September 11 found that a quarter of participants reported moderate to severe anxiety levels as measured by the Beck Anxiety Inventory (BAI), while half of the sample reported depression scores that met clinical caseness as assessed by the Center for Epidemiologic Studies-Depression Scale (CES-D). The sample of Arab Americans reported significantly higher levels of anxiety and depression compared to standardisation samples and community samples of four other minority groups. Kunst et al. (2013), in their publication on the development and validation of the perceived Islamophobia scale (PIS), note the lack of research on the psychological impact of Islamophobia on Muslims. In the development and testing of the PIS, they worked with samples of Muslims from Germany, France and the UK to validate their study. They found that perceptions of Islamophobia in two samples negatively predicted psychological distress after controlling for experiences of discrimination, suggesting the insufficient impact of anti-discrimination laws in protecting Muslim minorities from the negative effects of stigma on psychological wellbeing.

Islamophobia is a form of stigma. Though the psychological research on the effects of Islamophobia is limited, there is data on the impact of stigma on health. This includes O'Donnell et al. (2015), which found that there was an impact to both psychological and physical health in the context of actual and anticipated stigma. This brings us to the interactions between mental health and physical health particularly experienced in Muslim communities.

A substantial number of people with long-term conditions such as cardio-vascular disease (CVD) or diabetes also experience poor mental health, and specifically common mental problems or disorders, which may lead to poorer health outcomes and reduce life expectancy. Relative costs to healthcare are also significant as co-morbid mental health problems exacerbate physical illness and complicate its treatment. In the absence of faith-related health data with regard to long-term conditions, there are specific health inequalities experienced by ethnic minority communities that make up the bulk of Muslim communities in the UK. In general, South Asian groups showed higher rates of CVD, with Pakistani and Bangladeshi groups higher than Indian groups. South Asian men are 50 per cent more likely to have coronary heart disease than men in the general population. Bangladeshis have the highest rates (followed by Pakistanis, then Indians and other South Asians). With regard to diabetes, the 1999 and 2004 Health Surveys of England both reported that the observed prevalence was markedly higher in Bangladeshi and Pakistani patients. For the Bangladeshi and Pakistani population, this represents an almost five times higher prevalence than in the general population (Lowth and Jackson 2015).

Contributory factors to this may include the combined effects of:

- genetic variation
- socioeconomic differences (affecting poverty, nutrition and housing conditions)
- differences in social and cultural beliefs and lifestyle practices (e.g. dietary/food habits, exercise and treatment-seeking behaviour)

But with the lack of information on common mental health problems within Muslim communities, their related experiences of these and the lack of recognition of faith as a possible factor concerning life experience, as argued above, there is a lack of clarity as to the impact of:

- mental distress and common mental illnesses on physical health treatment non-compliance and religious fatalism

- faith as a defining factor concerning cultural beliefs, 'lifestyle practices' or emotional resilience
- the extent and nature of mental and physical ill-health co-morbidity in Muslim communities
- the role (positive or negative) that beliefs may play concerning such co-morbidity and/or related treatments

With regard to MUS, Mangwana et al. (2009), in their comparative study of White European and South Asian presentations to secondary care, did find relatively even presentations of 49 per cent and 52 per cent within these ethnic groups respectively. However, these figures were obtained from one location where patients from both ethnic groups were equally affected by relative deprivation. When one considers the disproportionate number of South Asians (specifically Muslims) living in relative deprivation compared with other ethnicities and faith groups it is feasible that there is a higher proportion of MUS in these communities.

Considering the significance of faith regarding Muslim mental health and the above data including the evaluation it can be said that:

- contributory factors to Muslim mental health inequalities include both the quality and form of statutory mental health provision and the experiences of being Muslim living in the UK at this time
- there is a lack of UK data on Muslim mental health, and sufficient indications from wider research that UK common mental health problems in Muslim communities are often linked to multiple or complex unaddressed social causes and are as such also complex
- this raises specific concerns regarding co-morbidity between mental health problems and long-term conditions or MUS in respect to their assessment and treatment in Muslim communities in line with Mir's (2005) and Mir and Sheikh's (2010) findings.

Conclusion

This chapter has explored the interaction between Muslims' beliefs derived from their faith in Islam and their interpretation of experience regarding wellbeing. It has also considered data on faith and spirituality and its impact on wellbeing, and data on Muslim mental health and wellbeing. The chapter has indicated ways in which mental health provision in the UK, in general, does not address the relationship between mental health and faith within Muslim communities. It has also demonstrated the impact of Islamic counselling in complex conditions where Muslims experience co-morbid physical and mental health problems.

The chapter has indicated that current therapeutic models miss core aspects of identity within this faith community impacting on mental health assessment and treatment. In this context, it has presented evidence from a long-term evaluation of the efficacy of an alternative approach to Muslim mental health: Islamic counselling, a faith-based therapeutic intervention practised with NHS patients with complex presentations of mental and long-term physical health problems. The research has shown an 82 per cent reduction in patient use of secondary care.

The chapter has presented available research relevant to understanding the complex nature of Muslim mental and physical health. This indicates that though faith is significant in Muslim understandings of personal experience, the lives of UK Muslims are impacted by factors such as relative deprivation, refugee status and histories of physical, psychological or domestic violence often within wider geopolitical contexts. Such socioeconomic and geopolitical factors may relate more to the causation of Muslim mental ill-health than 'culture'; however, these are experienced in the context of a faith identity.

This chapter, including the evaluation of Islamic counselling, has argued that faith is a significant factor in the mental wellbeing of Muslims in the UK but at present a factor that receives less consideration than it warrants. Muslims often have difficult, complex life experiences impacted by factors such as Islamophobia that can have a negative effect on mental wellbeing. However, common UK therapeutic practice appears ill-equipped to address the realities of contemporary Muslim life. But such experiences can be held in a therapeutic relationship that enables the client to come to an authentic understanding and reappraisal of their experience in the context of what they believe and know to be true. Islamic counselling provides such a therapeutic space.

The efficacy of Islamic counselling demonstrated above shows that when faith is appropriately engaged with Muslim clients therapeutically there are positive outcomes. This is evident in the context of complex co-morbidity. Muslims have significant influences that can lead to common mental health problems such as anxiety, depression or PTSD. There are also sufficient indications that the specific mental health needs of the Muslim community are not identified or effectively addressed in general by statutory provision. In the context of the combination of these factors, there are reasons why mental health inequalities within Muslim communities persist and why faith should be part of an appropriate response therapeutically with Muslims.

In considering the role of faith or belief in the maintenance of wellbeing, I have argued that the strategic lack of appropriate mental health policy in relation to faith within the health service in the UK and the evidence of the impact of Islamic counselling on secondary care attendance in co-morbid presentation and related evidence, demonstrates the complexity of Muslim mental health and calls for a paradigm shift in addressing Muslim mental health.

Data presented here shows evidence of the efficacy of Islamic counselling in the treatment of common mental health problems in complex presentations. This is not a typical initial efficacy trial but is responsive to the expressed need identified in the context of agencies on the ground. Further research is required on this model of Islamic counselling to verify both its efficacy and its effectiveness as a psychotherapeutic modality. Such research could be part of a strategic response to addressing Muslim mental health inequalities in the present context.

References

Altalib, H., Elzamzamy, K., Fattah, M., Ali, S. and Awaad, R. (2019). 'Mapping global Muslim mental health research: analysis of trends in the English literature from 2000 to 2015'. *Global Mental Health*, 6(6), 1–10.

Amer, M. M. and Hovey, J. D. (2012). 'Anxiety and depression in a post-September 11 sample of Arabs in the USA'. *Social Psychiatry and Psychiatric Epidemiology*, 47(3), 409–18.

American Psychiatric Association (2013). *Diagnostic and Statistical Manual of Mental Disorders*, 5th edn. Washington, DC: American Psychiatric Association Publishing.

Baron, N. (2002). 'Community based psychosocial and mental health services for southern Sudanese refugees in long-term exile in Africa', in J. T. V. M. de Jong (ed.), *Trauma, War, and Violence: Public Mental Health in a Socio-cultural Context*. New York: Kluwer.

BBC (2018). 'Religious hate crimes: Rise in offences recorded by police', 16 October. Available at: www.bbc.co.uk/news/uk-45874265 (last accessed 20 May 2022).

Belaire, C. and Young, J. (2000). 'Influences of spirituality on counsellor selection'. *Counseling and Values*, 44(3), 189–97.

Bhugra, B. (2002). 'Suicidal behaviour in South Asians in the UK'. *Crisis*, 23(3), 108–13.

Bhui, K., Bhugra, D., Goldberg, D., Dunn, G. and Desai, M. (2001). 'Cultural influences on the prevalence of common mental disorder, general practitioners' assessments and help-seeking among Punjabi and English people visiting their general practitioner'. *Psychological Medicine*, 31(5), 815–25.

Considine, C. (2018). *Islam, Race and Pluralism in the Pakistani Diaspora*. Studies in Migration and Diaspora. London: Routledge.

Cornah, D. (2006). 'The impact of spirituality on mental health. A review of the literature'. Mental Health Foundation. Available at: www.mentalhealth.org.uk/sites/default/files/impact-spirituality.pdf (last accessed 20 May 2022).

Davidson, G., Murray, K. and Schweitzer, R. (2008). 'Review of refugee mental health and wellbeing: Australian perspectives'. *Australian Psychologist*, 43(3), 160–74.

De Lusignan, S., Jones, S., McCrae, N., Cookson, G., Correa, A. and Chan, T. (2014). 'IAPT LTC/MUS Pathfinder Evaluation Project. Phase 1 Final Report'. Available at: https://www.academia.edu/36476694/IAPT_LTC_MUS_Pathfinder_Evaluation_Project_Interim_report (last accessed 11 July 2022).

Department of Health (2018). 'Service framework for mental health and wellbeing 2018–2021'. Available at: www.health-ni.gov.uk/sites/default/files/consultations/health/MHSF%20-%20Service%20Framework%20-%202018-2021.PDF (last accessed 20 May 2022).

Department of Human Services (2008). *Refugee Health and Well-being Action Plan: 2008–2010*. Melbourne: Department of Human Services.

Dharamsi, S. and Maynard, A. (2012). 'Islamic based interventions', in S. Ahmed and M. Amer (eds), *Counselling Muslims: A Handbook of Mental Health Issues and Interventions*. New York: Routledge, pp. 135–60.

Esposito, J. (ed.) (2014). *The Oxford Dictionary of Islam*. Oxford: Oxford University Press.

Faith in Allah (n.d.). 'Forty Hadith al-Nawawi in English and Arabic'. Available at: https://abuaminaelias.com/forty-hadith-nawawi (last accessed 20 May 2022).

Fazel, M., Wheeler, J. and Danesh, J. (2005). 'Prevalence of serious mental disorder in 7000 refugees resettled in western countries: a systematic review'. *The Lancet*, 365(9467), 1309–14.

Fazil, Q., Wallace, L., Singh, G., Ali, Z. and Bywaters, P. (2004). 'Empowerment and advocacy: reflections on action research with Bangladeshi and Pakistani families who have children with severe disabilities'. *Health and Social Care in the Community*, 12(5), 389–97.

Fink, P. (1992). 'Surgery and medical treatment in persistent somatizing patients'. *Journal of Psychosomatic Research*, 36, 439–47.

Frager, R. (1999). *Heart, Self, Soul: The Sufi Psychology of Growth, Balance and Harmony*. Wheaton, IL: Quest Books.

Gerritsen, A., Bramsen, I., Deville, W., van Willgen, L., Hoven, J. and van der Ploeg, H. (2006). 'Physical and mental health of Afghan, Iranian and Somali asylum seekers and refugees living in the Netherlands'. *Social Psychiatry and Psychiatric Epidemiology*, 41(1), 18–26.

Gillam, S., Jarman, B. and White, P. L. (1989). 'Ethnic differences in consultation rates in urban general practice'. *British Medical Journal*, 229, 953–7.

Greene, R., Pugh, R. and Roberts, D. (2008). 'SCIE Research Briefing 29. Black and minority ethnic parents with mental health problems and their children'. Available at: www.scie.org.uk/publications/briefings/briefing29 (last accessed 20 May 2022).

Guinee, J. P. and Tracey, T. J. G. (1997). 'Effects of religiosity and problem type counsellor description ratings'. *Journal of Counselling and Development*, 76, 65–73.

Gupta, J., Falb, K., Carliner, H., Hossain, M., Kpebo, D. and Annan, J. (2014). 'Associations between exposure to intimate partner violence, armed conflict and probable PTSD among women in rural Cote d'Ivoire'. *PLoS ONE*, 9(5), e96300.

Heath-Kelly, C. and Strausz, E. (2018). 'Counter terrorism in the NHS: evaluating Prevent Duty safeguarding in the NHS'. Available at: https://radical.hypotheses. org/files/2018/07/Warwick_project_report.pdf (last accessed 20 May 2022).

HM Government (2011). 'No health without mental health: a cross-government mental health strategy for people of all ages'. Available at: https://assets.publishing.service.gov.uk/government/uploads/system/uploads/attachment_data/file/213761/dh_124058.pdf (last accessed 20 May 2022).

Home Office (2018). 'Forced marriage unit statistics 2017'. Available at: https://assets. publishing.service.gov.uk/government/uploads/system/uploads/attachment_data/file/730155/2017_FMU_statistics_FINAL.pdf (last accessed 20 May 2022).

Kanwal Aslam, S., Zaheer, S. and Shafique, K. (2015). 'Is spousal violence being "vertically transmitted" through victims? Findings from the Pakistan demographic and health survey 2112–13'. *PloS ONE*, 10(6), e0129790.

Kelly, E. W. Jr (1995). 'Spirituality and religion in counselling education: a national survey'. *Counsellor Education and Supervision*, 33, 227–37.

Kim-Prieto, C. and Diener, E. (2009). 'Religion as a source of variation in the experience of positive and negative emotions'. *The Journal of Positive Psychology*, 4(6), 447–60.

Koenig, H. G. (2012). 'Religion, spirituality, and health: The research and clinical implications'. *International Scholarly Research Notices Psychiatry*, 278730.

Kulkens, M. (2009). 'Access to specialist services by refugees in Victoria'. Victorian Refugee Health Network. Available at: http://refugeehealthnetwork.org.au/wp-content/uploads/Specialist_access_reportNov301.pdf (last accessed 20 May 2022).

Kunst, J. R., Sam, D. L. and Ulleberg, P. (2013). 'Perceived islamophobia: scale development and validation'. *International Journal of Intercultural Relations*, 37(2), 225–37.

Lowth. M. and Jackson, C. (2015). 'Diseases in different ethnic groups'. *Patient*. Available at: https://patient.info/doctor/diseases-and-different-ethnic-groups (last accessed 20 May 2022).

Mangwana, S., Burlington, S. and Creed, F. (2009). Medically unexplained symptoms presenting at secondary care – a comparison of white European and of south Asian ethnicity. *International Journal of Psychiatry in Medicine*, 39(1), 33–44.

Maynard, A. (1998). 'Beginning at the beginning. Islamic counselling'. *Race and Cultural Education in Counselling Multi-Cultural Journal*, 16.

Maynard, S. (2007). 'Muslim mental health: a scoping paper on theoretical models, practice and related concerns in Muslim communities'. Available at: www.scribd.com/document/90324305/Muslim-Mental-Health-Stephen-Maynard (last accessed 20 May 2022).

Mernissi, F. (1975). *Beyond the Veil: Male-Female Dynamics in Muslim Society*. London: Saqi Books.

Mir, G. (2005). 'The impact of faith identity on the healthcare and health of Pakistani Muslims'. *Centre for Research on Ethnicity, Nationality and Multiculturalism*.

Mir, G. and Sheikh, A. (2010). '"Fasting and prayer don't concern doctors . . . they don't know what it is": communication, decision-making and perceived social relations of Pakistani Muslim patients with long term illnesses'. Ethnic Health, 15(4), 327–42.

Morrison, J., Clutter, S., Pritchett, E. and Demmitt, A. (2009). 'Perceptions of clients and counseling professionals regarding spirituality in counseling'. *Counseling and Values*, 53(3), 183–94.

Naylor, J., Parsonage, M., McDaid, D., Knapp, M., Fossey, M. and Galea, A. (2012). 'Long-term conditions and mental health. The cost of co-morbidities'. The Kings Fund. Available at: www.kingsfund.org.uk/sites/default/files/field/field_publication_file/long-term-conditions-mental-health-cost-comorbidities-naylor-feb12.pdf (last accessed 20 May 2022).

NHS England (2013). 'Adult Improving Access to Psychological Therapies programme'. Available at: www.england.nhs.uk/mental-health/adults/iapt (last accessed 11 July 2022).

NHS England (2016). 'The Five Year Forward View for mental health'. Available at: www.england.nhs.uk/wp-content/uploads/2016/02/Mental-Health-Taskforce-FYFV-final.pdf (last accessed 20 May 2022).

NICE (2005). 'Depression in children and young people: identification and management'. Available at: www.nice.org.uk/guidance/cg28/resources/depression-in-children-and-young-people-identification-and-management-pdf-975332810437 (last accessed 20 May 2022).

NICE (2018a). 'Depression in adults: treatment and management. A clinical guideline draft for consultation'. Available at: www.nice.org.uk/guidance/ng222/documents/html-content-2 (last accessed 11 July 2022).

NICE (2018). 'Promoting health and preventing premature mortality in black, Asian and other minority ethnic groups'. Quality Standard 167. Available at: www.nice.org.uk/guidance/qs167/resources/promoting-health-and-preventing-premature-mortality-in-black-asian-and-other-minority-ethnic-groups-pdf-75545605479877 (last accessed 20 May 2022).

Odell, S. M., Surtees, P. G., Wainwright, N. W. J., Commander, M. J. and Sashidharan, S. P. (1997). 'Determinants of general practitioner recognition of psychological problems in a multi-ethnic inner city health district'. *British Journal of Psychiatry*, 171, 537–41.

O'Donnell, A. T., Corrigan, F. and Gallagher, S. (2015). 'The impact of anticipated stigma on psychological and physical health problems in the under employed group'. *Frontiers in Psychology*, 6: 1263.

Office for National Statistics (2011). '2011 census data'. Available at: www.ons.gov.uk/census/2011census/2011censusdata (last accessed 20 May 2022).

Office for National Statistics (2012). '2011 census: key statistics for England and Wales, March 2011'. Available at: www.ons.gov.uk/peoplepopulationandcommunity/populationandmigration/populationestimates/bulletins/2011censuskeystatisticsforenglandandwales/2012-12-11#religion (last accessed 15 July 2022).

Oyserman, D. and Lee, S. W. S. (2008). 'Does culture influence what and how we think?: effects of priming individualism and collectivism'. *Psychological Bulletin*, 134, 311–42.

Platt, L., Smith, K., Parsons, S., Connelly, R., Joshi, H., Rosenberg, R., Hansen, K., Brown, M., Sullivan, A., Chatzitheochari, S. and Mostafa, T. (2014). *Millennium Cohort Study. Initial Findings from the Age 11 Survey*. London: Centre for Longitudinal Studies, Institute of Education.

Quackenbos, S., Privette, G. and Kelntz, B. (1985). 'Psychotherapy. Sacred or secular?'. *Journal of Counselling and Development*, 63, 290–3.

Reid, S., Wessely, S., Crayford, T. and Hotopf, M. (2001). 'Medically unexplained symptoms in frequent attenders of secondary health care: retrospective cohort study'. *BMJ*, 322, 767.

Richards, P.S. and Bergin, A. E. (1997). *A Spiritual Strategy for Counselling and Psychotherapy*. Washington, DC: American Psychological Association.

Rose, E., Westefield, J. and Ansley, T. (2001). 'Spiritual issues in counselling: clients' beliefs and preferences'. *Journal of Counselling Psychology*, 48(1), 61.

Scottish Government Population Health Directorate (2017). 'Mental health strategy 2017–2027'. Available at: www.gov.scot/publications/mental-health-strategy-2017-2027 (last accessed 20 May 2022).

Simon, G. E. and Von Korff, M. (1991). 'Somatization and psychiatric disorder in the NIMH Epidemiologic Catchment Area study'. *American Journal of Psychiatry*, 148(11), 1494–500.

Simon, G. E., Von Korff, M. and Lin, E. (2005). 'Clinical and functional outcomes of depression treatment in patients with and without chronic medical illness'. *Psychological Medicine*, 35, 271–9.

UK Government (2016). 'Improving Access to Psychological Therapies Report – Jul 2016 final, Aug 2016 primary'. Available at: www.gov.uk/government/statistics/improving-access-to-psychological-therapies-report-jul-2016-final-aug-2016-primary (last accessed 11 July 2022).

UK Government (2018). 'Ethnicity facts and figures'. Available at: www.ethnicity-facts-figures.service.gov.uk/uk-population-by-ethnicity/demographics/people-living-in-deprived-neighbourhoods/latest (last accessed 20 May 2022).

UNHCR (2017). 'Global trends forced displacement in 2017'. Available at: www.unhcr.org/globaltrends2017 (last accessed 20 May 2022).

Vijayakumar, L. and Jotheeswaran, A. T. (2010). 'Suicide in refugees and asylum seekers', in D. Bhurgra, T. Craig and K. Bhui (eds), *Mental Health of Refugees and Asylum Seekers*. Oxford: Oxford University Press, pp. 195–210.

Welsh Government (2019). 'Together for Mental Health Delivery Plan 2019–2022'. Available at: https://gov.wales/sites/default/files/consultations/2019-07/together-for-mental-health-delivery-plan-consultation-document.pdf (last accessed 20 May 2022).

World Health Organization and Calouste Gulbenkian Foundation (2014). *Social Determinants of Mental Health*. Geneva: World Health Organization.

Ysseldyk, R., Matheson, K. and Anisman, H. (2010). 'Religiosity as identity: toward an understanding of religion from a social identity perspective'. *Personality and Social Psychology Review*, 14(1), 60–71

13

THE MENTAL HEALTH OF MUSLIMS IN A NORTHERN CITY SUCH AS BRADFORD

*Aamnah Rahman**

General Overview of Mental Health in the UK

UK government statistics for the general population show that one in six people will experience a common mental health disorder during any given week (Baker 2018). Furthermore, one in four people in the UK will experience mental health issues at some point during their life (Mind 2019).

Mental health has various facets and is not stagnant, but rather is fluid and can change over time (depending on life circumstances). The impact will be different for each individual depending on their disposition and outlook on life. It can therefore be difficult to construct a whole picture without breaking it down into components by investigating the various causal and confounding factors (Abu-Raiya 2012). The complexity of mental health is intricately entwined into our health and wellbeing and can be in correlation with internal and external contributory factors that have an impact on mental ill-health. These include socioeconomic determinants of health such as poverty, inadequate housing, lack of employment opportunities, mental health, sense of self and belonging, relationships, culture, stigma, unrecognised individual potential, healthcare and access to services, appropriate service provision, diagnosis and treatment, and environmental factors including pollution and lack of green spaces (Perks 1987; McGhee 2003; Trueman et al. 2004; Pickett and Wilkinson 2008; Fink 2010; Shaw et al. 2010; Cook et al. 2013; Prady et al. 2013; Ciftci et al. 2012; Hall 2017; The Health Foundation 2018; Cronin-de-Chavez et al. 2019).

* This book chapter is funded for open access by Bradford Institute for Health Research. The views expressed are those of the author and not necessarily those of the Bradford Institute for Health Research or the Bradford Teaching Hospitals NHS Foundation Trust.

Baker (2018) suggests that there are disparities in the use of Improving Access to Psychological Therapies (IAPT) services and the rates of treatment and recovery, as 13 per cent of referrals for IAPT are from Black and Minority Ethnic (BME) communities, while the BME community makes up 20 per cent of England's total population. Furthermore, 40 per cent of Asian service users will complete their treatment, compared to 46 per cent of clients of White origin, and 61 per cent of Asian service users will improve compared to 66 per cent of White service users. Finally, only 44 per cent of Asian service users will recover fully, compared to 50 per cent of White service users. Whilst these figures do not include a breakdown of all BME and religious communities (they show statistics for Asian communities only),they provide an insight into the situation of BME mental health throughout the country.

Common mental health disorders including anxiety, depression, phobias, panic disorders and self-harm are all on the rise, along with less-known but more severe disorders such as schizophrenia and bipolar disorder. In addition to this young people aged 16 to 25 present with the highest incidence of mental health issues from all age groups but have the poorest access to mental healthcare services (NIHR 2018).

Overview of Muslim Mental Health

The mental health of Muslims is greatly under-researched (Dabbagh et al. 2012), although the concept of mental health is not new in the Islamic faith; the tradition of *hifdh al aql* (protection of mental state) consists of three paradigms of *jism* (body), *aqli* (sense of mind) and *roohi* (spiritual). *Ilm al nafs* (scientific knowledge of self) has been well documented in Islamic theology and philosophy by various Islamic scholars and *tabeeb* (doctors). Imam Abu Hamid Ghazali, a famous philosopher, scholar, theologian and Sufi mystic, wrote about mental health nearly a thousand years ago (Skinner 2010). However, the belief in these notions is lacking in modern-day Muslims and professionals working within mental health, perhaps due to a lack of knowledge or awareness. Islamic belief and having conviction can be split into three parts: *yaqein-ul-akal* (belief through common sense or rational sense), *yaqein-al-ain* (belief through seeing) and *yaqein-ul-ilm* (belief through knowledge).

Islamic sciences include *nafisyat* (the science of the self) and *nasiyat/tibb*, the medicine (advice) of the Prophet Muhammad (PBUH). *Nafisyat* and *nasiyat/tibb* are generally considered by Muslims as secondary sources to the teaching of the Holy Qur'an and *Sunnah* (practices of the prophet). Additionally, the Islamic model of the psyche is rooted in five main *muqasid al-Sharia* (objectives of law) which include protection of life, faith, family/lineage, intellect/society and property. There is no separation of the physical body from the mental and spiritual (Rothman and Coyle 2018); the body is like a gate to the spirit. Thus, an integrated and holistic approach is needed to deal with mental health as well as physical health. Surprisingly, some practices such as self-care are much more established in Islamic ideology and practice and were being implemented well before they became popular in Western models of psychology (Skinner 2010).

In practice, mental health issues can be more difficult to address within Muslim communities, and Muslims' health is often compromised by a lack of understanding, fear and suspicion, stigma, mistrust, beliefs in *sahr* (possession by supernatural forces or spirits known as jinn) and *jadoo* (sorcery and black magic), not knowing how to access services and negative connotations. In the Indian subcontinent and other parts of the Muslim world, mental health is often seen as a taboo subject that is not spoken about openly. People with mental health issues are often referred to as '*pagal*' (mad). Further, the notion of *izzat*, which is associated with shame and honour, means the affected person's family will not immediately seek professional help. Thus, they are in the position of dealing with something they are not equipped to deal with (Fazil and Cochrane 2003; Pilkington et al. 2012). Added to this, service provision is not always culturally or religiously appropriate, and so patients are prevented from being diagnosed correctly and treated appropriately.

Often cultural norms and lifestyles are in contradiction to Islamic theology and positive health behaviours. For example, the traditional cuisine in many South-East Asian communities is often heavily based on unhealthy saturated fats (Rawlins et al. 2013; Brown et al. 2015). Many Muslims are aware of this but find it difficult to adopt healthier cooking practices because of custom and family values. Similarly, Muslims are required to pray five times a day at set times (a spiritual and physical ritual). However, not all Muslims do this or conform in other ways to Islamic teachings on how to conduct their lives. Hence there is an imbalance between theology, belief and everyday practice.

While there are notable parallels between Western and Islamic models of psychology (Abu-Raiya 2012), there is also some disparity between Western psychological models and schools of thought and Islamic models of treatment for psychological distress (Skinner 2010). Practitioners of Islamic psychology argue that Muslim mental health can be dealt with through Islamic models of practice incorporating the concepts of mental and spiritual health. Practices that include the use of spiritual healing such as *ruqiah al-Shariah* (verses from the Qur'an recited in front of the person to relieve distress), *taweez* (amulets featuring either Qur'anic verses or a numbering system, given by spiritual healers to those affected by mental distress to wear around their neck) and exorcism to rid the body of jinn or their impact are unfamiliar. Considered strange and not therapeutic in Western models of psychology and by professional mental health practitioners, they are nonetheless commonly used in Islamic traditions. Western psychology and psychiatry have generally tended to be suspicious and downplay the effectiveness of Islamic healing methods, stating that they have no scientific basis. However, Western researchers do recognise the role that religion and spirituality plays in Islamic practice, and there has been a growing interest in the research (Raiya et al. 2007).

An increasing number of Muslims in the UK are from White British or European backgrounds (Jacobson and Deckard 2014). White converts are known as 'revert brother/sister' as in Islamic theology everyone is born a Muslim and has undertaken *aidhay als* (an oath of allegiance to Islam). However, the impact of upbringing and environment has shaped their lives and led them to become what they are. So when those brought up as non-Muslim become Muslim, they are reverts back to Islam and not converts. White reverts often lose their identity and the privileges attributed to 'Whiteness' in Britain, and the loss of contact with their birth family and familial culture can often be detrimental to their health. They may experience isolation and endure periods of loneliness (Moosavi 2015). However, perhaps the biggest challenge faced by White reverts to Islam is being accepted by the Islamic community and being able to practise their faith without prohibition. Again, the mental health of new Muslims is under-researched and not highlighted adequately (ibid.).

The Communities of Bradford

Currently, Bradford District has a population of 534,000, 129,000 of whom are of the Muslim faith, making up around 20 per cent of the total population (Northern Data Hub 2018). In Bradford District, 45.2 per cent of people live in areas that are considered to be in the 20 per cent most deprived wards in England, which is double the percentage of England as a whole (City of Bradford MDC 2016). Whilst the overall picture of health there may be falling behind national statistics, Bradford has many positive aspects and, true to the city's innovative style, many groundbreaking and progressive initiatives have been born out of the needs of the city's health.

Bradford has a rich history of migration over the last two centuries. Although people have migrated here from various parts of the Muslim world, the predominant communities are from the Indian subcontinent. The migration of South Asian Muslims to the UK goes back to the early 1950s and 1960s; they came to the UK to better themselves and their families economically and settled in the inner-city areas of Bradford and Keighley in close-knit communities (Communities and Local Government 2009). The majority of South Asian Muslims originate from the northern parts of Pakistan (Attock, Kamalpur, Gujar Khan and Rawalpindi divisions) and Azad Kashmir (Mirpur and Kotli divisions), along with smaller communities of Muslims of Indian and Bangladeshi origin.

A notable difference in the health of older Muslims who were first-generation migrants from that of migrants of subsequent generations can be observed through the 'healthy migrant effect' (Cabieses Valdes 2011). The first generation arrived in the UK as healthy, young and able-bodied people and were willing to work and earn money. This, however, this has not been without cost to their health and wellbeing. Over time their health deteriorated due to factors including loss of ties and disconnection with their motherland, feelings of isolation, the experience of abject poverty, the effects of direct racism and prejudice from the host nation (governmental, institutional and public) and the lack of access to service provision and appropriate diagnoses and treatment (Iley and Nazroo 2007; Jayaweera 2011; Joshi et al. 2014). Other factors such as stress, anxiety, and acculturation and assimilation (the process of settlement and adapting to a new way of life and culture and the systems governing it) had an impact upon their physical, social, emotional and mental health (Asghar 1980; Wu and Schimmele 2005; Dhadda and Greene 2017; Anwar 1991).

A significant proportion of Muslims in Bradford are also from other nationalities and ethnicities: they speak different languages and have cultures and subcultures divided into communities and sub-communities. Within the district, there are sixty-eight nationalities (Northern Data Hub 2018). Many Muslims living in these various communities will follow certain mosques and imams (religious leaders) who often have immense control over their congregation. Whilst the Muslims of the Middle East are known through their tribal heritage, those from the Indian subcontinent belong to *biraderi* systems (of castes and sub-castes) whereby the practice of religion and culture is deeply entwined into their everyday lives. Traditionally much of this structure has, intentionally or unintentionally, been used to exert the politics of *biraderi* systems and social control, making it difficult for those who do not wish to abide by such cultural norms and traditions.

Newer communities have settled in Bradford since the early 1990s from countries in the Middle East and Africa including Iran, Iraq, Afghanistan, Bosnia, Somalia and Sudan (Communities and Local Government 2009). Many of these communities have settled here having fled war and sought asylum so understandably the effect on their mental health is different from those who originally came to settle here for economic reasons (Warfa et al. 2011; Bartram 2013; Close et al. 2016). However, much of what was experienced concerning mental health by older Muslim communities applies to newer communities too, for many of the same reasons (Darlow et al. 2005; Stafford et al. 2011; Joshi et al. 2014; Gazard et al. 2015; Wohland et al. 2015; Close et al. 2016; Mindlis and Boffetta 2017).

Bradford is unique in that there is an active interest and a nexus of political activity in the Islamic community and it is often used as a 'test bed' for anything to do with policy or practice concerning Muslims (Sullivan and Akhtar 2019). Generally in the UK, BME communities' contribution to politics and the political debate is recognised but it has not been without the experience of political marginalisation (O'Toole et al. 2013; Ali 2013). Alongside this, there is also political marginalisation, segregation and the frustration at Muslims generally being portrayed as the 'Other' in this current climate of hostility and fearmongering (Hellyer 2009).

The Mental Health of Bradford's Muslims

The mental health of Muslims in Bradford is reflective of other communities within the UK with similar socioeconomic demographics and patterns of migration. However, there are some notable factors about health and wellbeing within Bradford District. Like many other cities, Bradford has seen massive economic, cultural, structural and societal changes since the 1970s and has adapted to the challenges these have posed. Many positive factors have had an impact on the city and its people, some of which may have some bearing on the overall mental health of the district. Thanks to the strong sense of community in the city, there is a very strong, proactive and coordinated voluntary and community sector that picks up a significant proportion of the work being done in the city around mental health, in areas such as early intervention, prevention, and promoting health and wellbeing.

As mentioned previously, Muslim and other migrant communities have traditionally settled in socially and economically deprived areas (with poverty, deprivation, higher rates of unemployment and lower rates of educational attainment, and environmental factors) which harm health and wellbeing. Poor environments are a detrimental contributing factor to mental health (Thompson and Kent 2014). Deprived inner cities are hardest hit by factors such as pollution, lack of quality green spaces, litter, damaged roadsides, broken glass, and noisy and busy main roads. The positive impacts of mental health in these communities have been attributed in general to the sense of community spirit and belonging.

Statistics indicate that overall Bradfordians are fairly happy and satisfied, and feel that their life has been worthwhile (ONS and Thriving Places Index 2019). These ratings are very slightly below the ratings for England as a whole apart from where anxiety is concerned, with 2.81 people out of 10 stating they were anxious compared to 2.9 people in England. Overall happiness, satisfaction and personal wellbeing have continued to increase since 2011–12 and are in line with the average for England. People reported that personal circumstances, including unemployment, long-term illness or disability, middle-age, not being in a relationship or being separated, widowed or divorced, renting a property as opposed to owning one and having a poor level of education were the main factors that affected their health and wellbeing. The Thriving Places Index (TPI) also showed that Bradford, whilst having improved from 2018 figures (3.8 out of 10 to 4.3 out of 10) is still ranked as a 'medium' in the scoring. The lowest scoring factors included safety, mortality and life expectancy, wellbeing, health and adult education.

Having spoken to a few professionals working in local organisations in the area of mental health within Bradford District, the most common mental health issues and causal factors that professionals deal with when working with Muslim clients include:

- anxiety and depression (usually resulting from poverty)
- isolation and loneliness
- lack of support
- jealousy
- negative experiences
- broken trust
- child abuse (neglect and sexual abuse – particularly for migrants)
- issues of interference from extended families (males and females)
- controlling mothers-in-law and other female in-laws (for females and particularly migrant women)
- coercive control, which is usually connected to domestic violence
- coping with either becoming a second wife or partner taking another wife (a relatively recent factor)
- lack of understanding of people and relationships which leads to a breakdown in relationships and further distress

Unfortunately, a lack of literature (unpublished and published) exploring these very real issues for local communities makes it difficult to explore further.

Young people are particularly exposed to mental health issues due to conflicting and confounding factors (Nadal et al. 2010; Islam 2011; Levin and Idler 2018; Mahboob 2018). Young Muslims are victims of popular assumptions that 'you can't be both British and Muslim' which adds to an internal and external crisis in terms of identity, belonging and place in society (Hankir et al. 2015).

In Bradford, certain disorders such as self-harm and panic disorders are on the rise in children too (City of Bradford MDC 2016). Statistics show that one in ten children are experiencing mental health issues and half of children's mental health issues begin by the age of 14 (Pitchforth et al. 2019; Roberts et al. 2019). Similarly to the adult population, a lack of awareness and knowledge of mental health, fear, stigma and perception of mental illness within the larger community can all be barriers to accessing appropriate help (Bradby et al. 2007)

Campbell and Carnevale (2020) report that a recent survey conducted by Kooth (an online mental health counselling service) of 7,482 BME children under the age of 18 highlights that the mental health of BME youngsters is disproportionally affected by the Covid-19 pandemic, with young BME people having contacted the service in much higher numbers than their White counterparts. The figures in Table 13.1 show the percentages of contacts made for various mental health issues by BME and White children:

Table 13.1 Percentages of contacts made for mental health issues by BME and White children under the age of 18.

Mental health issue	% BME	% White	Additional comments
Suicidal thoughts	26.6	18.1	
Anxiety and stress	11.4	3.00	Depression rates fell by 16.2 per cent for White children and increased by 9.2 per cent for BME children (almost 1 in 5)
Self-harm	29.5	24.9	

Kooth also reported that there was an increase of 44 per cent in the number of calls it received from BME youngsters, a 200 per cent increase compared to the previous year in those who reported issues with sleeping and a 159 per cent increase in those expressing concerns relating to school or college. Twenty-seven per cent reported issues with family relationships. Furthermore, while there was a 16.2 per cent fall in depression rates among White children, their BME counterparts reported a 9.2 per cent increase (almost one in five).

Previous studies on the mental health of young people in Bradford have noted that young people had a good understanding of mental health and the stigma attached to it, as well as its impact upon others (Islam 2011). Young people also endure added pressure around stigma and fear of being labelled as 'mad' which is rooted in concerns about their mental health conditions. The stigma will often prevent them from seeking or accessing appropriate help (Mahboob 2018), particularly outside their networks in Muslim communities (Ciftci et al. 2012).

Often people living in tight-knit and close communities will access help provided by trusted sources within their community. However, not all people have benefited from having strong community networks and organisations. In the past, the power dynamics within communities and gatekeeping tactics by some people within community organisations have been coercive in convincing the community to view statutory services with suspicion or to look for help within the community instead of mainstream services. But working practices are changing and there is a need to work more collaboratively (such as in the community, voluntary and statutory sector) to serve communities and provide culturally appropriate services. Many of these small voluntary and community sector organisations are being praised by statutory funders and commissioning streams for the valuable work they do for the local community.

Bradford District has a mental health and wellbeing strategy in place which enables the Clinical Commissioning Groups within the NHS to work in partnership with the voluntary and community sector to provide access to commissioned services that are provided by the voluntary and community sector organisations (City of Bradford MDC 2016). The ten-year long-term NHS plan for Bradford has seen an uplift of 10 per cent in spending on mental health (mainly for staffing costs) with promises that there will be additional service provision.

Interestingly, several sources state that not all health is accessed through healthcare (Bunker et al. 1995; Kuznetsova 2012, cited in Buck and Maguire 2012). Local NHS commissioners also show that whilst GPs are the first port of call for many people with mental health issues and physical ailments in Bradford District, only around 10 per cent of health and wellbeing issues overall are being accessed through healthcare (Bradford Clinical Commissioning Group 2020). Further clarity and analysis are needed about how the other 90 per cent of health issues are being addressed in the city. Lifestyles, health behaviour, self-care, genetics, social capital and networks, general socioeconomic situation and environmental factors all impact health (Bunker et al. 1995; Kuznetsova 2012, cited in Buck and Maguire 2012), so these could be confounding impact factors.

Muslim Women and Mental Health

There are notable differences in the mental health of young Muslim women from that of their mothers. Whilst their way of life can be impacted by the *biraderi* systems of the Indian subcontinent (Knott and Khokher 1993), their life experience will be more varied due to being in education or employment, while older Muslim women have been mainly confined to the home (Communities and Local Government 2009). In an analysis of the 1991 and 2011 UK Population Census, Simpson et al. (2006) found that disparities in occupation in people originating from the Indian subcontinent were for reasons including language proficiency, skill sets, cultural acceptance of certain occupations and the connection to living in close-knit communities. Similarly, in Bradford many older Muslim women (particularly those of Bangladeshi/Pakistani/Kashmiri origin) have traditionally tended not to work because of living in close-knit cultural communities, the perceptions of working in mixed environments and language issues. Where older women of Indian origin have been employed, it has been in low-skilled and semi-manual roles in local industries where women have tended to dominate, such as clothing manufacturers.

Having a British education and language proficiency, younger Muslim women have broken traditional norms and excelled (although usually not without struggle) in the professional and educational sectors (particularly higher education) and have even outclassed their male counterparts (Samie and Sehlikoglu 2015; Khattab and Modood 2018). Similarly to other women, however, this has come at a cost to their personal and family life (Ahmad 2001; Samie and Sehlikoglu 2015; Baig 2016; Lewicki and O'Toole 2017).

The mental health of younger Muslim women is impacted further by the experience of racism and prejudice (in education and employment), from institutional, governmental, hierarchal and societal structures, being sidelined or neglected, and suffering a lack of aspiration and underachievement in these fields due to being from BME communities (Communities and Local Government 2009; Nadal et al. 2010; Elahi and Khan 2017; Levin and Idler 2018). Furthermore, negative perceptions of Muslim women by mainstream British society where they are viewed as 'traditionally submissive', suppressed, marginalised and not confident about speaking or standing up for their rights can have a detrimental effect and cause feelings of frustration and being undermined. Muslim women are often confronted by a two-way battle of recognition and acceptance between their own culture and that of the mainstream and being recognised as valued members of society who have a lot to contribute.

Added to the above, Gunson et al.'s (2019) study of Muslim women and their spiritual beliefs in Glasgow showed that these women believed that some issues around Muslim women's mental health are caused by transnational marriages to men from the Indian subcontinent or the impact of being in consanguineous marriage (married to blood relations) and marriages to men of the same *biraderi*. Difficulties arise due to differences in levels of understanding about cultural norms, roles within the household and what is acceptable or not. Other factors include sense of self (balancing Western values and Eastern cultural/religious influences), fear of stigma and reprisals for acting in a way that does not conform to the family and cultural norms, such as wearing Western clothing, having male friends or being in a relationship before marriage.

Muslim women, like other women, have been subject to patriarchal control and victims of domestic violence (Macey 1999), leaving them feeling demoralised and worthless (Coid et al. 2008; Dutt and Webber 2010). In addition to domestic abuse, a significant number of Muslim women will fall prey to 'honour-based violence' (Utz-Billing and Kentenich 2008; Fernandez 2009) and can be forced into marriage if they step outside their cultural and perceived religious norms. Some Muslim countries (mainly in Africa) practise female genital mutilation which can have a detrimental effect on health and wellbeing, often leaving women feeling incomplete, fearful, inferior and suppressed (Utz-Billing and Kentenich 2008).

Bradford's single-parent households are more common due to rising divorce rates, so mental health can be impacted due to isolation. Neesie, a Bradford organisation set up to support single mothers, states its WhatsApp group is most active from 8 p.m. to 10 p.m. as that is the time when single mothers feel most isolated as the children have gone to sleep (Neesie 2019).

Locally, despite their negative stereotyping, Muslim women are represented in many platforms – ranging from academia and politics to management and sport – which have been set up to represent their cause and counteract the negative narrative attributed to them. Initiatives such as the Professional Muslims Forum and the Muslim Women's Council, together with committees, working groups, local initiatives in promoting sports, health and wellbeing, and tackling Islamophobia, and social media platforms within Bradford District have as their main aim to support, upskill and empower women through education, training and enterprise.

Differences in Thinking and Practice

Similar to other South-East Asian and Middle Eastern communities, the notions of *sahr*, *jadoo* and *hasad* (the evil eye) are popular beliefs in some spheres of Muslim culture (Aloud and Rathur 2009; Dein and Illaiee 2013) and can impact how communities deal with the situation. The understanding of Islam and Islamic practice among the majority of older Muslims from the Indian subcontinent is rooted in a mix of influences of ancestral, cultural and religious practices of that region.

Jinns are mentioned in the Qur'an and understood to be spiritual and generally invisible creatures that can present in various forms and are mainly considered harmful to people (Ameen 2005, cited in Gunson et al. 2019). The South Asian Muslim community have traditionally tended to rely upon *peers* (spiritual healers) and *taweez* to deal with mental health. These practices are familiar to them as access to psychiatric services would be limited in their countries of origin due to the lack of professionals and service provision (Brown et al. 2015; Bubandt et al. 2019; Mittermaier 2019).

In the UK, older people are not always understood by professionals and services due to the difficulties in their expression (language, terminology and understanding) of mental health which can discourage people from seeking professional help (Krause 1989). Older people from minority backgrounds face additional difficulties in expressing mental health issues as much of the terminology used to describe problems such as anxiety, depression and panic disorders in English does not exist in Asian languages. This is the main reason why older South Asian communities use terminology such as 'heavy heart' or 'sinking heart' to describe their symptoms, which are not understood by the medical profession in the UK (Krause 1989).

The resilience of the older generations is different too. Considering the level of hardship they have endured to establish themselves in the UK, they tend to present much more positively. Sometimes the attitude of older people is seen by non-Muslims as passive as they tend to attribute all of their life experiences to the will of Allah SWT. In contrast to this, younger people are more open about mental health and proactively seek answers by trying to analyse life events that may have contributed to the demise of their mental health. Islam's (2011) paper on Bradford youngsters and mental health states that young people can also experience mental health issues due to family interference by being pressured into family wishes to approach religious/spiritual healers instead of professionals. This difference in opinion adds to the barriers to access and means that young Muslim people are often not accessing the services they need.

Many are of the view that people are responsible for their destiny, so life is what you make it. Hence, their understanding and perceptions of mental health and mental health issues, the notion of seeking help, and fears about confidentiality, the desire to keep it within the family, and using faith and spiritual healers are all different from those of their elders (Islam 2011; Mahboob 2018). This change in thinking can be attributed to increased knowledge and a growing understanding of the Qur'an and Qur'anic *ayah* (scriptures), such as: 'Indeed, Allah SWT will not change the condition of a people until they change what is in themselves' (Qur'an: 13:11).

Younger people tend to interpret this *ayah* (scripture) as meaning that Allah SWT does not help those who do not help themselves. So as such they will take heed of the message and try to change from being passive to proactive. Thus, having a different approach to dealing with health and other issues including accessing mental healthcare services and self-help is pertinent. Young people are much more familiar with the terminology used for mental health issues; this can help them to navigate the path of care and treatment.

Whilst younger Muslims have faced similar issues to older generations, they are also dealing with issues around identity and allegiance. Like other minority populations living in the West, they have also experienced racism and prejudice in more subtle and complex forms (Nadal et al. 2010). This includes social exclusion and being stereotyped as 'terrorists' along with other issues such as underachievement in education and employment. They are often not selected for jobs which they are capable of doing. It is not always possible for them to recognise or prove that what they have experienced is racism and/or prejudice. This added complexity is in part due to a rise in Islamophobia, which is a form of bigotry and racism specific to the Muslim faith (Elahi and Khan 2017).

Within this complexity, along with facing common mental health disorders such as depression, anxiety and suicidal thoughts, it is understandable that the younger generations also experience mental health issues due to confusion about identity, allegiance and belonging in British society, with up to 78 per cent stating that they were confused about identity and belonging (Mahboob 2018) and affinity with their belief systems (Muslim Youth Helpline 2019). This has a bigger impact on how they view themselves as members of society in the UK (Dabbagh et al. 2012; Mahboob 2018).

Younger generations, with their upbringing and understanding of Islam, have a broader scope than that of their elders. They have grown up in multicultural societies and live with Muslims from other parts of the world. Their influences come from both the Muslim culture and beliefs of their parents (conduct, clothing, social influences and so on) and the Western society they have been brought up in. This shapes their identity and aspirations as third- and fourth-generation Muslims within the UK, thus making them subject to greater acculturation.

Younger generations are usually fluent in English and articulate, and can acquire and express knowledge of mental health issues differently from their parents. However, barriers to seeking correct diagnoses and accessing appropriate interventions (fear of family, the stigma of diagnosis and so on) remain at varying levels, further complicating matters (Islam 2011; Muslim Youth Helpline 2019).

There are differences in prevalence in mental health issues for males and females (Muslim Youth Helpline 2019). A survey of 1,077 Muslim girls and women aged 16 to 30 reported that they had either suffered themselves or knew someone who had a mental health issue such as anxiety, exam stress, depression, family issues, suicidal thoughts, identity struggles, self-harm, eating disorders or post-traumatic stress disorder. Young Muslim males reported issues such as pornography addiction, sex addiction, and alcohol and drug abuse slightly higher than young females (Muslim Youth Helpline 2019). Overall, around 50 per cent of participants reported that they had approached friends the last time they had experienced an issue affecting their wellbeing. However, 40 per cent of the males in the survey reported that they did not approach anyone the last time they had a mental health issue. The survey also showed differences in seeking help among the younger age group, with 37 per cent of 16-to-22-year-olds reporting that they did not speak to anyone, compared to 29 per cent of the 23-to-30-year-olds.

Another study, by Bristol charity Sharing Voices (2019), found that a large and growing number of young people are turning to alternative or non-traditional methods of seeking help, such as social media. A survey on young Muslim people's mental health in Bradford carried out as part of this study reported that 26 per cent of young people would reach out on social media platforms for help. The same survey reported that 22 per cent would ask their family, but only 7 per cent would seek help from faith healers. However, young people feel uneasy about stating their identity when accessing social media due to the negative narratives portrayed in the mainstream media of Muslims being involved with crime and being at risk of radicalisation (Mahboob 2018).

There are some factors to explain lower rates of mental ill health in South Asians, including strong and protective cultures, social networks and supportive extended family networks (Bhui et al. 2003; Fink 2010; Islam 2011). Similarly, in a study of Muslim adolescence and mental health centred around two secondary schools to measure whether psychological distress is associated with 'Westernisation', a sense of 'Britishness' and perceived discrimination, the results showed that Muslims were less likely to experience psychological distress (Dabbagh et al. 2012). Living with both biological parents and within extended networks, joint family systems, religious and ethnic cohesion, and having social capital (community networks and structures) along with religious beliefs were protective factors having a positive impact, thus leading to better mental health (Pilkington et al. 2012). However, caution was also raised as further research needed to be conducted.

Similar scenarios can be applied to the mental health of Bradford's children. However, there are concerns that there are children displaying symptoms that do not fit the Diagnostic and Statistical Manual of Mental Disorders (DSM) scale, which does not include religious and cultural beliefs in *jaddo*, *hasad*, *nazr* and *sahr*, and will therefore not receive appropriate diagnoses and treatment (Toseeb et al. 2017).

Observations and Discussion

To gain a full overview of the mental health of Muslims in the UK and locally, certain confounding and/or contributory factors in addition to those mentioned in the previous sections need to be discussed. Firstly, there are external factors in how Islam and Muslims are perceived by mainstream society, mainly due to Islamophobia (Hussain 2009; Hankir et al. 2015). Islam is seen as dangerous and a threat to mainstream UK culture and identity by the national media and in its reporting of Muslims. Muslims are increasingly perceived as and labelled as the 'Other', making them different and at odds with other communities (Lewis et al. 2013). This has an impact on how Muslim mental health is experienced and treated (Shah and Sonuga-Barke 1995).

In reality, Islam and Muslims have much in common with British and European culture and religious identity (Hellyer 2009). Common values such as doing good deeds, being polite, showing love and care towards neighbours, having strong community connections, earning an honest living and so on are as much Islamic as they are British. However, in practice issues arise owing to several factors including perception and misunderstanding of each other's religion and culture, and Islamophobia (Samari et al. 2018). Other factors such as segregation of certain communities and general lack of desire to integrate add to the situation.

Secondly, and perhaps more importantly for Muslims, the understanding of mental health and how it relates to theology and practice in Islam is required to put things into perspective. Health and wellbeing are important to Muslims as health is considered as an *amanat* (guardianship and gift), and so Muslims are responsible for looking after their health by upholding this trust and fulfilling obligations to Allah SWT. If someone does not look after their health, the concept of *khianat* (betraying the trust or safekeeping of the *amanat* of Allah SWT) is implied. *Khianat* is disliked by Allah SWT and can take the form of tongue, ears, eyes and body misuse (alcohol, smoking and substance abuse). Muslims also have a belief in *al-Qadar* (destiny and fate) and so many Muslims believe that everything in a person's life is written for them by Allah SWT. Furthermore, mental health can be seen as either a test or a punishment from Allah SWT.

As mentioned earlier in the chapter, Muslims are from various ethnicities and communities, speak different languages, and have individual traits, personalities and dispositions. There are differences in the way mental health is perceived and dealt with between the younger and older generations, men and women, cultures and ethnicities, and people's levels of awareness of mental health vary. Whilst overall health inequalities in Bradford remain high compared to other cities of similar demographics, protective factors have been linked to living in strong, close-knit communities and having social capital along with having a set code of conduct under Islamic jurisdiction (Connor 2012; Bhui et al. 2003).

In addition to this, having a supportive and vibrant community and voluntary sector (even with the pressures of austerity and current cuts in service provision) has meant that Muslims in Bradford District experiencing mental health issues have been better supported with service provision. At a 2017 conference in Birmingham on mental health and stigma in Muslims in England, one discussion was on the need to have culturally bespoke mental health services for Muslims (Hankir et al. 2017). Bradford District has several culturally and religiously specific services providing interventions in BME communities, such as Ihsaan, Roshni Ghar, Naye Subah and Sharing Voices. These organisations pick up a significant amount of work from NHS primary care, particularly for mild to moderate mental health issues, which reduces the anxiety around access to services. Further, it eases the barriers to accessing healthcare as people do not always feel comfortable going to see professionals in mental health hospital settings. Evidence shows that this type of robust service provision, reaching out to marginalised and isolated communities where mainstream services have lagged behind, combined with culturally and religiously led appropriate interventions, are better received (Knifton et al. 2010; Mahboob 2018; Mir 2012) and result in positive effects.

This type of service provision is, however, only one element of the total provision, and for some people from minority groups this type of service provision may be a hindrance, especially for those who do not fit the norms of Muslim society, i.e. minority Muslim communities and those who are living on the fringes of Muslim society, and those who have little faith or have left the Islamic faith. So it is important to be able to offer a choice of providers and provision.

The disadvantages of these services are that they are often limited in resources and staff. Funding remains a huge issue and the uncertainty of future funding means they often work on time-limited projects. Furthermore, there is a danger that if the balance of provision in services is unequal it could split service provision into an 'us and them' scenario whereby services for Muslims and other minorities are provided by these organisations and the rest is with statutory care. It is therefore important to have therapists or mental health professionals who understand the clients' perspective so that people can work congruently. The main primary and secondary care providers should invest in cultural competency training for their staff (Clegg et al. 2016; Herring et al. 2019). Such training provides an insight into understanding specific communities and their function for professionals who may not otherwise come into contact with them if their work is limited to statutory settings. So all therapists and frontline staff should be encouraged to seek training in how to approach clients using culturally and religiously appropriate methods. A large number of people have expressed the need to have professionals who have an understanding of the clients' culture and religion or are from the same background (Islam 2011; Mahboob 2018). There is also a need to encourage and support more young Muslims to train in mental health and work as frontline professionals to serve their local communities.

Statutory care is still the biggest provider of healthcare in general (due to finances, capacity and resource); there have nonetheless been calls to work more collaboratively with the third sector (community and voluntary). In attempting to work differently, initiatives around mental health in Bradford have tried to engage with various groups by offering interventions such as out-of-hours support as people often hit low points when services are not available to support them. Mind in Bradford offers a number of services which are available 365 days a year along with face-to-face sessions for young people in the evenings in local GP practices. The initiatives include 'One You', a healthy minds portal that aims to connect all mental health services in one directory, the objective being that accurate and appropriate information will enable appropriate and timely intervention which leads to positive mental health (Mind 2019). Health trainers and social prescribing services have been established in the district for a decade and provide valuable low-intensity interventions.

More solutions are required to benefit the local community. It may mean that a combination of various approaches and methods helps to improve the health and wellbeing of Muslims. All sectors and funding streams need to work collaboratively and cohesively in partnerships to deliver the portfolio. More consideration also needs to be given as to how mental health services are being delivered. For example, alongside primary care locations for service provision in communities, places of worship and other public buildings can also be used as venues to provide support for health and wellbeing needs (Tomalin and Sadgrove 2016). In addition, local children's centres and school community rooms are accessible to Muslim communities, who will utilise them to their maximum potential. The weakness of one sector can be the strength of another and vice versa. However, for this to happen on a broader level, a shift in policy and practice needs to take place. It is important to have equal partnerships based upon an agreed criterion with proportionate representation from the communities affected.

The City Collaboratory initiative for ActEarly currently being pioneered at the Bradford Institute for Health Research envisages this, whereby there is a whole-systems approach with various contributing and confounding factors to health and wellbeing (Wright et al. 2019). This is a research collaboration involving statutory services, commissioners, arts and culture, academics, child development, environmentalists, housing, policy makers, social justice, transport, urban design, and so on with the aim of reducing health inequalities. It is still in its early stages but the thinking and will are there to ignite this catalyst of change.

Another possibility may be through raising the profile of mental health and its importance by using references to the Qur'an and hadith. Once people are more familiar with concepts around mental health and religious scriptures, some Muslims may choose to look at health and wellbeing differently. Here it is important to stress that it is not just about looking after the body physically and mentally but also about caring for the neighbourhood and environment, which also has an impact upon mental health.

On another note, there is also a continuing motion to encourage mainstream providers not to fear political correctness and work with issues such as faith (which for some is a determinant of health) or clients' cultural perspectives. The therapeutic relationship will not be congruent if therapists have apprehensions or are extra cautious about enforcing certain aspects of the therapeutic process such as either imposing Western models of treatment upon clients or are reluctant to challenge aspects of the client's case due to fear of offending the client (Mir 2012). The definition of cultural competency is not always consistent and can add to health inequalities (Beck et al. 2019). Cultural competency training for mental health workers can be seen as the way forward. It should also include religious awareness training and ongoing diversity competencies of existing staff, with new staff employed who already have these competencies (Kumas Tan et al. 2007, cited in Morgan 2019). Furthermore, having staff members who are interpreters with additional skills or appropriate interpretation training to serve local community languages is also advantageous (Beck et al. 2019).

Whilst it appears that Bradford is on track to achieving better mental health outcomes through adequate and timely service provision, so much more needs to be done jointly by the local authority, health, education and community services, the voluntary sector and private industry to tackle structural inequalities, deprivation and neglect, which in turn lead to health inequalities including mental health. Minorities usually bear the brunt of neglect so must be included and involved from the onset of service planning, design and delivery models. Co-production methods that enable active participation and community ownership are key elements for the development and provision of services. In Bradford, Muslim communities are involved with organisations such as Health Watch, Maternity Voices (a collaboration of all organisations dealing with maternal health), Women's Health Network and the NHS Trust Board of Governors, alongside various community and voluntary sector networks. A positive aspect of mental health in Bradford is that community voices and, more importantly, those of service users are being heard by the organisations and people who need to hear them. More work, however, remains to be done.

References

Abu-Raiya, H. (2012), 'Western psychology and Muslim psychology in dialogue: comparisons between a Qura'nic theory of personality and Freud's and Jung's ideas'. *Journal of Religion and Health*, 53, 326–38.

Ahmad, F. (2001) 'Modern traditions? British Muslim women and academic achievement'. *Gender and Education*, 13(2), 137–52.

Ali, S. (2013). 'Identities and sense of belonging of Muslims in Britain: using survey data, cognitive survey methodology, and in-depth interviews'. PhD thesis, Oxford University.

Aloud, N. and Rathur, A. (2009). 'Factors affecting attitudes toward seeking and using formal mental health and psychological services among Arab Muslim populations'. *Journal of Muslim Mental Health*, 4(2), 79–103.

Anwar, M. (1991). 'Ethnic minorities' representation: voting and electoral politics in Britain, and the role of leaders', in P. Werbner and M. Anwar (eds), *Black and Ethnic Leaderships in Britain*. London: Taylor & Francis, pp. 28–42.

Asghar, M. (1980). 'Book review: *The Myth of Return: Pakistanis in Britain* by Muhammad Anwar (London, Heinemann, 1979). 278pp. £8.50', *Race & Class*, 22(1), 103–5.

Baig, R. B. (2016). 'The power to change: Muslim women's rights movement and the resistance towards gender-based violence'. *China Journal of Social Work*, 9(3), 200–17.

Baker, C. (2018). Mental health statistics: prevalence, services and funding in England'. Available at: https://commonslibrary.parliament.uk/research-briefings/sn06988 (last accessed 23 May 2022).

Bartram, D. (2013). 'Happiness and "economic migration": a comparison of Eastern European migrants and stayers'. *Migration Studies*, 1(2), 156–75.

Beck, A., Naz, S., Brooks, M. and Jankowska, M. (2019). 'Improving Access to Psychological Therapies (IAPT)'. Available at: https://lewishamtalkingtherapies.nhs.uk/wp-content/uploads/2021/10/IAPT-BAME-PPG-2019.pdf (last accessed 23 May 2022).

Bhui, K., Stansfeld, S., Hull, S., Priebe, S., Mole, F. and Feder, G. (2003). 'Ethnic variations in pathways to and use of specialist mental health services in the UK', *British Journal of Psychiatry*, 182(2), 105–16.

Bradby, H., Varyani, M., Oglethorpe, R., Raine, W., White, I. and Helen, M. (2007). 'British Asian families and the use of child and adolescent mental health services: a qualitative study of a hard to reach group'. *Social Science & Medicine*, 65(12), 2413–24.

Bradford Clinical Commissioning Group (2020). 'New online mental health support service for adults'. Available at: www.bradfordcravenccg.nhs.uk/news/new-online-mental-health-support-service-for-adults (last accessed 11 July 2022).

Brown, T. J., Smith, S. and Summerbell, C. D. (2015). 'A systematic review of diet and physical activity interventions to prevent or treat obesity in South Asian populations', *Appetite*, 87(1), 403.

Bubandt, N., Rytter, M. and Suhr, C. (2019). 'A second look at invisibility: Al-Ghayb, Islam, ethnography', *Contemporary Islam*, 13(1), 1–16.

Buck, D. and Maguire, D. (2012). 'Inequalities in life expectancy: changes over time and implications for policy'. The King's Fund. Available at: www.kingsfund.org.uk/sites/default/files/field/field_publication_file/inequalities-in-life-expectancy-kings-fund-aug15.pdf (last accessed 23 May 2022).

Bunker, J. P., Frazier, H. S. and Mosteller, F. T. (1995). 'The role of medical care in determining health: creating an inventory of benefits.', in B. C. Amick, III, S. Levine, A. R. Tarlov and D. Chapman Walsh (eds), *Society and Health*. New York: Oxford University Press, pp. 305–41.

Cabieses Valdes, B. B. (2011). 'The living conditions and health status of international immigrants in Chile: comparisons among international immigrants, and between them and the Chilean-born'. PhD thesis, University of York.

Campbell, S. and Carnevale, F. A. (2020). 'Injustices faced by children during the COVID-19 pandemic and crucial next steps'. *Canadian Journal of Public Health*, 111(5), 658–9.

Ciftci, A., Jones, N. and Corrigan, P. W. (2012). 'Mental health stigma in the Muslim community'. *Stigma*, 7(1), 17–32.

City of Bradford MDC (2016). 'Mental wellbeing in Bradford district and Craven: a strategy 2016–2021'. Available at: www.bradford.gov.uk/media/3578/mental-wellbeing-strategy-in-bradford-district-craven.pdf (last accessed 23 May 2022).

Clegg, S., Heywood-Everett, S. and Siddiqi, N. (2016). 'A review of cultural competence training in UK mental health settings'. *British Journal of Mental Health Nursing*, 5(4), 176–183.

Close, C., Kouvonen, A., Bosqui, T., Patel, K., O'Reilly, D. and Donnelly, M. (2016). 'The mental health and wellbeing of first generation migrants: a systematic-narrative review of reviews', *Globalization and Health*, 12(1), 47.

Coid, J. W., Kirkbride, J. B., Barker, D., Cowden, F., Stamps, R., Yang, M. and Jones, P. B. (2008). 'Raised incidence rates of all psychoses among migrant groups: findings from the East London first episode psychosis study'. *Archives of General Psychiatry*, 65(11), 1250–8.

Communities and Local Government (2009). 'The Pakistani Muslim Community in England. Understanding Muslim Ethnic Communities'. Available at: https://webarchive.nationalarchives.gov.uk/ukgwa/20110202173123/http://www.communities.gov.uk/publications/communities/pakistanimuslimcommunity (last accessed 11 July 2022).

Connor, P. (2012). 'Balm for the soul: immigrant religion and emotional well-being'. *International Migration*, 50(2), 130–57.

Cook, B., Wayne, G.F., Valentine, A, Lessios, A and Yeh, E. (2013). 'Revisiting the evidence on health and health care disparities among the Roma: a systematic review 2003–2012'. *International Journal of Public Health*, 58(6), 885–911.

Cronin-de-Chavez, A., Islam, S. and McEachan, R. R. C. (2019). 'Not a level playing field: a qualitative study exploring structural, community and individual determinants of greenspace use amongst low-income multi-ethnic families'. *Health & Place*, 56, 118–26.

Dabbagh, N., Johnson, S., King, M. and Blizard, R. (2012). 'Muslim adolescent mental health in the UK: an exploratory cross-sectional school survey', *International Journal of Culture and Mental Health*, 5, 202–18.

Darlow, A., Bickerstaffe, T., Burden, T., Green, J., Jassi, S., Johnson, S., Kelsey, S., Purcell, M., South, J. and Walton, F. (2005). 'Researching Bradford: a review of social research on Bradford District'. Available at: http://eprints.leedsbeckett.ac.uk/882/1/Researching Bradford.pdf (last accessed 23 May 2022).

Dein, S. and Illaiee, A. S. (2013) 'Jinn and mental health: looking at jinn possession in modern psychiatric practice'. *The Psychiatrist*, 37(9), 290–3.

Dhadda, A. and Greene, G. (2017). 'The healthy migrant effect for mental health in England: propensity-score matched analysis using the EMPIRIC Survey'. *Journal of Immigrant and Minority Health*, 20(4), 799–808.

Dutt, K. and Webber, M. (2010). 'Access to social capital and social support among South East Asian women with severe mental health problems: a cross-sectional survey'. *International Journal of Social Psychiatry*, 56(6), 593–605.

Elahi, F. and Khan, O. (2017). 'Islamophobia: still a challenge for us all. A 20th-anniversary report'. The Runnymede Trust. Available at: www.runnymedetrust. org/publications/islamophobia-still-a-challenge-for-us-all (last accessed 23 May 2022).

Fazil, Q. and Cochrane, R. (2003). 'The prevalence of depression in Pakistani women living in the West Midlands'. *Pakistani Journal of Women's Studies*, 10(1), 21–30.

Fernandez, S. (2009). 'The crusade over the bodies of women'. *Patterns of Prejudice*, 43(3–4), 269–86.

Fink, G. (ed.) (2010). *Stress Consequences: Mental, Neuropsychological and Socioeconomic*. Oxford: Academic Press.

Gazard, B., Frissa, S., Nellums, L., Hotopf, M. and Hatch, S. L. (2015). 'Challenges in researching migration status, health and health service use: An intersectional analysis of a South London community', *Ethnicity and Health*, 20(6), 564–93.

Gunson, D., Nuttall, L., Akhtar, S., Khan, A., Avian, G. and Thomas, L. (2019). 'Spiritual beliefs and mental health: a study of Muslim women in Glasgow'. UWS-Oxfam Partnership: Collaborative Research Reports Series, no. 4. Available at: https://mwrc.org.uk/wp-content/uploads/2020/07/Spiritual-Beliefs-and-Mental-Health.pdf (last accessed 24 May 2022).

Hall, B. C. (2017). 'Local insight profile for "Bradford Local Authority" area'. Prepared for Third Sector Trends event, Bradford City Hall, 29 June 2017.

Hankir, A., Carrick, F. R. and Zaman, R. (2015). 'Islam, mental health and being a Muslim in the West', *Psychiatria Danubina*, suppl., 27(1), 53–9.

Hankir, A., Carrick, F. R. and Zaman, R. (2017). 'Part I: Muslims, social inclusion and the west. Exploring challenges faced by stigmatized groups', *Psychiatria Danubina*, 29, 164–72.

Hellyer, H. (2009). *Muslims of Europe: The 'Other' Europeans*. Edinburgh: Edinburgh University Press.

Herring, C., Brown, S. K., Morgan, B. T., Thompson, J., Kullmar, A. and Blood-Siegfried, J. (2019). 'Virtual orientation of volunteer short-term international health teams to increase self-confidence and cultural and global health competence'. *The Journal of Continuing Education in Nursing*, 50(1), 35–40.

Hussain, F. (2009). 'The mental health of Muslims in Britain: relevant therapeutic concepts', *International Journal of Mental Health*, 38(2), 21–36.

Iley, K. and Nazroo, J. Y. (2007). 'Ethnicity, mental health', in G. Fink (ed.), *Stress Consequences Mental, Neuropsychological and Socioeconomic*. Oxford: Elsevier.

Islam, S. (2011). 'Square pegs in round holes: the mental health needs of young adults and how well these are met by services. An explorative study.' *Journal of Public Mental Health*, 10(4), 211–24.

Jacobson, D. and Deckard, N. D. (2014). 'Surveying the landscape of integration: Muslim immigrants in the United Kingdom and France'. *Democracy and Security*, 10(2), 113–31.

Jayaweera, H. (2011). 'Health of migrants in the UK: what do we know?'. The Migrant Observatory briefing. Available at: www.bl.uk/collection-items/health-of-migrants-in-the-uk-what-do-we-know (last accessed 24 May 2022).

Joshi, S., Jatrana, S., Paradies, Y. and Priest, N. (2014). 'Differences in health behaviours between immigrant and non-immigrant groups: a protocol for a systematic review', *Systematic Reviews*, 3, 61.

Khattab, N. and Modood, T. (2018). 'Accounting for British Muslim's educational attainment: gender differences and the impact of expectations'. *British Journal of Sociology of Education*, 39(2), 242–59.

Knifton, L., Gervais, M., Newbigging, K., Mirza, N., Quinn, N., Wilson, N. and Hunkins-Hutchison, E. (2010). 'Community conversation: addressing mental health stigma with ethnic minority communities'. *Social Psychiatry and Psychiatric Epidemiology*, 45(4), 497–504.

Knott, K. and Khokher, S. (1993). 'Religious and ethnic identity among young Muslim women in Bradford'. *Journal of Ethnic and Migration Studies*, 19(4), 593–610.

Krause, I.-B. (1989). 'Sinking heart: a Punjabi communication of distress'. *Social Science & Medicine*, 29(4), 563–75.

Kuznetsova, D. (2012). Healthy places: councils leading on public health'. New Local. Available at: www.newlocal.org.uk/publications/healthy-places-councils-leading-on-public-health (last accessed 24 May 2022).

Levin, J. and Idler, E. L. (2018). 'Islamophobia and the public health implications of religious hatred'. *American Journal of Public Health* 108(6), 718–19.

Lewicki, A. and O'Toole, T. (2017). 'Acts and practices of citizenship: Muslim women's activism in the UK', *Ethnic and Racial Studies*, 40(1), 152–71.

Lewis, J., Mason, P. and Moore, K. (2013). 'Pointing the finger: images of Islam in the UK', in J. Petley and R. Richardson (eds), *Pointing the Finger: Islam and Muslims in the British Media*. Oxford: Oneworld, pp. 40–65.

Macey, M. (1999). 'Religion, male violence, and the control of women: Pakistani Muslim men in Bradford, UK', *Gender & Development*, 7(1), 48–55.

Mahboob, M. (2018). 'Young people's mental health in a changing world'. A report by Sharing Voices. Available at: https://sharingvoices.net/wp-content/uploads/2019/07/Report_SVB_YPeople_2018_01.pdf (last accessed 24 May 2022).

McGhee, D. (2003). 'Moving to "our" common ground: a critical examination of community cohesion discourse in twenty-first century Britain', *Sociological Review*, 51(3), 376–404.

Mind (2019). 'Mental health facts and statistics'. Available at: www.mind.org.uk/ information-support/types-of-mental-health-problems/statistics-and-facts-about-mental-health/how-common-are-mental-health-problems/#.Xa71qtL0mUk (last accessed 24 May 2022).

Mindlis, I. and Boffetta, P. (2017). 'Mood disorders in first- and second-generation immigrants: systematic review and meta-analysis'. *The British Journal of Psychiatry*, 210(3), 182–9.

Mir, G. (2012). 'Addressing depression in Muslim communities'. University of Leeds School of Medicine. Available at: https://medicinehealth.leeds.ac.uk/dir-record/ research-projects/980/addressing-depression-in-muslim-communities%0A (last accessed 24 May 2022).

Mittermaier, A. (2019). 'The unknown in the Egyptian uprising: towards an anthropology of al-Ghayb'. *Contemporary Islam*, 13(1), 17–31.

Moosavi, L. (2015). 'White privilege in the lives of Muslim converts in Britain'. *Ethnic and Racial Studies*, 38(11), 1918–33.

Muslim Youth Helpline (2019). 'What's the issue?'. Available at: https://myh.org.uk/ resources/research-report (last accessed 24 May 2022).

Nadal, K. L., Griffin, K. E., Hamit, S., Leon, J., Tobio, M. and Rivera, D. P. (2010). 'Subtle and overt forms of Islamophobia: microaggressions toward Muslim Americans', *Journal of Muslim Mental Health*, 6(2).

Neesie (2019). 'Facilitating prosperity for single mums and women'. Available at: https://neesie.org.uk (last accessed 24 May 2022).

NIHR (2018). 'Annual Report Year 4 April 2017– March 2018'. Available at: www. nihr.ac.uk/documents/partners-and-industry/NIHR_Impact_and_Value_ report_ACCESSIBLE_VERSION.pdf (last accessed 11 July 2022).

Northern Data Hub (2018). 'Bradford population – City of Bradford Metropolitan District Council'. Available at: https://datahub.bradford.gov.uk/ebase/datahubext. eb?search=Bradford+population&ebd=0&ebp=10&ebz=1_1572347600121 (last accessed 24 May 2022).

Office of National Statistics and Thriving Places Index (2019). 'Annual Population Survey: personal well-being scores 2019'. Available at: www.centreforthriving-places.org/wp-content/uploads/2020/02/HC-TP19-full-report_FINAL.pdf (last accessed 11 July 2022).

O'Toole, T., Nilsson DeHanas, D., Modood, T., Meer, N and Jones, S. et al. (2013). 'Taking part. Muslim participation in contemporary governance'. Available at: www. bristol.ac.uk/ethnicity/projects/muslimparticipation/documents/mpcgreport.pdf (last accessed 24 May 2022).

Perks, R. B. (1987). 'Immigration to Bradford: the oral testimony'. *Immigrants & Minorities*, 6(3), 362–8.

Pickett, K. E. and Wilkinson, R. G. (2008). 'People like us: ethnic group density effects on health'. *Ethnicity & Health*, 13(4), 321–34.

Pilkington, A., Msetfi, R. M. and Watson, R. (2012). 'Factors affecting intention to access psychological services amongst British Muslims of South Asian origin'. *Mental Health, Religion and Culture*, 15(1), 1–22.

Pitchforth, J., Fahy, K., Ford, T., Wolpert, M., Viner, R. and Hargreaves, D. (2019). 'Mental health and well-being trends among children and young people in the UK, 1995–2014: analysis of repeated cross-sectional national health surveys'. *Psychological Medicine*, 49, 1–11.

Prady, S. L., Pickett, K. E., Croudace, T., Fairley, L., Bloor, K., Gilbody, S., Kiernan, K. E., & Wright, J. (2013). 'Psychological distress during pregnancy in a multi-ethnic community: findings from the Born in Bradford cohort study', *PLoS ONE*, 8(4), 60693.

Raiya, H. A., Pargament, K. I., Stein, C. and Mahoney, A. (2007). 'Lessons learned and challenges faced in developing the psychological measure of Islamic religiousness'. *Journal of Muslim Mental Health*, 2(2), 133–54.

Rawlins, E., Baker, G., Maynard, M., & Harding, S. (2013). 'Perceptions of healthy eating and physical activity in an ethnically diverse sample of young children and their parents: the DEAL prevention of obesity study'. *Journal of Human Nutrition and Dietetics*, 26(2), 132–44.

Roberts, S., Arseneault, L., Barratt, B., Beevers, S., Danese, A., Odgers, C. L., Moffitt, T. E., Reuben, A., Kelly, F. J. and Fisher, H. L. (2019). 'Exploration of NO2 and PM2.5 air pollution and mental health problems using high-resolution data in London-based children from a UK longitudinal cohort study'. *Psychiatry Research*, 272, 8–17.

Rothman, A. and Coyle, A. (2018). 'Toward a framework for Islamic psychology and psychotherapy: an Islamic model of the soul'. *Journal of Religion and Health*, 57(5), 1731–1744.

Samari, G., Alcalá, H. E. and Sharif, M. Z. (2018). 'Islamophobia, health, and public health: a systematic literature review'. *American Journal of Public Health*, 108(6), e1–e9.

Samie, S. F. and Sehlikoglu, S. (2015). 'Strange, incompetent and out-of-place'. *Feminist Media Studies*, 15(3), 363–81.

Shah, Q. and Sonuga-Barke, E. (1995). 'Family structure and the mental health of Pakistani Muslim mothers and their children living in Britain'. *British Journal of Clinical Psychology*, 34(1), 79–81.

Sharing Voices (2019). 'Young people's mental health in a changing world'. Available at: https://sharingvoices.net/news/reports (last accessed 11 July 2022).

Shaw, R. J., Pickett, K. E. and Wilkinson, R. G. (2010). 'Ethnic density effects on birth outcomes and maternal smoking during pregnancy in the US linked birth and infant death data set'. *American Journal of Public Health*, 100(4), 707–13.

Simpson, M., Purdam, K., Tajar, A., Fieldhouse, E., Gavalas, V., Tranmer, M., Pritchard, J. and Dorling, D. (2006). 'Ethnic minority populations and the labour market: an analysis of the 1991 and 2001 census'. Department for Work and Pensions. Research report no. 333. Available at: https://webarchive.nationalarchives.gov.uk/ukgwa/20130128102031/http://www.dwp.gov.uk/asd/asd5/rports2005-2006/Report333.pdf (last accessed 24 May 2022).

Skinner, R. (2010). 'An Islamic approach to psychology and mental health'. *Mental Health, Religion and Culture*, 13(6), 547–51.

Stafford, M., Newbold, B. K. and Ross, N. A. (2011). 'Psychological distress among immigrants and visible minorities in Canada: a contextual analysis'. *International Journal of Social Psychiatry*, 57(4), 428–41.

Sullivan, P. and Akhtar, P. (2019). 'The effect of territorial stigmatisation processes on ontological security: a case-study of Bradford politics', *Political Geography*, 68, 46–54.

The Health Foundation (2018). 'Do young people have the assets for a healthy future?'. Available at: www.health.org.uk/blogs/do-young-people-have-the-assets-for-a-healthy-future (last accessed 11 July 2022).

Thompson, S. and Kent, J. (2014). 'Connecting and strengthening communities in places for health and well-being', *Australian Planner*, 51(3), 260–71.

Tomalin, E. and Sadgrove, J. (2016). 'Places of worship as minority ethnic public health settings in Bradford'. Available at: www.faithaction.net/portal/wp-content/uploads/FA-PoW-PH-Bradford.pdf (last accessed 24 May 2022).

Toseeb, U., Pickles, A., Durkin, K., Botting, N. and Conti-Ramsden, G. (2017). 'Prosociality from early adolescence to young adulthood: A longitudinal study of individuals with a history of language impairment'. *Research in Developmental Disabilities*, 62, 148–59.

Trueman, M., Klemm, M. and Giroud, A. (2004). 'Can a city communicate? Bradford as a corporate brand'. *Corporate Communications: An International Journal*, 9(4), 317–330.

Utz-Billing, I. and Kentenich, H. (2008). 'Female genital mutilation: an injury, physical and mental harm'. *Journal of Psychosomatic Obstetrics & Gynecology*, 29(4), 225–9.

Warfa, N., Curtis, S., Watters, C., Carswell, K., Ingleby, D. and Bhui, K. (2011). 'Migration experiences, employment status and psychological distress among Somali immigrants: a mixed-method international study'. *BMC Public Health*, 12, 749.

Wohland, P., Rees, P., Nazroo, J. and Jagger, C. (2015). 'Inequalities in healthy life expectancy between ethnic groups in England and Wales in 2001'. *Ethnicity and Health*, 20(4), 341–53.

Wright, J., Hayward, A., West, J., Pickett, K., McEachan, R. M., Mon-Williams, M., Christie, N., Vaughan, L., Sheringham, J., Haklay, M., Sheard, L., Dickerson, J. et al. (2019). 'ActEarly: a City Collaboratory approach to early promotion of good health and wellbeing'. *Wellcome Open Research*, 4, 156.

Wu, Z. and Schimmele, C. M. (2005). 'The healthy migrant effect on depression: variation over time?'. *Canadian Studies in Population*, 32(2), 271–95.

14

THE CULTURAL ADAPTATION OF ACCEPTANCE AND COMMITMENT THERAPY FOR PAIN MANAGEMENT SERVICES

Razia Bhatti-Ali and Mohammad Shoiab

Introduction

Research on the healthcare of Muslim families in the UK has shown them to have the poorest overall health profile in Britain, with Pakistani Muslims reporting lower psychosocial wellbeing and reduced ability to manage long-term conditions compared to other religious groups (Mir and Sheikh 2010). This trend appears to be perpetuated by the focus of professionals attributing health disparities to socioeconomic factors, a 'community mindset' and the patient's lack of understanding of long-term conditions (Muslim Health Network 2004).

Moreover, discrimination and exclusion are also salient factors which may also have a role in maintaining health inequalities (Commission of British Muslims on Islamophobia 2004). A report by Public Health England (2018) states that the prevalence of racist discrimination directly impacts the health of minority groups. For Muslims, with the rise of Islamophobia there are further barriers to equitable health services.

The role of broader sociopolitical and economic factors is undoubtedly significant in creating and maintaining inequalities in health (Public Health England 2018). However, it is essential to recognise that the management of health and wellbeing is also impacted upon by cultural beliefs and illness perceptions which are often shaped by traditional and religious practices (Taheri 2008). Reduced access to services for Muslim patients has been attributed to poor communication and a lack of cultural sensitivity from healthcare staff who have little understanding of how culture and religion may help address inequalities more efficiently (Ikezi et al. 2015).

Mir and Sheikh (2010) contend that the stereotypical perceptions of Muslim patients held by professionals serve as a barrier to delivering equitable services. When addressing health disparities, much of the public health literature focuses on ethnicity rather than religion (Public Health England 2018). However, for many Muslims, religious identity may be more meaningful than ethnicity as the predominant UK Muslim population regard religion as their identity (Modood 2008).

For the Muslim community, Islam is 'a complete way of life' as taught in the Qur'an and the *Sunnah* (teachings of the Prophet Muhammad (PBUH) and therefore cannot be separated from culture. Thus, culture, language, religion and traditions are central to tackling the prevalent disparities in health and wellbeing in Muslim populations.

Thus, many of the health inequalities commonly observed in Muslim groups could be better addressed by professionals if their interventions were culturally and religiously sensitive and incorporated the teachings of the Quran and *Sunnah* to engage the patients in addressing underlying risk factors such as poor diet and lack of physical activity. For example, maintaining good physical health as a means of respecting the body is advocated in both the Holy Qur'an and the prophetic teachings (hadith) for the benefit it brings to one's emotional, psychological and, more importantly, spiritual life (Al Khayat 2004).

The Prophet Muhammad (PBUH) promoted physical activities such as walking, archery, horse riding and swimming along with engaging in family activities as necessary for maintaining health and wellbeing (hadith). From an Islamic perspective, observing the basic tenets of Islam (prayer, fasting, *Hajj* or the Holy Pilgrimage to Mecca) and consuming a healthy diet enables one to achieve a state of physical and mental balance which in itself is intrinsically a form of worship.

For example, performing the five daily prayers involves movement of all muscles and joints of the body and includes being in a state of presence before God. Fasting in the month of Ramadan and the performance of the *Hajj* are physically and mentally exerting tasks requiring dedication and willpower. Physical exercise, prayer and ablution, the pilgrimage, moderation in diet, good manners and healthy relationships are all critical activities promoted in Islam as contributing to reverence to God and spiritual elevation as well as maintaining a balance in health and wellbeing (Al Khayat 2004).

Chronic Pain Management and Culture

The International Association for the Study of Pain (2020) defines pain as 'an unpleasant sensory and emotional experience associated with, or resembling that associated with, actual or potential tissue damage' (Raja et al. 2020). This definition suggests that the human body can experience pain without any real physical tissue damage or injury. Furthermore, the definition goes on to note that 'through their life experiences, individuals learn the concept of pain'. Cross-cultural investigations evidence that the experience of pain can be powerfully influenced by cultural attitudes and health beliefs and may determine the emotional, physiological and spiritual construction of the pain experience (Brady et al. 2015; Lipton and Marbach 1984). Beliefs and values can also mediate other pain coping strategies such as stoicism, spiritual coping, hypervigilance and catastrophising (Brady et al. 2015).

Research on the association between culture and the effect on the pain experience is not a new concept. In 2002, researchers in Greater Manchester recruited over 2,000 South Asian and African-Caribbean patients with chronic musculoskeletal pain to assess the presence of pain in specific joints and the level of physical function. The main findings were that the pain profile of the South Asian and African-Caribbean patients differed from that of Caucasian populations. Pain in multiple sites was considerably more prevalent among different ethnic groups when compared to the local Caucasian population, suggesting a prevalence of social, cultural and psychological differences in pain expression (Allison et al. 2002).

The Centre for Applied Research and Evaluation-International Foundation (2016) has criticised current interventions for mental and physical health disorders as being West-centric and not in tune with diverse cultural beliefs. The development of interdisciplinary pain management programmes (PMPs) based on the biopsychosocial model has been a cost-effective endeavour aimed at supporting the patient with chronic pain to regain function and improved quality of life.

However, as beliefs about pain and expectations of treatment are likely to be influenced by cultural values, which often differ from the Western models of service delivery, these programmes have not always been effective when delivered to minority populations (Shoiab et al. 2016; Ehrlich et al. 2016). Perhaps this may explain why people from diverse cultural backgrounds are often reluctant to engage with standard treatment programmes and instead manifest alternative help-seeking behaviours.

The Health and Care Professions Council (HCPC 2012), which is the regulatory body for fifteen different professions in the UK, sets specific 'standards of proficiency'. It stipulates that professionals need to 'be aware of the impact of culture, equality and diversity on practice' and 'be able to communicate effectively' and 'understand the key concepts of the knowledge base relevant to their profession'. These standards stress the importance of clinicians having cultural awareness and the ability to adapt their practice to the needs of patients from diverse cultural backgrounds.

From a societal perspective, global changes in migration and movement of populations necessitate the cultural competence of health services to be improved, enabling them to provide evidence-based care without bias and stereotypes about an individual's majority or minority cultural status, and influenced by respect for their values and world view. An evidence-based cultural adaptation has the potential to provide a methodology to modify treatments systematically so that the culture and context of diverse groups are considered in the intervention.

Bernal et al. (2009) have described cultural adaptation as 'the systematic modification of an evidence-based treatment (EBT) or evidence-based intervention (EBI) protocol which considers language, culture, and the context in such a way that it is compatible with the individual's cultural patterns, meanings, and values'. Peacock and Patel (2008) found that primary care practitioners within the UK, particularly GPs, acknowledge the need for culturally grounded pain management services for both physical therapy and psychological and behavioural management of pain. Furthermore, for non-English speaking patients, health practitioners often depend upon interpreting services. While the interpreting service may be linguistically equivalent, it may not always be conceptually applicable, thereby leaving the service delivery lacking in quality and effectiveness (Fletcher 2006). Furthermore, the dearth of high-quality, evidence-based studies further confounds the issue of effectively addressing self-management and multidisciplinary interventions for chronic pain in culturally and linguistically diverse populations and migrant populations (Brady et al. 2015).

Hence there is an imperative for developing culturally grounded pain management services which can enhance the understanding of the individual pain experience and disability within minority populations so that equitable treatment interventions can be implemented (Torres-Cueco 2018). It can be argued that recognition by professionals that patients with chronic pain from a diverse cultural group may have different concepts about health and illness, and different expectations from consultations and delivery of care, will have the benefit of increasing the confidence and motivation of service users and improving compliance with health advice and treatment interventions (Hopkins and Bahl 1993).

Culturally Adapted Psychological Interventions

The nature of chronic pain as a musculoskeletal, physical health condition is well established (Morley et al. 1999). However, with the advancement of biopsychosocial perspectives, it is integral to consider the interplay of emotional distress and the appropriate management of these processes as they conjointly contribute to the development and maintenance of persistent pain and thus require due consideration in developing a culturally adapted intervention for pain management (Dahl and Lundgren 2006).

There is a growing body of evidence indicating the usefulness of adapting mental health interventions, particularly cognitive behaviour therapies (CBT) to manage the psychological health of Muslim communities (Naeem et al. 2011, 2015; Mir et al. 2010, 2012). Research on culturally adapted psychological interventions in Pakistan, China and England concur that for non-Western populations, successful patient-centred health interventions can only be achieved by taking cultural, religious and spiritual aspects into account (Bernal 2009; Hwang et al. 2015; Naeem et al. 2015; Algahtani et al. 2019).

Algahtani et al. (2019) carried out a study adapting CBT for local patients experiencing depression and anxiety in Saudi Arabia and Bahrain. The results indicate that CBT may need to be altered for those from non-Western backgrounds to incorporate the role of cultural factors and their influence on assessment, formulation and interventional techniques. The researchers highlighted the importance of cultural sensitivity and the impact it has on improved engagement. They also emphasised the role religion may have on health beliefs and the need to develop the appropriate use of language and translation of psychological concepts for a culturally adapted CBT intervention to be useful.

Naeem et al. (2009) investigated the extent to which CBT was consistent with the personal, religious, family, social and cultural values of Pakistani patients. They evaluated a brief, culturally adapted CBT intervention in a primary care setting and following a larger randomised controlled trial (RCT). They concluded that the tailored intervention was more effective than 'treatment as usual' (Naeem et al. 2015).

Likewise, Mir et al. (2019) developed and piloted a culturally adapted behavioural activation (BA) treatment for depression based on 'positive religious coping' to increase service uptake and recovery in Muslim communities. The programme was delivered over twelve weeks by a minimally trained mental health worker and instructed the participants to use culturally adapted CBT skills and principles. This study also showed promising results and accentuated the importance of delivering culturally relevant psychological interventions.

In terms of pain management, since the early 1990s CBT has become the leading psychological treatment strategy supported by substantial research trials examining evidence for the benefits of CBT for pain management (Morley et al. 1999; Williams et al. 2012). CBT for pain management is based upon the principle that individual beliefs and attitudes affect behaviour and thereby affect the pain experience. By teaching individuals to adopt new ways of thinking and feeling, their behavioural responses to pain can also be adapted to increase tolerance. A variety of psychological strategies are used to improve pain control with an emphasis on self-management. However, its applicability to managing pain in minority groups remains an area requiring further research.

Cardosa et al. (2012) examined the effects of a two-week CBT pain programme in Malaysia in which cultural adaptation was improved by encouraging family members to attend at least once to enlist their support for the self-management approach and to enable post-programme gains in conjunction with relaxation techniques such as Islamic prayer and meditation. This study demonstrated that Western-orientated behavioural interventions for pain could be successfully adapted to be used with people from a non-Western cultural background.

Sagheer et al. (2013) examined the prevalence of anxiety and depression in a chronic low back pain (LBP) population at a tertiary care centre in Pakistan. They found that of the 140 patients recruited, over half of the participants were experiencing abnormal levels of anxiety (55–77 per cent) and depression (48–57 per cent). The study concluded that individuals with chronic LBP were at a higher risk of experiencing anxiety and depression with the risk being higher for females.

In addressing cultural and religious themes specifically for Muslim patients with pain conditions, Maki et al. (2014) carried out a qualitative research study exploring the beliefs and expression of Arabic patients experiencing LBP, to help inform the design of a pain management programme acceptable within the Arab culture. The study enlisted eighteen patients who attended three focus groups each. The results from the study identified four main themes. These were: maintaining independence and identity within the family unit (e.g. female role within the household); self-management strategies for LBP (e.g. religious coping statements, the importance of pacing, etc.); acceptance of the impact of long-term LBP (e.g. cyclical nature of pain); and patient expectations of healthcare professionals involved in their care (e.g. sympathy, provision of exercise and information sheets). Maki et al. (2014) concluded that insight into family roles could inform how patients are taught to pace household chores or communicate their pain experience to others.

Addressing culture-specific psychological (e.g. coping mechanisms) and social (family roles) themes in a pain management programme for Arabic patients may help develop insights into delivering PMPs for Muslim populations in the United Kingdom.

A later study by Edwards et al. (2016) aimed to explore the relationships between chronic pain and religious faith among older adults from five different faith groups (Christians, Hindus, Sikhs, Jews and Muslims) using semi-structured qualitative interviews. They stressed the importance of understanding faith/belief and how it is articulated within the context of other aspects of their identity in response to the experience of pain.

Irrespective of faith, Edwards et al. (2016) established that the direct use of religious activities such as prayer formed an essential part of the self-management of pain and served the function of maintaining a relationship with God at a time of uncertainty to induce a calming effect and increase coping. For Muslim patients, as well as their relationship with God (spirituality), the ritualistic aspects of worship such as prayer and Qur'anic recitation served as an additional source of strength and a means for coping and resilience.

Edwards et al. (2016) found that association with a faith group for most participants in their study facilitated wellbeing and provided an additional tool to self-manage pain. Furthermore, they found that individual interpretations of religious scripture/doctrine were enmeshed in personal judgements (religious and otherwise) which were useful in determining how pain can be understood within the framework of each specific religious faith.

This study concluded that while there are aspects of the self-management of pain that are common across faiths (e.g. distraction, social support and alternative therapies), there are also characteristics unique to particular doctrines (e.g. prayer, the meanings of suffering and karma). Therefore, it is expedient for religious, spiritual and psychological permeations to be considered equally important as the physical aspects of pain when considering cultural adaptations of health interventions to address the multifaceted essence of pain experience and expression.

Acceptance and Commitment Therapy for Chronic Pain in Muslim Patients

Following on from the success of CBT as a therapeutic modality for pain management, acceptance and commitment therapy (ACT) has developed momentum as an innovative and evidence-based psychological intervention in the management of pain and chronic health conditions (Feliu Soler 2018; Lin 2019). ACT is a third-wave behavioural approach developed by Hayes et al. (1999). It emphasises values-based living as a way of increasing functionality for those individuals who may have lost direction in life due to their struggle with their specific chronic pain condition.

ACT is based on the premise that it is the 'struggle' with pain that causes suffering rather than the pain itself. By reversing unhelpful behaviours that maintain pain, one can find meaning in life by committing to reconnect with personal values rather than putting life on hold. While CBT works by helping the patient identify and change negative or unfavourable thoughts, ACT fundamentally emphasises that suffering is normal and allows the experience of uncomfortable feelings and thoughts while acting on what is important to the individual (Dahl et al. 2004).

ACT processes enable the development of psychological flexibility or a set of skills that help empower people to accept whatever unwanted thoughts, feelings or experiences manifest while persisting in moving towards valued goals or whatever matters most to the individual (Biglan et al. 2008). Harris (2019) describes psychological flexibility as the ability to be present in the moment with full awareness and being open to whatever experience occurs with a willingness to be guided by core values on the action taken (Harris 2019). This process can be achieved by paying attention, interacting with thoughts differently and practising acceptance of issues that are out of the individual's control, thus increasing quality of life and enhancing ways of living (Dahl and Lundgren 2006).

For many people from the Muslim community, their religious belief systems are the guiding point to living a values-based life, which is why the ACT approach may be a congruent intervention when managing pain conditions and may also help address the barriers faced by Muslim patients in accessing equitable pain management services. ACT as a therapeutic modality may be more likely to engage patients from the Muslim community due to its principles being more congenial to an Islamic approach to life and particularly for those who may find engaging with the collaborative nature of a CBT approach challenging.

Yavuz (2016) elegantly delineates the parallels between ACT's psychological flexibility model and Islam. He argues that ACT shares conceptual and practical commonalities with Islam, particularly with the six processes described by Hayes (2004) that foster psychological flexibility (Nieuwsma et al. 2016). These include (1) acceptance of one's condition; (2) defusion of thoughts (which means noticing thoughts rather than being caught up in them); (3) being present in the moment; (4) using self-as-context which means having an awareness of awareness; and living a (5) values-based life as guidance to taking (6) committed action to improve a condition. These six processes can be used as a helpful framework for developing an Islamic-based PMP and may be valuable in increasing cultural and religious sensitivity within the standardised PMPs.

Acceptance

Acceptance is an integral part of the ACT therapeutic model built on the premise that progress can only be made if the individual is prepared to experience some pain while still living a life based on their values. Instead of trying to escape from pain and its unwelcome effects, the patient learns to see it as a normal part of their life. Acceptance does not mean having to tolerate the unpleasant stimuli but to give painful thoughts and feelings space without struggling against them. Developing acceptance of the unpleasant experience opens the patient's willingness to engage in goal-directed actions.

Acceptance is the opposite of 'experiential avoidance', which means trying to get away from unpleasant thoughts, feelings and memories rather than being willing to face the experience and learn to live with the discomfort. There are perceptible similarities with stoicism in the view that a person is not confined, constricted or defined by their health condition, as health is only one facet of them as a person. Chronic pain may affect the body, but not the choice or ability to pursue goals and values (Stephens 2007). Patients living with persistent pain are provided with methods that encourage them to let go of the struggle with pain to help them develop effective coping strategies and a re-engagement with their values.

Acceptance in the Islamic faith can be illustrated by examining the concept of *sabr* in times of difficulty. *Sabr* is an Arabic word that may be translated as patience, persistence, self-discipline and perseverance in the face of hardship. It does not refer to a state of being passive but rather being able to stand firm (Ali ibn Abu Talib 2014). This concept inspires individuals to strive for a meaningful life by developing acceptance of the affliction instead of struggling with aversive situations. The Holy Qur'an makes several references to the connection between being patient and persevering in doing right to attain relief and deliverance from Allah.

> Seek God (Allah)'s help with patient perseverance and prayer. It is indeed hard, except for those who are humble. (Holy Qur'an 2:45)

> Oh, you who believe! Seek help with patient perseverance and prayer, for God is with those who patiently persevere. (Holy Qur'an 2:153)

> Be sure We shall test you with something of fear and hunger, some loss in goods, lives, and the fruits of your toil. But give glad tidings to those who patiently persevere. Those who say, when afflicted with calamity, 'To Allah we belong, and to Him is our return.' They are those on whom descend blessings from their Lord, and mercy. They are the ones who receive guidance. (Holy Qur'an 2:155–7)

The notion of *sabr* is often conjoint with the concept of *shukr*, or gratitude. A hadith (narratives based on the teachings of the Prophet (PBUH)) narrated by a companion of the Prophet (PBUH) said:

> How excellent is the case of a faithful servant – there is good for him in everything and this is not the case with anyone except him. If prosperity attends him, he expresses *shukr* (gratitude) to Allah (SWT), and that is good for him. If adversity falls on him, he endures it patiently (with *sabr*), and that is good for him. (Pervez 2014)

Research shows that gratitude or *shukr* is a universally rewarding process for increasing happiness and emotional wellbeing (Emmons and Crumpler 2000). Noor (2016) carried out a study of students to assess the effects on levels of happiness when an Islamic-based expressive gratitude strategy was used. The practice of being mindful of the blessings of Allah in a gratitude exercise was compared to the happiness level of Muslims practising a secular-based gratitude exercise and a control group who did not practise gratitude. Results showed that Islamic-based gratitude increased participants' happiness level due to the fit it had with their beliefs and values. Thus, Muslims encouraged to engage in *sabr* and *shukr* while making *dhikr* (remembrance of God, meditation) and taking actions based on their values are more likely to experience increased levels of wellbeing.

The focus on long-term consequences rather than immediate positive outcomes such as experiential avoidance of aversive situations helps guide patients towards acceptance and commitment to change. Islamic teachings discourage avoidance of committed actions when faced with aversive situations. The hadith 'Trust in Allah but also tether your camel' reflects the idea that patients should act and engage in self-management rather than take the fatalistic view of relying on God alone to provide a solution. This hadith helps motivate patients to engage in self-management of pain rather than viewing their fate as assured.

Cognitive defusion

Cognitive defusion is the process which allows the individual to step back and detach themselves from their thoughts, images and memories by 'making closer contact with verbal events as they really are, not merely as what they say they are' (Hayes et al. 2012). Cognitive fusion is when we respond to our thoughts as being factual. When this happens, an individual automatically becomes caught up in perceiving their thoughts as literal truths and becomes tangled in them like being caught in a spider's web. In this, the thought itself is not the target issue, but the entanglement with the thought becomes the issue of concern as it allows cognition to dominate behaviour.

The spider's web metaphor can usefully illustrate this. When walking into a room with spider's webs, we may try our best to ignore them but this does not stop the discomfort that they may give rise to. Defusion can be achieved by disentangling ourselves from the intricate webs whenever we notice ourselves getting caught in them. Defusion skills help the individual notice thoughts that are unhelpful and to detach from them rather than placing power and belief in them. Another common metaphor for defusion is to view the mind as the sky with thoughts being like passing clouds, transient and not permanent, and as they pass on, new thoughts will rise into and out of awareness until they disappear. This metaphor resonates with the Qur'anic verse 'For indeed, with hardship will be ease' (Holy Qur'an 94:5) as the thought or state of discomfort is not everlasting.

From an Islamic perspective, cognitive fusion also has parallels with the concept of *wasawasa*, which is referred to as persistent unsubstantiated fears, doubts or 'whispers' in which people often become entwined. Islam views unhelpful thinking processes as a distraction and hindrance from living a life based on values, and warns against *wasawasa*. The Holy Qur'an guides humans to take perspective of their cognitions, metacognitions and behaviours and to take actions based on values, rather than changing thinking styles: 'And We have already created man and know what his self [*nafs*] whispers [*waswasa*] to him, and We are closer to him than [his] Jugular vein' (Holy Qur'an 50:16).

In Islam, remembrance of God is recommended as a means of overcoming *wasawasa*: 'Verily in the remembrance of Allah, there is contentment of the heart' (Holy Qur'an 13:28). Therefore, teaching Muslim patients how to defuse from their thoughts using an Islamic perspective may help validate the intervention and give people the incentive to act on the process.

Furthermore, 'The Guest House', a poem by 13th-century Sufi mystic Jalaluddin Rumi, is a useful tool to defuse from unhelpful thoughts as it creates a metaphor for life as a voyage filled with both pleasing and unwelcome experiences. The core message is that whatever life's journey brings, whether it is happiness or great difficulty, it is one's imperceptible faith, attitude and commitment to greet the experience without worry or dislike that will help foster enlightenment and compassion towards others and the self. Inexorably, life's sojourn will entail good and bad experiences, but the bad experiences may be opportunities for growth while the good events are not necessarily conducive to spiritual and personal growth: 'But perhaps you hate a thing, and it is good for you, and perhaps you love a thing, and it is bad for you. And Allah Knows, while you know not' (Holy Qur'an 2:216).

Being present

ACT promotes ongoing non-judgemental contact with psychological and environmental events as they occur to experience the world more directly, be it good or bad. Mindfulness is used to tune in to what is happening around the individual instead of them being caught up in worry and rumination. Focusing attention on the task at hand helps the individual experience more of life rather than missing each precious moment. Similarly, from an Islamic viewpoint appreciating the Almighty's moment-by-moment creation by being present in mind is the path to experiencing the real meaning of life and living it with true purpose.

The Sufi-based approach of *muraqabah*, which metaphorically means meditation, enables the individual to watch and take care of their soul and gain a closeness to their Creator. Therefore, practising mindfulness and being present in the moment without attachment to the past and the future is a central principle in Islam. Furthermore, the concept of *tawba*, which refers to repentance or returning to the right path, is a process that leads to developing awareness of the present and working towards a values-based existence.

When becoming overwhelmed in a state of illness and suffering, patients may attribute responsibility for their behaviour to their illness; however, the verses repeatedly referred to in the Qur'an: 'we burden not any person but that which he can bear' (Holy Qur'an 6:152) and 'Allah does not charge a soul except with that within its capacity' (Holy Qur'an 2:286) motivate individuals who find it difficult to cope with life situations to practise prayer as a way of developing a state of being present. Mindfulness, in this context, is becoming aware of thoughts rather than suppressing them and learning to let them pass rather than becoming overwhelmed by them (Hussain 2011).

The Holy Qur'an recommends mindfulness and remembrance instead of trying to fight unhelpful thoughts by engaging in them or trying to conquer them: 'Those who have faith and whose hearts find peace in the remembrance of God- truly it is in the remembrance of God that hearts find peace' (Holy Qur'an 13:28). When the mind is allowed space and silence, then any thought entering the mind can be seen for what it is: just a thought, to be observed and understood rather than the defining factor of an individual's sense of self.

Within the context of pain management, the use of mindfulness to create a space in which the individual can step back from the pain and learn to cultivate a tolerance resonates with the Islamic practice of using prayer and praise of God during hard times to attempt to release an individual from cognitive entanglement and bring the individual into present moment awareness. The Prophet Muhammad (PBUH) advised a companion, 'Constantly be mindful of Allah, and you will find Him Omnipresent' (hadith).

Self as context

Within the ACT model, self as context refers to self-awareness or the 'observing self' in that it is the part of the individual that notices experienced sensations, thoughts, feelings and the images that pass through the mind. The French philosopher René Descartes famously said in his biographical treatise in 1637, 'I think; therefore, I am', suggesting that our sense of self is based on our thinking mind. However, the self as context refers to humans as being more than just thoughts and feelings. When individuals are entangled in the content of their lives, they find it challenging to step back and observe. ACT regards the language of the mind as a double-edged sword as, despite its advantages, if not mastered it can become painful and problematic for the individual (Harris 2019). The key that opens the door to self as context is mindfulness as it enables one to pay attention to the present moment and to thoughts and feelings without judgement.

Within the Islamic faith, the concept of *nafs* (the self) can be understood in relation to the self and the soul: 'And remember your Rabb inside your-self' (Holy Qur'an 7:205). The more frequent use of the *nafs* is the reference to a specific part of the self that consists of a conglomeration of wants, desires, fears and tendencies that attempts to protect even at the cost of misrepresenting the true nature of reality.

In order to cultivate a state of mind where the realities of both mental and emotional states become clear without the individual becoming swept away on a wave of entangled thoughts and internal sensations, it is important to become more mindful of what is happening within, to prevent action that is likely to increase distress: 'Indeed, the *nafs* that overwhelmingly commands a person to do sin' (Holy Qur'an 12:53). Learning to control the *nafs* or the ego allows the individual to find direction to free themselves from being attached to erroneous self-stories or limiting beliefs and to develop the resilience to use self-management techniques from a faith-based approach.

The act of *tawba* (repentance) is a process of behaviour change devoid of the need to remain attached to self-stories (even if those self-stories are linked to unacceptable past actions). The Holy Qur'an states, 'Indeed, Allah will not change the condition of a people until they change what is in themselves' (Holy Qur'an 13:11). *Tawba* may allow patients who are struggling with the belief that their pain condition is a punishment for past sins to be able to dispense with such restrictive cognitions or the tug of war that often occurs between the thought and the distress it may cause. When the mind is allowed space and silence through the practice of mindfulness, then any thought entering the mind materialises as a transient entity and not the defining factor of an individual's sense of self.

Values and committed action

Persistent chronic pain conditions often lead to the sufferer chasing short term and limiting methods of alleviation. In the process, there is a compromise on valued activities such as exercise, socialisation, intimacy in relationships, involvement in family and community events, prayer and practice of faith. A valued action is likely to be personal even though cultural, religious and moral factors may underpin it. A values-based life can only be achieved when the individual decides to take committed actions to pursue those values even in the face of adversity.

The Islamic faith reinforces the importance of taking decisive action (committed action) even when one is inclined to act towards avoiding pain as a means of attaining spiritual growth. The Holy Qur'an states: 'Allah does not burden a soul beyond that it can bear' (Holy Qur'an 2:286) and 'No misfortune ever befalls except by permission of Allah. And whoever has faith in Allah – he will guide his heart. And Allah is knowing of all things' (Holy Qur'an 64:11)

The remembrance of Allah (*dhikr*) which equates to mindfulness and meditation is recommended as a way of moving towards values-based actions that reflect what the situation requires. The Muslim faith discourages people from engaging in avoidance behaviours in the face of an aversive experience or situation and encourages acting on values even when the natural urge is to avoid pain (Hussain 2011).

The Prophet Muhammad (PBUH) said, 'If the Resurrection were established upon one of you while he has in his hand a sapling, then let him plant it' (hadith), which suggests the importance of acting towards values without any attachment to the past or the future regardless of the level of adversity. The bus metaphor often used in ACT illustrates this well. While driving the bus of life, thoughts and feelings can be regarded as unruly passengers travelling in the back of the bus making disparaging comments that distract the individual from pursuing their desired route in life. If the driver sticks to the normal course, then the commotion caused by the passengers ceases while when the bus turns towards a road of valued activities, the mind noise can become loud and upsetting.

These disruptive passengers can, at times, become more than a nuisance and chip away at resilience by causing distraction and distress with their constant barrage of unhelpful comments and criticisms. The useful lessons from this metaphor are that for optimum health and wellbeing it is essential to remain focused on driving the bus in the direction that truly matters to the individual regardless of the mental noise by using values as the compass bearing that helps steer the bus onto the right path (Hayes et al. 2004).

When considering values, it is not uncommon to confuse them with goals. It may be helpful to distinguish the two by seeing values as the way we travel on our journey of life and goals as our destination. Yavuz (2016) argues that there is a strong compatibility between the ACT concept of values and Islam. Islamic guidance states that this world is temporary and fragile and can inevitably be snuffed out like a candle in the wind. A successful afterlife will be attained according to every individual's actions and deeds in life following judgement day; hence the way people conduct themselves during life's journey will determine their outcome.

Thus, the goal may be to attain a successful afterlife while the values-based actions in achieving this goal will be to live a life of *ihsan* (excellence) which the Prophet Muhammad (PBUH) described as 'To worship Allah as if you see Him, and if you do not see Him, He sees you' (Al-Bukhari 1978). From this perspective, it is incumbent in Islam to be observant and committed to pursuing values, as each individual will leave behind a legacy based on their actions and will be questioned upon these on the day of judgement.

Committed action means a productive and mindful life congruent with one's values while accepting the pain and suffering that is inescapably part of life. From an Islamic standpoint, following moral, social and behavioural principles is seen as an integral part of committed actions. This concept is congruent with the tombstone metaphor often used in ACT which explores what people would want their life to stand for after they have left this world and to promote a values-based life. Hayes suggests a useful way to frame this is to ask the individual what they would to want to hear if they could attend their own funeral (Hayes et al. 2012).

The Islamic practice of regularly performing charitable acts is a means of laying down the foundations for a positive legacy and a way of striving towards a values-based existence which supports wellbeing in both material life and the hereafter. The Holy Qur'an recommends working towards values and righteous actions in a paced and graded manner to allow for change to be implemented effectively without overwhelming the individual. An example of this can be seen in the way the total prohibition of alcohol was achieved in a graded manner by revealing the following three verses in order of the change required.

First:

They ask you about intoxicants and games of chance. Say: In both of them, there is a great sin and means of profit for men, and their sin is greater than their profit. And they ask you as to what they should spend. Say: What you can spare. Thus, does Allah make clear to you the communications, that you may ponder. (Holy Qur'an 2:219)

Then:

O you who believe! do not go near prayer when you are Intoxicated until you know (well) what you say. (Holy Qur'an 4:43)

Finally:

O ye who believe! Wine and the game of chance and idols and divining arrows are only the abomination of Satan's handiwork. So shun each one of them that you may prosper. (Holy Qur'an 5:90)

Similarly, ACT advocates any change to be implemented gradually in a mindful and values-based manner (Hayes et al. 2004).

Within the ACT model, the absence of sadness is not a 'normal' state, but instead, pain, difficulties and unpleasant experiences are inevitable and natural consequences of life (Hayes et al. 2012). Likewise, Islam acknowledges that pain or uncomfortable experiences are tests of life and are inevitably fluid. For Muslim patients who are experiencing pain and suffering, this approach allows an appropriate rationale for the individual to take responsibility for their psychological and physical wellbeing, recognising that pain and suffering may be a test from the Almighty. Still, it comes with the responsibility of taking committed action based on values to alleviate suffering: 'Indeed, Allah will not change the condition of a people until they change what is in themselves. And when Allah intends for a people ill, there is no repelling it' (Holy Qur'an 13:11). And: 'Whenever a Muslim is afflicted by harm from sickness or other matters, God will expiate his sins, like leaves drop from a tree' (hadith from Bukhari and Muslim).

Application of the Culturally Adapted Pain Management Programme

Given that ACT has parallels with an Islamic approach to health and illness, it was considered appropriate to use this in the adaptation of a PMP that would address the cultural/religious and language needs of Muslim patients referred to the Living with Pain Team. The first intervention was undertaken in Bradford, where one-fifth of the population are Pakistani Muslims. The Living with Pain Team highlighted that many patients from this community found it difficult to engage in a PMP delivered in English and struggled to relate to concepts that were not congruent with their cultural values. Some patients held the view that long-term pain was the result of a punishment or a test from Allah (God) and therefore took a fatalistic view of their pain condition. As a result, they found it challenging to engage in a self-management approach towards dealing with their chronic pain (Shoiab et al. 2016).

Furthermore, cultural practices of relying on relatives to become carers in times of ill health reinforced dependence and physical deconditioning. Acceptance of the chronic illness replaced by resignation and external attributions for health conditions become a significant obstacle in engaging with this patient group. As examined above, the lack of understanding of cultural and religious beliefs often leads to an inequitable service provision for chronic pain patients from the Muslim community (ibid.).

Health professionals have consistently attributed the lack of engagement from the Muslim community to reduced motivation and failure to identify that the healing process is embedded within their cultural belief system (Hopkins and Bahl 1993). Therefore, it was compelling to utilise cultural and religious factors as the key to breaking down barriers and enabling a person-centred, holistic approach to the management of chronic pain.

Consequently, a culturally adapted PMP (CA-PMP) incorporating the ACT model was delivered to a group of Muslim patients referred to the chronic pain management service in Bradford. The content of the PMP was adapted from the standardised model and included ACT and Islamically revised concepts of psychological flexibility (Shoiab et al. 2016). The CA-PMP was delivered in the Urdu language and included a session from the hospital's Muslim chaplain who was able to reinforce Islamic teachings that promoted self-management, compassion, mindfulness, physical activity, and the dispersing of cultural and religious myths. A GP with a special interest (GPwSI) in pain management was also able to provide an educational session on the use of medication and the associated costs and benefits as there was a notable reliance on medication as opposed to self-management.

The ACT framework for pain management was delivered by a consultant clinical psychologist and adapted with metaphors and stories relevant to the religious and cultural background of the group based on the six core processes of ACT. In terms of outcomes, objectively, the participants made statistically significant improvements in self-efficacy, anxiety and depression following the programme. Subjectively the participants reported a clearer understanding of their persistent pain for the first time within their cultural context with an increased motivation to put the self-management techniques into practice. There was also a tangible appreciation of the religious aspects of the PMP with the participants demonstrating a strong incentive to use their learning to improve quality of life.

Bhatti-Ali et al. (2019) undertook a further evaluation of the CA-PMP. They carried out a pilot study incorporating the ACT model of learning to live with pain which was also delivered in the Urdu language. The participants were a non-randomised sample of seven patients (two male and five female) referred to the chronic pain management team who had found it hard to engage in the standard PMP. The programme was carried out over six weeks with a one-month follow-up session.

The weekly sessions included some didactic teaching, individual work and homework review, as well as group discussions around values, goal setting and mindfulness. Video and audio material presented in the Urdu language was also incorporated in the sessions to reinforce the benefits of mindfulness and relaxation techniques in the management of pain. Islamic teachings promoting a values-based life through Qur'anic stories and metaphors based on authentic hadith sources reinforced self-management, relaxation and physical activity to help cultivate psychological flexibility and resilience.

The outcome measures revealed a significant decrease in the level of depression and anxiety and a significant increase in the functional level of patients at post-intervention. Further qualitative data collected from this study at the end of the programme yielded positive responses and indicated that the patients perceived the CA-PMP as enlightening and beneficial. They also reported that the CA-PMP had helped increase their motivation to adopt a self-management approach to managing their pain condition. The follow-up session indicated that the patients were continuing to maintain their self-management and were confident about applying the skills and techniques taught during the programme.

The results from both pilot evaluations indicate a substantial value in delivering a language-specific and CA-PMP for Muslim patients. The cultural adaptation of the standard PMP techniques enabled the successful engagement of the patient group by not only breaking down cultural and language barriers but enabling the patients to use a holistic approach to the management of their pain while increasing awareness of how cultural myths and perceptions may be playing a significant role in perpetuating the experience of persistent pain. The participants responded well to ACT and reported enjoying the discussions on self-management using the six core processes of ACT and, more importantly, the religious content of the sessions.

The pilot evaluations are a promising step towards the development of culturally competent plans of care for managing pain by taking the context of the Muslim patients' spiritual beliefs, values, coping strategies and life experiences. With the dearth of research in this area, future research involving larger samples and a randomised controlled design is warranted to shed more light on the effectiveness of using a CA-PMP as well as using an ACT-based approach for managing chronic pain. There is a strong need for an evidence base for such interventions and evaluation data that is relevant and applicable to British Muslim communities.

Conclusions

There is an ethical imperative to provide culturally sensitive and culturally appropriate interventions in health services to minimise health disparities. Health service providers are required to aspire towards the provision of an effective and inclusive healthcare system. This requires healthcare staff to be sensitive to the influence of culture and religion on perceptions of and expressions of pain and illness as patients who find meaning in their pain are more likely to manage their suffering better than those who find the pain to be a burden (Kodiath 1998). Culturally competent care can be designed by increasing knowledge, changing attitudes and fostering sensitivity amongst healthcare professionals who are delivering pain management services.

Culturally adapted interventions for Muslim patients require practitioners to have some familiarity with Islamic teachings and beliefs. Essentially, Islam is a way of life, and Muslim patients' values are invariably based on these teachings. For example, from a Western perspective there may be an underlying narrative of individualism and secularism while Islam emphasises community and spirituality. Consequently, values such as self-actualisation, self-expression, independence and assertive communication styles expressing individual opinion may contradict with Islamic values of interdependence, self-control and community-actualisation, and contain communication styles for the protection of others' opinions (Williams 2005).

This insight is essential, given the cultural diversity of the population in the UK. Furthermore, the influx of refugee populations from Muslim countries who may have suffered war and conflict-related injuries will also provide new challenges and opportunities in the provision of pain management services, making the need for Islamically based culturally adapted services crucial.

Finally, in terms of future directions, though cultural adaptations are a positive move towards promulgating inclusivity, it is necessary to be conscious of the fact that cultural adaptations and cultural competencies alone are inadequate if they do not function alongside other initiatives aimed at reducing discrimination and health inequalities within the Muslim community. This includes addressing implicit bias within the healthcare system and socioeconomic disadvantages, and adopting policies and practices that tackle cultural and structural racism whilst being responsive to the demand for all-encompassing health services.

References

Al-Bukhari, M. (1978). *Sahih al-bukhari*. Dar Ul-Hadith.

Algahtani, H., Almulhim, A., AlNajjar, F., Ali, M., Irfan, M., Ayub, M. and Naeem, F. (2019). 'Cultural adaptation of cognitive behavioural therapy (CBT) for patients with depression and anxiety in Saudi Arabia and Bahrain: a qualitative study exploring views of patients, carers, and mental health professionals'. *The Cognitive Behaviour Therapist*, 12, e44.

Ali ibn Abu Talib (2014). *Nahjul-Balagha* [Path of Eloquence], vol. 1, trans. Y. T. Al Jabour. Newington, VA: Yasin Publications.

Al Khayat, M.H. (2004). *The Right Path to Health: Health Education through Religion.* Health as a Human Right in Islam. World Health Organization Regional Office for the Eastern Mediterranean. Available at: https://applications.emro.who.int/dsaf/dsa217.pdf (last accessed 25 May 2022), pp. 11, 18, 21.

Allison, T.R., Symmons, D.P., Brammah, T., Haynes, P., Rogers, A., Roxby, M. and Urwin, M. (2002). 'Musculoskeletal pain is more generalised among people from ethnic minorities than among white people in Greater Manchester'. *Annals of the Rheumatic Diseases,* 61, 151–6.

Bernal, G., Jimenez-Chafey, M. I. and Domenech Rodriguez, M. M. (2009). 'Cultural adaptation of treatments: a resource for considering culture in evidence-based practice'. *Professional Psychology: Research and Practice,* 40(4), 361–8.

Bhatti-Ali, R., Shoiab, M. and Hussain, R. (2019). 'Delivering a culturally adapted Pain Management Programme'. A pilot study presented at the British Pain Society ASM 2019.

Biglan, A., Hayes, S.C. and Pistorello, J. (2008). 'Acceptance and commitment: implications for prevention science'. *Prevention Science*, 9(3), 139–52.

Brady, B., Veljanova, I. and Chipchase, L. (2015). 'Are culturally and linguistically diverse populations responsive to chronic pain interventions?' *Physiotherapy*, 101, e168.

Cardosa, M., Osman, Z. J., Nicholas, M., Tonkin, L., Williams, A., Aziz, K. A., Ali, R. M. and Dahari, N. M. (2012). 'Self-management of chronic pain in Malaysian patients: effectiveness trial with 1-year follow-up'. *Translational Behavioural Medicine*, 2(1), 30–7.

Centre for Applied Research and Evaluation-International Foundation (2016). 'Global position statement: culturally adapted interventions in mental health'. Available at: https://careif.org/wp-content/uploads/2017/12/CAREIF-Global-PS-Culturally-Adapted-Interventions-in-Mental-Health.-Series-1.pdf (last accessed 30 May 2022).

Commission of British Muslims on Islamophobia (2004). *Islamophobia, Issues, Challenges and Action*. Stoke-on-Trent: Trentham Books.

Dahl, J. and Lundgren, T. (2006). *Living Beyond Your Pain: Using Acceptance and Commitment Therapy to Ease Chronic Pain*. Oakland, CA: New Harbinger.

Dahl, J., Wilson, K. G. and Nilsson, A. (2004). 'Acceptance and commitment therapy and the treatment of persons at risk for long-term disability resulting from stress and pain symptoms: a preliminary randomized trial'. *Behaviour Therapy*, 35(4), 785–801.

Edwards, R. R., Dworkin, R. H., Sullivan, M. D., Turk, D. C. and Wasan, A. D. (2016). 'The role of psychosocial processes in the development and maintenance of chronic pain'. *The Journal of Pain*, 17(9), T70–T92.

Ehrlich, C., Kendall, E., Parekh, S. and Walters, C. (2016). 'The impact of culturally responsive self-management interventions on health outcomes for minority populations: a systematic review'. *Chronic Illness*, 12(1), 41–57.

Emmons, R. A. and Crumpler, C. A. (2000). 'Gratitude as a human strength: appraising the evidence'. *Journal of Social and Clinical Psychology*, 19, 56–69.

Feliu Soler, A., Montesinos, F., Gutiérrez-Martínez, O., Scott, W., McCracken, L. and Luciano, J. (2018). 'Current status of acceptance and commitment therapy for chronic pain: a narrative review'. *Journal of Pain Research*, 11, 2145–59.

Fletcher, G. (2006). 'Enhancing care for Muslim patients in Bradford'. *Diversity in Health & Social Care*, 3(2), 154–5.

Hadith narrations. Available at: https://sunnah.com (last accessed 25 May 2022).

Harris, R. (2019). *ACT Made Simple*. Oakland, CA: New Harbinger Publications, Inc.

Hayes, S. C. (2004). 'Acceptance and commitment therapy, relational frame theory, and the third wave of behavioral and cognitive therapies'. *Behavior Therapy*, 35, 639–65.

Hayes, S. C., Follette, V. M. and Linehan, M. (eds) (2004). *Mindfulness and Acceptance: Expanding the Cognitive-behavioral Tradition*. New York: Guilford Press.

Hayes, S. C., Pistorello, J. and Levin, M. E. (2012). 'Acceptance and commitment therapy as a unified model of behavior change'. *The Counseling Psychologist*, 40(7), 976–1002.

Hayes, S. C., Strosahl, K. D. and Kelly, G. W. (1999). *Acceptance and Commitment Therapy: An Experiential Approach to Behavior Change*. New York: Guilford Press.

Health and Care Professions Council (2012). 'Standards'. Available at: www.hcpc-uk.org/standards (last accessed 15 July 2022).

Hopkins, A. and Bahl, V. (1993). *Access to Health Care for People from Black and Ethnic Minorities*. London: Royal College of Physicians.

Hussain, F. A. (2011). *Therapy from the Quran and Hadith: A Reference Guide for Character Development*. Riyadh: Darrusalam.

Hwang, W.-C., Myers, H., Chiu, E., Mak, E., Butner, J., Fujimoto, K. and Miranda, J. (2015). 'Culturally adapted cognitive behavioral therapy for depressed Chinese Americans: a randomized controlled trial'. *Psychiatric Services*, 66, 1035–42.

Ikezi, S., Campbell, N. and Frost, E. (2015). 'Impact of socioeconomic, ethnic, cultural, and sociobehavioral differences on management of chronic pain syndromes'. *Topics in Pain Management*, 31(2), 1–7.

International Association for the Study of Pain (1994). 'IASP terminology'. Available at: www.iasp-pain.org/Taxonomy (last accessed 30 May 2022).

Kodiath, M. F. (1998). 'Cultural influence on the assessment and treatment of chronic pain'. *Home Health Care Management & Practice*, 11(1), 46–51.

Lin, J., Scott, W., Carpenter, L., Norton, S., Domhardt, M., Baumeister, H. and McCracken, L. M. (2019). 'Acceptance and commitment therapy for chronic pain: protocol of a systematic review and individual participant data meta-analysis'. *Systematic Reviews*, 8(1), 140.

Lipton, J. A. and Marbach, J. J. (1984). 'Ethnicity and the pain experience'. *Social Science and Medicine*, 19(12), 1279–98.

Maki, D., Critchley, D., Watson, P. and Lempp, H. (2014). 'An exploration of Arab patients' experiences and beliefs of long-term lower back pain in Bahrain'. Rheumatology, 53 (issue suppl. 1), i121.

Mir, G., Ghani, R., Meer, S. and Hussain, G. (2019). 'Delivering a culturally adapted therapy for Muslim clients with depression'. *The Cognitive Behaviour Therapist*, 12, E26.

Mir, G., Kanter, J. W., Meer, S., Cottrell, D., McMillan, D. and House, A. (2012). 'BA-M treatment manual: addressing depression in Muslim communities'. University of Leeds. Available at: https://medicinehealth.leeds.ac.uk/download/downloads/id/290/ba-m_manual_february_2016.pdf (last accessed 30 May 2022).

Mir, G. and Sheikh, A. (2010). '"Fasting and prayer don't concern the doctors . . . they don't even know what it is": communication, decision-making and perceived social relations of Pakistani Muslim patients with long-term illnesses'. *Ethnicity & Health*, 15(4), 327–42.

Modood, T. (2008). 'Muslims, Equality and Secularism', in B. Spalek and A. Imtoual (eds), *Religion, Spirituality and the Social Sciences: Challenging Marginalisation*. Bristol: Policy Press.

Morley, S., Eccleston, C. and Williams, A. (1999). 'Systematic review and meta-analysis of randomized controlled trials of cognitive behaviour therapy and behaviour therapy for chronic pain in adults, excluding headache'. *Pain*, 80(1–2), 1–13.

Muslim Health Network (2004). 'It's official: British Muslims have the worst state of health'. Available at: www.muslimhealthnetwork.org/news_8.shtml (accessed June 2004).

Naeem, F., Gobbi, M., Ayub, M. and Kingdon, D. (2009). 'University students' views about compatibility of cognitive behaviour therapy (CBT) with their personal, social and religious values'. *Mental Health, Religion & Culture*, 12(8), 847–55.

Naeem, F., Phiri, P., Munshi, T., Rathod, S., Ayub, M., Gobb, M. and Kingdon, D. (2015). 'Using cognitive behaviour therapy with South Asian Muslims: findings from the culturally sensitive CBT project'. *International Review of Psychiatry*, 27(3), 233–46.

Naeem, F., Waheed, W., Gobbi, M., Ayub, M. and Kingdon, D. (2011). 'Preliminary evaluation of culturally sensitive CBT for depression in Pakistan: findings from developing culturally-sensitive CBT Project (DCCP)'. *Behavioural and Cognitive Psychotherapy*, 39(2), 165–73.

Nieuwsma, J. A., Walser, R. D. and Hayes, S. T. (eds) (2016). *ACT for Clergy and Pastoral Counselors*. Oakland, CA: Context Press.

Noor, N. (2016). 'Effects of an Islamic-based gratitude strategy on Muslim students' level of happiness'. *Mental Health, Religion & Culture*, 19(7), 686–703.

Peacock, S. and Patel, S. (2008). 'Cultural influences on pain'. *Reviews in Pain*, 1(2), 6–9.

Public Health England (2018). 'Local action on health inequalities. Understanding and reducing ethnic inequalities in health'. Available at: https://assets.publishing. service.gov.uk/government/uploads/system/uploads/attachment_data/file/730917/local_action_on_health_inequalities.pdf (last accessed 30 May 2022).

Raja, S. N., Carr, D. B., Cohen, M., Finnerup, N. B., Flor, H., Gibson, S., Keefe, F. J., Mogil, J. S., Ringkamp, M., Sluka, K. A., Song, X.-J., Stevens, B., Sullivan, M. D., Tutelman, P. R., Ushida, T. and Vader, K. (2020). 'The revised International Association for the Study of Pain definition of pain: concepts, challenges, and compromises'. *Pain*, 161(9), 1976–82.

Pervez, A. (2014). 'Sabr is key to jannah'. The Message International. Available at: https://messageinternational.org/family/sabr-is-key-to-jannah (last accessed 30 May 2022).

Sagheer, M. A., Khan, M. F. and Sharif, S. (2013). 'Association between chronic low back pain, anxiety and depression in patients at a tertiary care centre'. *Journal of the Pakistan Medical Association*, 63(6), 688–90.

Shoiab, M., Sherlock, R., Bhatti-Ali, R., Suleman, A. and Arshad, M. (2016). 'A language-specific and culturally adapted pain management programme'. *Physiotherapy Journal*, 102(suppl. 1), e197–e198.

Stephens, W. O. (2007). *Stoic Ethics: Epictetus and Happiness as Freedom*. London: Continuum.

Taheri, N. (2008). 'Overview of health care in Islamic history and experience'. Available at http://ethnomed.org/cross-cultural-health/religion/health-care-in-islamic-history-and-experience (last accessed 30 May 2022).

Torres-Cueco, R. (2018). 'Pain culture health-care system in the postmodern society'. *Pain and Rehabilitation*, 44, 5–9.

Williams, V. (2005). 'Working with Muslims in counselling – identifying sensitive issues and conflicting philosophy'. *International Journal for the Advancement of Counselling*, 27(1), 125–30.

Williams, A. C., Eccleston, C. and Morley, S. (2012). 'Psychological therapies for the management of chronic pain (excluding headache) in adults'. *The Cochrane Database of Systematic Reviews* (11), CD007407.

Yavuz, K. F. (2016). 'ACT and Islam', in J. A. Nieuwsma, R. D. Walser and S. T. Hayes (eds), *ACT for Clergy and Pastoral Counselors*. Oakland, CA: Context Press.

PART 4

BRITISH MUSLIMS PROMOTING HEALTH

15

WHERE'S THE DADDY? THE MUSLIM FATHER'S ROLE IN RAISING HIS CHILDREN – A CRITICAL SOCIAL POLICY PERSPECTIVE

*Shahid Islam**

Background

Whilst Muslims in Britain are not a homogeneous group, the largest pro-portion identifies with Pakistani and Bangladeshi background, with over 90 per cent of people from these backgrounds belonging to the Muslim faith (Elahi and Khan 2017). Young people make up the bulk of this population as a third of Muslims from these backgrounds are under the age of 15, compared to one-fifth of the general population (Hussain 2017). Data pertaining to edu-cational and economic outcomes about Muslim adolescents from the last two census counts shows that there are persistent inequalities which are detrimental to their life chances and developmental outcomes across a range of spheres. By way of example, Hussain's work (2017) highlights that Muslims are more likely than any other faith group to leave education at 16 with no qualifications, and as a consequence this adversely affects their employment prospects as employment data for 16–24-year-olds shows that only 29 per cent of Muslims are employed, compared to 51 per cent for all other religious groups.

Policy directives since the year 2000 in particular have established the potential impact of missed opportunities during young adulthood and how this may initiate the first steps towards an adult life marked out with disad-vantages (Graham 2000; Wilkinson and Marmot 2003; Social Exclusion Unit

---

* This book chapter is funded for open access by Bradford Institute for Health Research. The views expressed are those of the author and not necessarily those of the Bradford Institute for Health Research or the Bradford Teaching Hospitals NHS Foundation Trust.

2005). One crucial characteristic often found with disadvantage is that it rarely confines itself to a single domain but instead has a tendency to cluster with other disadvantages. In that way young adults who face serious problems in their education, for example, will also face difficulties in the labour market (Social Exclusion Unit 2005; Kiernan and Mensah 2011), and are more likely to become involved in crime or antisocial behaviour (Rutter 1989) or drug abuse (Newell et al. 2005) and face mental health problems (Islam 2011). Transmitted deprivation is a further associated risk; in other words, without appropriate support there is an increased possibility of these disadvantages being passed from one generation to the next.

Major studies across the world that follow families over time testify that the seeds of positive social and emotional health development are sown in early childhood, and fathers' involvement with their children during these formative years are inextricably linked with positive development at a number of levels which can ameliorate some of the above identified issues (Ramchandani et al. 2013; Panter-Brick et al. 2014). A systematic review completed by Sarkadi et al. (2008) found that across twenty-two out of twenty-four studies, fathers who were actively involved in nurturing and raising their children during the early years found such children to have fewer problems associated with behavioural and psychological wellbeing, and this investment in parenting enhanced their children's cognitive development. Research looking at the other side of this coin shows disengaged interactions by fathers as early as the first three months of life were associated with a five-times increase in later behavioural problems resulting in problematic social and emotional development (Ramchandani et al. 2013).

The thesis of this chapter is to bring into sharp focus the role of the Muslim father as a force for good during the early years to positively influence their children's social and emotional health and thus prevent the abovementioned issues and give their child the best possible start. This is juxtaposed alongside a discussion of the policy and practice directives that Muslim fathers experience which act as either barriers or enablers to them taking an active role in their children's lives. As we will see, creating contexts where fathers are encouraged to take an active role in all aspects of their children's lives warrants serious consideration by policy makers and practitioners.

Intervening Early to Improve Social and Emotional Health

There is an established body of knowledge highlighting that the quality of interactions in the first few years of life can affect children well into adulthood (Nores and Barnett 2010; Sandler et al. 2015; Branjerdporn et al. 2017). In consequence, early intervention programmes that equip families with the skills to parent in an effective way are promoted as a blueprint for a healthy and happy society (Field 2010; Allen 2011). The primary aim of parenting programmes is to motivate change within the parent's behaviour, perception, communication and understanding, so that desirable changes occur within the child's behaviour (Lundahl et al. 2006). Learning these skills early is crucial as the optimum time to influence developmental trajectories recedes with age (Grantham-McGregor et al. 2007). It is worth defining early intervention as it is a common enough term in the literature but specifically during the early years it means:

> [I]dentifying and providing early support to children and young people who are at risk of poor outcomes, such as mental health problems, poor academic attainment, or involvement in crime or antisocial behaviour. Effective early intervention works to prevent problems occurring, or to tackle them head-on before they get worse. (Early Intervention Foundation 2018)

Do We Need Early Intervention?

Crucially, data about Muslims living in the UK from a number of sources highlights the disproportionate rates of contact with mental health and criminal justice services and poor educational outcomes. Figure 15.1, for example, shows that the number of Muslims in prison in 2016 is 15.2 per cent, which is more than three times higher than the commensurate population which at the time was 4.0 per cent. Figure 15.2 shows similar disparities for mental health detentions for the years 2016–18. The difference in rates by ethnicity for the largest Muslim groups in UK compared to the White British population highlights that identity is likely to be a crucial issue. Of course it would not be possible to reduce

	Number	% of prison population	% pt. change on 2002	% general population aged 15+
Christian	40,919	48.5%	-9.5%	61.3%
Muslim	12,825	15.2%	+7.5%	4.0%
Hindu	400	0.5%	+0.1%	1.5%
Sikh	759	0.9%	+0.3%	0.7%
Buddhist	1,529	1.8%	+1.2%	0.5%
Jewish	449	0.5%	+0.3%	0.5%
No religion	25,749	30.5%	-0.9%	24.1%
Other	1,547	1.8%	+1.3%	0.5%
Not recorded	130	0.2%	+0.1%	7.0%
Total	**84,307**			

Figure 15.1 Prison population by religious group, December 2016.
(Source: UK Government (2017).)

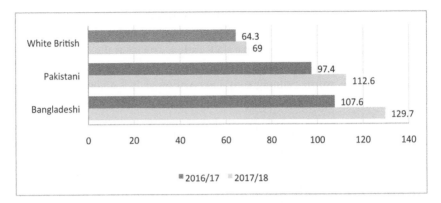

Figure 15.2 Number of detentions under the Mental Health Act per 100,000 people, by specific ethnic group.
(Source: NHS Digital (2017). Graph adapted from this source.)

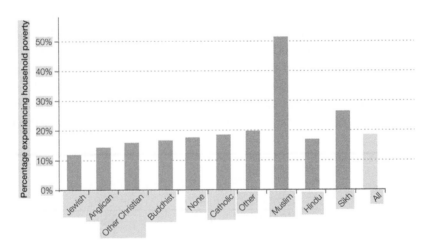

Figure 15.3 Overall poverty rate by religious affiliation in the UK.
(Source: Heath and Mustafa (2017).)

these outcomes to any single cause as there are usually multiple disadvantages that 'act in concert' to lead to a cluster of poor outcomes (Marmot 2012). Space precludes a detailed discussion on why so many people who share this religious identity experience disproportionate rates of contact with these services though one possible explanation is discussed under the heading of 'growing up in a hostile society' further in this writing.

On this point, Nazroo's (1998) work cautions us to remember that where the possible causal pathways for ill health or indeed other undesirable outcomes are not made clear then we risk generating 'un-theorised ethnicity', which can lead to the pathologising of minority ethnic status in itself which is both stigmatising and reinforcing of stereotypes (ibid.). It is worth pointing out that the causes and consequences debate is a complicated spider's web which cannot ignore the role of poverty and how this affects so many other parts of a person's existence (Wilkinson and Pickett 2010). There is no denying that the majority of the Muslims in the UK live in a context of poverty, with some reports suggesting over 50 per cent of British Muslims experience household poverty compared with the national average of 18 per cent (Heath and Mustafa 2017). Figure 15.3 highlights the marked differential levels of poverty experienced by members of different faith groups in which Muslims are shown to be particularly affected.

This notwithstanding, even in contexts of poverty there is evidence to show that early interventions such as parenting programmes which improve knowledge and capability can contribute to later positive child outcomes regardless of social disadvantage and deprivation (Kiernan and Mensah 2011). Similar relationships have been noted in Helen Pearson's (2016) book *The Life Project* in which data from several birth cohort studies were collectively discussed to discover that parenting made all the difference to children's development even when poverty was a pertinent issue. In Pearson's words: 'Parents offer the first and strongest buffer against disadvantage (. . .) parenting appears to be important independent of socioeconomic status and, crucially, that interested parents appear to be able to compensate partly for the disadvantages concomitant with a difficult start' (Pearson 2016).

Growing Up in a Hostile Society

None of the above should suggest parenting and early intervention measures presents us with a universal panacea that will vanquish problems for Muslim children in spite of widespread prejudicial attitudes. This point about prejudice had famously reached a zenith when Baroness Saeeda Warsi expressed her concerns by saying 'prejudice against Muslims has now passed the dinner table test', meaning it is now acceptable to hold such views openly and in polite company (BBC 2011). Equally, this writing should not imply that the involvement of fathers will make young people immune to the consequences that might stem from the negative portrayal of Muslims in the media. Such thinking would be simplistic and misplaced as all of these matters need addressing in their own right if we wish to create a fair and equal society. However, these points notwithstanding and with all options considered, the impact of fathers and their potential to pave a positive path for their children whilst shielding them from being pushed down a troubled route warrants serious policy consideration.

Policy makers and interventionists concerned with improving children's developmental trajectory through better inclusion of their fathers will find the social and psychological mechanisms through which young people navigate adulthood particularly useful. This will be discussed later in this section but first it is worthwhile defining a term that will appear in the course of this discussion; that term is 'life course'. Sometimes referred to as 'life cycle', it means 'the development of a person through childhood, adolescence, mid-life, old-age and death' (Pearson 2016); in other words, everything we encounter in our lives through birth, childhood and adulthood contributes to our state of health and to our eventual destination in life (ibid.). This next section examines the potential impact of growing up in a hostile and unwelcoming society and, if this is likely to be problematic, what role the father can play to ameliorate some of the problems.

When and How Did Muslims Become the 'Other'?

From the early 1960s until the mid 1990s Muslims were considered 'to be unthreatening, law abiding and unproblematic' (Marranci 2011), but with the advent of the Rushdie affair in 1989 this changed and introduced the idea of the Muslim stereotype which was based on the notion of the Muslim community's inability to adjust to British values. The principal cause for this transformation were the disturbances and riots during this period across a number of cities with sizeable Muslim populations. This new narrative gave rise to the idea of high levels of criminality among this demographic, and concepts such as 'Asian gangs' were coined to describe the perpetrators. This broad stereotype has gradually funnelled down to the concept of 'Muslim gangs' (Alexander 2000). This construct is widely used and perpetually reinforced through alarmist media headlines on a regular basis. Analysis of research data reveals a strong relationship between negative media reporting and corresponding increases in race hate crimes perpetrated against Muslims across the globe (Awan and Zempi 2017). Analysis of media material completed by the Centre for Media Reporting looked at more than 10,000 articles and TV clips from the last three months of 2018 and found that 59 per cent of print articles linked Muslims with negative behaviour (Faisal 2019). A similar study some years earlier reached a similar conclusion. This time it was found that media outputs were denunciating in their portrayal of Muslims. The authors described the portrayals as 'informed often by a virulent, racialised islamophobic discourse' (Sian et al. 2012).

The consequences of such a discourse allow us to understand and describe the milieu where hate crimes, negative opinion polls and discrimination are on the rise. These variables are tangible and lend themselves to research analysis and policy discussions. However, what is less visible but equally crucial is the insidious threat posed by Islamophobic constructs and the impression they leave on young people's sense of self and identity.

The Young Impressionable Mind

A body of research highlights that children become aware of their own identity as early as aged 5 and soon after begin to attach positive or negative feelings to their own and other people's ethnicity (Davey 1983). While growing up, young people cannot remain neutral to political events, media coverage about people who they share an identity with, and the policy and institutional responses towards members of their community. Growing up in circumstances where a person's self-image is portrayed in a negative light or under a constant vilified spotlight can be detrimental to the process of identity formation which social psychologists agree takes place during early adolescence. Ghuman (1999) describes the process as follows – 'some of the questions which the growing adolescent begins to ask about himself/herself are related to the quest for personal identity, such as, who am I? What sort of person am I? Who do I belong to?' – and goes on to explain that the Freudian school of psychology posits that young people explore and experiment with their inner feelings and thoughts as they undergo rapid and substantial physiological and psychological development in the quest to develop an identity.

The desirable and positive outcome from this identity formation is that of coherent identity which essentially means growing into an adult without having to face any major upheavals or troubles. This is possible if the young person is able to place their trust in others and through channelling their energies in a positive and constructive manner. The absence of these support mechanisms increases the risk of the formation of identity diffusion which is the direct opposite of coherent identity and paves the way towards criminal activity, social exclusion and a pathway towards a life course marked out with deprivation.

When we consider the above processes and place them side by side with the images and narrative young Muslims are exposed to about their identity, then it should raise a cause for concern about the potential impact this may have on their life course. Alexander (2000) paints a picture of what young people will often see and hear:

> It is this racist 'common-sense' (. . .) that Michael Gove so memorably termed 'the swamp' within which extremist 'crocodiles' swim (. . .) This has positioned 'the Muslim community' as homogeneous, outside of and opposed to Britishness, and understood through stereotypes of poverty and the underclass, criminality, misogyny, cultural and generational conflict, identity crisis,

and the clash of civilizations. These older racial and ethnic stereotypes have been dusted down and recycled to explain everything from the 2001 'riots' to grooming, 'gangs', forced marriage [and] mythical Trojan horses.

We need to place identity formation in the above context of otherness and inferiority alongside the concept of what psychologists have described as 'stereotype threat' to appreciate the difficult waters Muslim adolescents must wade through during these formative years. Stereotype threat constitutes a pervading 'sense that one can then be judged or treated in terms of the stereotype or that one might do something that would inadvertently confirm it' (Steele et al. 2002). The most widely cited example of this is the experiment in north India where low-caste Hindu children (Dalits) took part in a test along with other children who did not share the same status. The results were similar for all children when social identity was not a factor. However, when the test was repeated and the children were this time deliberately pigeonholed into their respective caste groupings, the Dalit children were found to perform more poorly than the others. This led the investigators to conclude that these results were

> of interest because they suggest the possibility that if there is a belief system that stigmatizes members of a particular social group and if individuals are publicly identified as members of that group, their behaviour responds by conforming to the belief system. (Hoff and Pandey 2004)

The threat is not specific to a particular type of task or a particular social category, and it is not necessary that one has to believe the stereotype for it to impede performance or affect self-esteem (Steele et al. 2002). Previous research has shown that stereotype threat impairs the performance of the group the threat is associated with, for example African-Americans or lower-income people on verbal tests, Latino students on spatial ability tests, and women on tests of political knowledge and mathematics (McIntyre et al. 2011).

Higher rates of educational failure and the disproportionate rate of mental health detentions alongside contact with criminal justice systems by members of the Muslim communities cannot be separated from the psychological zeitgeist that pervades the society they grow up in. An ethnographic study by Alam (2006) which engaged young Muslim men in Bradford shows this subject raised its head a number of times during the course of his study. One young man shared his anxieties as follows:

> [All] this 9/11 has really put pressure on us, not because we're Pakistani, but as Muslims. Government's always questioning everything we do, these days.

It's like us, as Muslims, we're Public Enemy Number One. It gets to you. It's bound to get to you. You try to shrug it off but it keeps coming back at you, keeps getting worse. (Alam 2006)

Indeed, in the intervening years since this quotation was published many high-profile incidents have taken place which show the recurrence of this narrative that places the Muslim as 'public enemy number one'. It is not possible or desirable to recount all such instances but a few high-profile ones include President Donald Trump's attempted ban on Muslims entering the USA, and the academic scholar Richard Dawkins describing Islam as 'the most evil of all religions' (Goins-Phillips 2017). All of these go towards reinforcing the message that members of this religious community are the 'Other' and, as we have seen, such divisive and discriminatory remarks carry the potential to adversely affect a young person's sense of worth and self-esteem. Every parent would wish to seek protection from the undesirable outcome of stereotype threat (i.e. lowered self-esteem and poorer performance) and the problems associated with identity diffusion which is why understanding the usefulness of the father's role and then pressing this into use becomes paramount.

Birth Cohort Studies and Dads – Can Involved Fathers Make a Difference to their Children?

Published evidence highlights that children with involved fathers are more likely to be resilient, handle stress effectively, have a higher sense of self-control and self-esteem, have a greater respect for authority and display a greater amount of empathy (Allen and Daly 2007), all of which will be helpful in creating a buffer against the negative consequences outlined above when considering identity formation.

Several birth cohort studies have followed the lives of many thousands of children and shown the correlation between 'positive parenting' and 'good outcomes'. These studies have helpfully broken down behaviours and exposures that are either present or absent to try to explain their impact on health and developmental outcomes during childhood and across the lifespan. For example, one set of data collected during the 1970s and analysed in 2006 by Blanden found that 'children whose parents had read to them when they were five and showed an interest in their education when they were ten were significantly less likely to be in poverty at age thirty' (Pearson 2016).

Other studies have found behaviours such as instituting regular mealtimes and bedtimes, talking to children, responding to them warmly and setting appropriate boundaries for behaviour all help children to a positive start in life. Not surprisingly, these are the content materials that go into most parenting programmes that are considered to have a significant impact reaching beyond the childhood years. One study, for example, states that the social and developmental benefits of attending parenting programmes can be felt as long as twenty years after attendance (Sandler et al. 2015). Panter-Brick et al. (2014), in their systematic review, have helpfully summarised what the cohort studies tell us about the impact of involved fathers on their children:

> Cohort studies have revealed the overall protective and positive effect of father involvement on offspring social, educational, behavioral, and psychological outcomes through-out infancy, childhood, adolescence and adulthood. Short and long-term positive outcomes include those pertaining to psychological health, externalizing and internalizing behavioural problems, substance misuse, criminality or delinquency, economic disadvantage, capacity for empathy, peer relationships, non-traditional attitudes to earning and child care, satisfaction with adult sexual partnerships, and self-esteem and life-satisfaction.

Whether taken collectively, as above, or individually, the studies exemplify that fathers are central to their children's future health and wellbeing. The Avon Longitudinal Study of Parents and Children cohort, for example, which recruited families in the 1990s, recently explored the impact of fathers' attitudes towards involvement with their children and whether this had any notable influence on children when they reached their teenage years. Opondo et al. (2016), reporting in the *BMJ*, found that children of confident fathers who embraced parenthood (i.e had a positive and involved attitude towards parenting) were less likely to show behavioural problems before their teenage years.

Sometimes datasets generate findings that are both unexpected and crucially important. Laubenthal et al. (2012), for example, when examining blood samples taken from parents and babies to screen for damaged DNA, found that fathers who smoked were more likely to pass on damaged DNA to their children than mothers who smoked, and the damage was seen as a predictor for a variety of cancers. The recommendations from this study advised expectant fathers to stop smoking several months prior to conception to reduce the risk of passing on damaged DNA. Until now the advice about smoking during pregnancy, much like the rest of parenting and raising a family, has centred on the mother. The emerging evidence is highlighting the need to be more inclusive of fathers.

Policy and Practice

Whilst knowledge about the impact of fathers on children's development has been rapidly growing, this has not yet made any significant inroads into policy or practice. This is not only the case for Muslim fathers but fathers across the board. Panter-Brick et al. (2014), in their systematic review, found that very few references to engaging fathers were made in policy documents that reviewed the economic, health and education benefits for investing in early child development programmes. Fathers remain marginal to the bulk of parenting programmes and on the outside of the circle of inclusion when families are engaged about parenting-related programmes. Part of the problem is that too often the very word 'parenting' is subsumed into 'mothering' because in most societies the involvement of fathers in childrearing has traditionally been framed as the role of 'provider' (Nystr and Kerstin 2004; Opondo et al. 2016).

This practice which leads to excluding fathers is inconsistent with the evidence of what fathers can bring to the family and as such there is a need for remedial action which would make parenting programmes more accessible for fathers to improve the chances of their children gaining the best start in life. A case could be made that this would apply to all fathers irrespective of marginalised status or religious background. Although this would be broadly correct, to reduce the extant inequalities previously mentioned there is a compelling case that improved opportunities for Muslim fathers to attend such programmes warrants concerted efforts, especially when we consider the data relating to material poverty, poor educational outcomes and the disproportionately higher rates of contact with psychiatric and criminal justice services.

Fathers Attending Parenting Programmes

Data for fathers across all ethnic and religious groups suggests uptake of parenting programmes is low and many interventions do not even report father participation (Tully et al. 2017). And while research is growing that explores the reasons behind this inequity, there is concern that current UK policy aimed at supporting fathers remains primarily informed by dominant White middle-class values and experiences, and therefore fails to respond adequately to the needs of Britain's diverse fathers (Chowbey et al. 2013). Research exploring lack of father participation identifies a range of interrelated factors that act as barriers to participation. Tully et al. (2017) list these as follows:

1. practical factors, such as fathers' work commitments and availability of childcare
2. programme factors, such as content not being relevant for fathers
3. personal factors, such as fathers' beliefs about seeking help or awareness of parenting interventions
4. family factors, such as mothers' facilitation of father engagement, known as 'maternal gate-keeping'
5. practitioner factors, such as the skills and confidence of people employed in the relevant organisations in engaging fathers
6. organisational factors, such as offering sessions outside working hours, and the policies and practices regarding father inclusion

We could add to this list by including cultural and religious values and how these affect men's attitudes towards participation. In common with many other religious beliefs, Islam is patriarchal – that is, it defines the father's 'proper' role as the head of the household, moral guide, custodian of tradition and provider (Seto et al. 2010; Khan 2006) and this will have a bearing on how the father perceives his parenting role. There are numerous verses from religious Islamic texts which hold this position; for example, one proverbially likens the father to a responsible shepherd who takes care of his flock as shown in the following hadith:

> Every one of you is a shepherd and is responsible for his flock. The leader of people is a guardian and is responsible for his subjects. A man is the guardian of his family and he is responsible for them (. . .) No doubt, every one of you is a shepherd and is responsible for his flock. (Ṣaḥīḥ al-Bukhārī 6719, cited in Ahmed 1985)

The influence of religious identity and cultural values presents a crucial source for motivation and behaviour and yet is largely ignored in policy and practice discussions on this subject. Khan's (2006) study, for example, found Muslim fathers were, by and large, only actively searching online for information on fatherhood or parenting via Islamic websites. Qualitative research completed by Chowbey et al. (2013) noted similar findings in terms of aspirations for a religious identity for their children and how they valued fatherhood as a route to securing this. A key finding from their study is worth quoting:

> The majority of the fathers in this study talked about providing a religio-ethnic identity to their children through teaching them their religion, language and culture. Knowledge of traditional food, clothing and appropriate greetings were considered important. Many fathers identified obedience, respect for elders and conformity as highly desirable qualities in children, suggesting a divergence from the dominant White middle-class perspective which may value inquisitiveness.

This should not imply a division between Islamic values and desire for integration into mainstream society, as the same authors found that a primary theme emerging from their empirical data was the need to adequately prepare their children for active and successful participation in UK society. This was particularly acute among fathers who were less well off (i.e. unemployed or in low-skilled employment). While fathers wanted to raise their children to become confident and aspirational citizens they did not wish to compromise their ethnic and religious identity in the process. The following extract from Chowbey et al. (2013) illuminates this point:

Parents who failed to inculcate a religio-ethnic identity were considered a poor example. Those who produced children who were confident and successful within mainstream UK society, but at the same time were adept and comfortable interacting within the private spaces of their religio-ethnic community, were held as role models.

For Muslim parents, faith and religion are seen as a force for good in family life in both their own personal development and the development of their children's self-esteem and confidence (Khan 2006). Thus, interventions that harmonise with men's religious commitments whilst sharing evidence-based practices to equip them with the necessary toolkits to support their parenting skills are likely to be most productive (Khan 2006; Seto et al. 2009).

An important consideration to include for programme planners is to understand what Muslim fathers desire to gain from parenting programmes and the concerns that preoccupy them about their children. In the same way as we cannot expect children to be neutral to hostile and defamatory messages about their identity, the same is true for parents, which is why they fear that discrimination may affect their children. Chowbey et al. (2013), for example, found that the majority of the fathers in their study

> reported providing inputs aimed at addressing additional obstacles faced by their children due to their minority ethnic status as part of their key responsibilities. For example, dealing with racism and the perceived hostile external environment was a priority for many fathers. Some respondents recognised these inputs from their own fathers as very significant and responsible for their own success in life.

In light of the earlier discussion, this is a particularly noteworthy observation as it seems fathers are aware of the dangers associated with living in a hostile environment while also recognising the role of the father in ameliorating the problems.

Bridging the Gap

Attracting fathers from any background to parenting programmes is a perennial challenge and is particularly acute when trying to engage fathers from minority ethnic backgrounds. Tully et al.'s (2017) work is important in this discussion as they explored 'what works well' in terms of engaging fathers. When asking fathers what they valued most they found respondents gave highest ratings to understanding what is involved in the programme; knowing the facilitator is trained; knowing the programme is effective; and the training being held at a convenient location and time. Worth mentioning is the fact that 'what is involved' is not restricted to the evidence base and scientific quality of an intervention; equally important is how far the programme is aligned with the father's values and to what extent it addresses their concerns. If fathers can see the programme will be in line with their religio-ethnic identity and will not undermine their perspective of what fatherhood entails then it is likely to be positively received.

Researchers have explored practical considerations and delivery preferences, finding that fathers favoured less intensive delivery formats involving seminars, father-only groups, television series and online programmes rather than weekly or more intensive programmes (Tully et al. 2017). These are likely to be of particular importance to fathers who find long and irregular working hours a daily reality, which may apply to a large proportion of families who experience household poverty. Whilst there are several studies suggesting poverty is a factor that often crowds out health and wellbeing concerns (Grantham-McGregor et al. 2007; Dermott 2012; Goisis et al. 2016), Tully et al.'s (2017) findings are more optimistic, as they found sociodemographic variables did not predict attendance at parenting programmes in the way that might be expected. They describe this as an 'encouraging finding as it suggests that fathers from a range of sociodemographic backgrounds are seeking help for parenting and child behaviour problems'.

Furthermore, researchers have examined the topics fathers rated as most important when it comes to considering attendance and found that at the top end of their priorities were building a positive parent–child relationship, increasing children's confidence and social skills, and positively influencing children's development (Frank et al. 2015). These, indeed, are the same skillsets and aspirations that will help Muslim fathers lay the foundation for a healthy and happy future which avoids the pitfalls associated with dependency, deprivation and social exclusion.

Concluding Remarks

This chapter provides a theoretically informed discussion on parenting programmes and places it next to the underexplored area of participation by Muslim fathers. In summary, while there is a robust evidence base for positively engaged fathers influencing children's developmental outcomes, there are also challenges which result in a lower uptake among Muslim men of such programmes. Improved attendance, it is argued, is likely to lead to better outcomes for young Muslims across a range of measures including health, education, self-esteem and the general life course. Addressing this inequity is likely to help people from this background avoid the traps of deprivation, social exclusion and criminality. It must be stressed that the issues identified here are not unique to Muslims; there are numerous studies that report similar concerns in other communities, such as children growing up in White working-class estates (Holloway and Pimlott-Wilson 2012), the Eastern

European Roma (Islam et al. 2018) and the Gypsy and Traveller communities (McFadden et al. 2018).

Whilst there may be some parallels in problematic engagement of fathers in parenting programmes among other marginalised communities, what is unique with Muslim fathers is the hope and possibility that they are likely to participate in programmes if there is provision to treat their world-views respectfully and in an inclusive manner. There are now programmes designed with such principles, and evaluation of their effectiveness is offering promising results (see Thomson et al.'s (2018) evaluation of the '5 Pillars of Parenting' programme).

On this point of diversity and inclusiveness and looking back on our earlier discussion on growing up in a hostile environment, it seems appropriate to share an African proverb here: 'the child who is not embraced by the village will burn it down to feel its warmth'. In other words, the path of marginalisation and otherness that results from the pernicious portrayals of marginalised communities in media and policy circles must bear some responsibility for how young people locate their sense of self and the lifestyle and choices they make as a result. When large numbers of a particular community consistently experience negative outcomes across a broad range of measures then the societal attitudes they grow up in while they are impressionable should be placed in the spotlight to assess what role this may have played in these outcomes.

Interlineated throughout this discussion is the connection between young Muslims in the UK and their predisposition to the conditions that are fertile grounds for delinquency, criminality and mental health problems. Discussions on ways to improve these matters have rarely made the connection between the positive and protective influence fathers can have on their children. And whilst we accept this alone cannot eliminate all the issues we have discussed it would be an omission to not press into gear the usefulness of the father's role in helping achieve the best start in life for their children.

Parenting programmes need to seek ways to engage Muslim fathers to increase rates of participation. Too often, low rates of participation have been viewed through the lens of logic models and process evaluations with minimal policy considerations directed towards context. If we take process evaluation to be concerned with questions about the intended delivery of the intervention, context evaluation pertains to the natural events and influences in the environment of the intervention that might act to contribute to or impede intervention success (Hawe et al. 2004). As we have seen, there are many variables that come into play that affect rates of participation, and any concerted effort to increase participation amongst Muslim fathers will need to take into account factors such as the levels of readiness, attitudes towards fatherhood and content of programme material if genuine progress is sought in increasing rates of participation.

Improving availability and encouraging access to relevant parenting programmes for Muslim fathers can augment efforts to reduce inequalities for future generations. If delivered effectively, such programmes carry the potential to improve children's life courses, which is good for individuals and for society as a whole. In a world of increasing hostility and negativity towards Muslims which can elevate the dangers of identity diffusion and stereotype threat, the application of methods that can counteract these negative outcomes is ever more pressing.

References

Ahmed, Z. U. D. (1985). *The Translation of the Meaning of Summarized Sahih Al-Bukhari. Arabic–English*, trans. M. M. Khan. Riyadh: Maktaba Dar-us-Salam.

Alam, Y. (2006). *Made in Bradford*. Pontefract: Route.

Alexander, C. (2000). *The Asian Gang: Ethnicity, Identity and Masculinity*. Oxford: Berg.

Allen, G. M. (2011). 'Early intervention: the next steps'. Independent report to Her Majesty's Government. Available at: https://assets.publishing.service.gov.uk/government/uploads/system/uploads/attachment_data/file/284086/early-intervention-next-steps2.pdf (last accessed 30 May 2022).

UK Government (2017). 'Prison population figures 2017'. Available at: www.gov.uk/government/statistics/prison-population-figures-2017 (last accessed 11 July 2022).

Allen, S. and Daly, K. (2007). 'The effects of father involvement: an update research summary of the evidence'. Centre for Families, Work & Well-Being, University of Guelph. Available at: www.fatherhood.gov/sites/default/files/resource_files/effects_of_father_involvement.pdf (last accessed 30 May 2022).

Awan, I. and Zempi, I. (2017) 'The impacts of anti-Muslim hate crime', in F. Elahi and O. Khan (2017). 'Islamophobia: still a challenge for us all. A 20th-anniversary report'. The Runnymede Trust. Available at: www.runnymede-trust.org/publications/islamophobia-still-a-challenge-for-us-all (last accessed 30 May 2022).

BBC (2011). 'Baroness Warsi says Muslim prejudice seen as normal', 20 January. Available at: www.bbc.co.uk/news/uk-politics-12235237 (last accessed 30 May 2022).

Branjerdporn, G., Meredith, P., Strong, J. and Garcia, J. (2017). 'Associations between maternal-foetal attachment and infant developmental outcomes: a systematic review'. *Maternal and Child Health Journal*, 21(3), 540–53.

Chowbey, P., Salway, S. and Clarke, L. (2013). 'Supporting fathers in multi-ethnic societies: insights from British Asian fathers'. *Journal of Social Policy*, 42(2), 391–408.

Davey, A. (1983). *Learning to Be Prejudiced: Growing Up in Multi Ethnic Britain*. London: Edward Arnold.

Dermott, E. (2012). 'Poverty versus parenting: an emergent dichotomy'. *Studies in the Maternal*, 14(2), 1–13.

Early Intervention Foundation (2018). 'Realising the potential of early intervention'. Report. Available at: www.eif.org.uk/report/realising-the-potential-of-early-intervention (last accessed 31 May 2022).

Elahi, F. and Khan, O. (2017). 'Islamophobia: still a challenge for us all. A 20th-anniversary report'. The Runnymede Trust. Available at: www.runnymedetrust.org/publications/islamophobia-still-a-challenge-for-us-all (last accessed 30 May 2022).

Faisal, H. (2019). 'State of media reporting on Islam & Muslims'. Quarterly report, Oct–Dec 2018. Available at: https://mcb.org.uk/report/state-of-media-reporting-on-islam-and-muslims (last accessed 31 May 2022).

Field, F. (2010). 'The Foundation Years: preventing poor children becoming poor adults'. The report of the Independent Review on Poverty and Life Chances. Available at: http://www.complexneeds.org.uk/modules/Module-1.1-Under-standing-the-child-development-and-difficulties/All/downloads/m01p040d/the_foundation_years_preventing_poor_children_becoming_poor_adults.pdf (last accessed 31 May 2022).

Frank, T. J., Keown, L., Dittman, C. and Sanders, M. (2015). 'Using father preference data to increase father engagement in evidence-based parenting programs'. *Journal of Child and Family Studies*, 24(4), 937–47.

Ghuman, P. S. (1999). *Asian Adolescents in the West*. Loughborough: British Psychological Society.

Goins-Phillips, T. (2017). 'Famed atheist Richard Dawkins: Islam is the "most evil religion in the world"'. Blaze Media. Available at: www.theblaze.com/news/2017/06/12/famed-atheist-richard-dawkins-islam-is-the-most-evil-religion-in-the-world (last accessed 30 May 2022).

Goisis, A., Sacker, A. and Kelly, Y. (2016). 'Why are poorer children at higher risk of obesity and overweight? A UK cohort study'. *European Journal of Public Health*, 26(1), 7–13.

Graham, H. (2000). 'Introduction: the challenge of health inequalities', in H. Graham (ed.), *Understanding Health Inequalities*. Maidenhead: Open University Press.

Grantham-McGregor, S., Cheung, Y. B., Cueto, S., Glewwe, P., Richter, L. and Strupp, B. (2007). 'Developmental potential in the first 5 years for children in developing countries'. *Lancet*, 369(9555), 60–70.

Hawe, P., Shiell, A., Riley, T. and Gold, L. (2004). 'Methods for exploring implementation variation and local context within a cluster randomised community intervention trial'. *Journal of Epidemiology and Community Health*, 58(9), 788–93.

Heath, A. and Mustafa, A. (2017). 'Poverty and the labour market', in F. Elahi and O. Khan (eds), 'Islamaphobia: still a challenge for us all. A 20th-anniversary report'.

The Runnymede Trust. Available at: www.runnymedetrust.org/publications/islamophobia-still-a-challenge-for-us-all (last accessed 30 May 2022).

Hoff, K. and Pandey, P. (2004). 'Belief systems and durable inequalities: an experimental investigation of Indian caste'. Policy Research Working Paper No. 3351. Washington, DC: The World Bank.

Holloway, S. and Pimlott-Wilson, H. (2012). 'Research summary: who wants parenting classes and why? The primary years'. A report for the ESRC and British Academy. Available at: www.lboro.ac.uk/service/publicity/news-releases/2012/94_Primary%20Parenting%20Classes%20Research%20Summary.pdf (last accessed 31 May 2022).

Hussain, S. (2017). 'British Muslims: an overview', in F. Elahi and O. Khan (eds), 'Islamaphobia: still a challenge for us all. A 20th-anniversary report'. The Runnymede Trust. Available at: www.runnymedetrust.org/publications/islamophobia-still-a-challenge-for-us-all (last accessed 30 May 2022).

Islam, S. (2011). 'Square pegs in round holes: the mental health needs of young adults and how well these are met by services – an explorative study'. *Journal of Public Mental Health*, 10(4), 211–24.

Islam, S., Small, N., Bryant, M., Yang, T., Cronin de Chavez, A., Saville, F. and Dickerson, J. (2018). 'Addressing obesity in Roma communities: a community readiness approach'. *International Journal of Human Rights in Healthcare*, 12(2), 77–90.

Khan, H. (2006). 'In conversation with Muslim dads'. Report from a series of regional workshops held between May 2004 and July 2006. Available at: www.fatherhoodinstitute.org/uploads/publications/268.pdf (last accessed 31 May 2022).

Kiernan, K. E. and Mensah, F. K. (2011). 'Poverty, family resources and children's early educational attainment: the mediating role of parenting'. *British Educational Research Journal*, 37(2), 317–36.

Laubenthal, J., Zlobinskaya, O., Poterlowicz, K., Baumgartner, A., Gdula, M. R., Fthenou, E., Keramarou, M., Hepworth, S. J., Kleinjans, J. C., van Schooten, F. J., Brunborg, G., Godschalk, R. W., Schmid, T. E. and Anderson, D. (2012). 'Cigarette smoke-induced transgenerational alterations in genome stability in cord blood of human F1 offspring'. *FASEB Journal*, 26(10), 3946–56.

Lundahl, B., Risser, H. and Lovejoy, M. (2006). 'A meta-analysis of parent training: moderators and follow-up effects'. *Clinical Psychology Review*, 26(1), 86–104.

Marmot, M. (2012). 'The Marmot Review: fair society, healthy lives. Strategic review of health inequalities in England post-2010'. Available at: www.parliament.uk/globalassets/documents/fair-society-healthy-lives-full-report.pdf (last accessed 31 May 2022).

Marranci, G. (2011). *Faith, Ideology and Fear: Muslim Identities Within and Beyond Prisons*. Abingdon: Routledge.

McFadden, A., Siebelt, L., Gavine, A., Atkin, K., Bell, K., Innes, N., Jones, H., Jackson, C., Haggi, H. and MacGillivray, S. (2018). 'Gypsy, Roma and Traveller access to and engagement with health services: a systematic review'. *European Journal of Public Health*, 28(1), 74–81.

McIntyre, R. B., Paulson, R., Taylor, C., Morin, A. and Lord, C. (2011). 'Effects of role model deservingness on overcoming performance deficits induced by stereotype threat'. *European Journal of Social Psychology*, 41(3), 301–11.

Nazroo, J. Y. (1998). 'Genetic, cultural or socio-economic vulnerability? explaining ethnic inequalities in health'. *Sociology of Health and Illness*, 20(5), 710–30.

Newell, R., Seabrook, T. and Torn, A. (2005). *Problematic Drug Use by Under 25's in Bradford: The Experiences and Opinions of Drug Users*. Bradford: University of Bradford.

NHS Digital (2017). 'Mental Health Act statistics, annual figures: 2016–17, experimental statistics'. Available at: https://digital.nhs.uk/data-and-information/publications/statistical/mental-health-act-statistics-annual-figures/mental-health-act-statistics-annual-figures-2016-17-experimental-statistics (last accessed 12 July 2022).

Nores, M. and Barnett, W. S. (2010). 'Benefits of early childhood interventions across the world: (under)investing in the very young'. *Economics of Education Review*, 29, 271–82.

Nystr, K. and Kerstin, O. (2004). 'Parenthood experiences during the child's first year: literature review', *Journal of Advanced Nursing*, 46(3), 319–30.

Opondo, C., Redshaw, M., Savage-McGlynn, E. and Quigley, M. A. (2016). 'Father involvement in early child- rearing and behavioural outcomes in their pre-adolescent children: evidence from the ALSPAC UK birth cohort', *BMJ Open*, 6(11), 1–8.

Panter-Brick, C., Burgess, A., Eggerman, M., McAllister, F., Pruett, K., & Leckman, J. F. (2014). 'Practitioner review: engaging fathers – recommendations for a game change in parenting interventions based on a systematic review of the global evidence'. *Journal of Child Psychology and Psychiatry and Allied Disciplines*, 55(11), 1187–212.

Pearson, H. (2016). *The Life Project: The Extraordinary Story of Our Ordinary Lives*. London: Penguin Books.

Ramchandani, P. G., Domoney, J., Sethna, V., Psychogiou, L., Vlachos, H. and Murray, L. (2013). 'Do early father-infant interactions predict the onset of externalising behaviours in young children? Findings from a longitudinal cohort study'. *Journal of Child Psychology and Psychiatry, and Allied Disciplines*, 54(1), 56–64.

Rutter, M. (1989). 'Pathways from childhood to adult life'. *Journal of Child Psychology and Psychiatry*, 30(1), 23–51.

Sandler, I., Ingram, A., Wolchik, S., Tein, J. Y., & Winslow, E. (2015). 'Long-term effects of parenting-focused preventive interventions to promote resilience of children and adolescents'. *Child Development Perspectives*, 9(3), 164–71.

Sarkadi, A., Kristiansson, R., Oberklaid, F. and Bremberg, S. (2008). 'Fathers' involvement and children's developmental outcomes: a systematic review of longitudinal studies'. *Acta Paediatrica, International Journal of Paediatrics*, 97(2), 153–8.

Seto, A., Becker, K. and Narang, N. (2009). 'Working with Asian American fathers', in C. Z. Oren and D. C. Oren (eds), *Counseling Fathers*. New York: Routledge, pp. 101–20.

Sian, K., Law, I. and Sayyid, S. (2012). 'The media and Muslims in the UK'. Centre for Ethnicity and Racism Studies, University of Leeds. Available at: www.ces.uc.pt/projectos/tolerace/media/Working%20paper%205/The%20Media%20and%20Muslims%20in%20the%20UK.pdf (last accessed 31 May 2022).

Social Exclusion Unit (2005). 'Transitions: young adults with complex needs'. Office of the Deputy Prime Minister, London.

Steele, C. M., Spencer, S. J. and Aronson, J. (2002). 'Contending with group image: the psychology of stereotype threat and social identity theory threat'. *Advances in Experimental Social Psychology*, 34, 379–441.

The Wave Trust (2015). 'The 1001 critical days: the importance of the conception to age two period'. Available at: www.wavetrust.org/1001-critical-days-the-importance-of-the-conception-to-age-two-period (last accessed 11 July 2022).

Thomson, K., Hussein, H. and Roche-Nagi, K. (2018). 'Evaluating the impact of the 5 pillars of parenting programme: a novel parenting intervention for Muslim families'. Community Practitioner. Available at: www.communitypractitioner.co.uk/resources/2018/03/evaluating-impact-5-pillars-parenting-programme-novel-parenting-intervention (last accessed 31 May 2022).

Tully, L. A., Piotrowska, P. J., Collins, D. A. J., Mairet, K. S., Black, N., Kimonis, E. R., Hawes, D. J., Moul, C., Lenroot, R. K., Frick, P. J., Anderson, V. and Dadds, M. R. (2017). 'Optimising child outcomes from parenting interventions: fathers' experiences, preferences and barriers to participation', *BMC Public Health*, 17(1), 550.

Wilkinson, R. and Marmot, M. (eds) (2003). *Social Determinants of Health: the Solid Facts*. 2nd edn. World Health Organization.

Wilkinson, R. G. and Pickett, K. (2010). *The Spirit Level: Why Equality is Better for Everyone*. London: Penguin Books.

16

HEALTH PROMOTION THROUGH MOSQUES AND MUSLIM HEALTH PROFESSIONALS: A CASE STUDY OF THE BRITISH ISLAMIC MEDICAL ASSOCIATION'S LIFESAVERS

Salman Waqar and Aqib Khan

Introduction

Muslim communities in the West come from diverse backgrounds and are a growing population cohort. These communities are heterogeneous and represent a rich tapestry of cultural, denominational and socioeconomic mixing. Reports of Muslims in Britain date back to the 1300s, with references in *The Canterbury Tales*, the first large groups then arriving over 300 years ago as subjected during the British Raj in India, followed by another large influx of economic immigrants during the mid-twentieth century. Today, the majority of British Muslims hail from the diaspora of the Commonwealth – mainly from South Asia, with smaller but significant numbers of those with Sudanese, Nigerian and Malaysian heritage, as well as those from the various nations of the Arab world. According to the 2011 census, the British Muslim community is almost split down the middle by way, with 47 per cent of Muslims born in the UK. The Muslim Council of Britain (MCB) reports that one in three Black and Minority Ethnic (BME) people in the UK are from a Muslim background (MCB 2015).

British Muslims and Health

The rituals and practices of Muslim communities lend themselves to certain behaviours and beliefs which can present unique challenges and opportunities for public health. For instance, fasting during Ramadan is observed by most Muslims across the globe, and many Muslim patients report that their religious beliefs play an important part in how they approach their health and their lives more generally (Ghani 2013; Rasool 2014; Sheikh 2007).

Despite being a relatively young population (33 per cent under the age of 15 and 4 per cent over 65), the self-reported quality-of-life measures and health outcomes of these communities are not good. Long-term conditions, which are costly to health systems and livelihoods alike, are poorly managed in this patient population (Ali 2015; Mir and Sheikh 2010; Lynch et al. 2000; Karlsen and Nazroo 2002; Harriss 2007). Furthermore, the MCB analysis of the 2011 census (MCB 2015) reports that 24 per cent of Muslims aged over 50 claim to be in 'bad' or 'very bad' health, and in approximately fifty local authorities 40 per cent of Muslim women aged over 65 report 'bad health'.

Health inequalities are not born out of a vacuum, and it is no surprise that Muslim communities also report socioeconomic deprivation with 48 per cent of the Muslim population residing in the bottom centile of deprived local authority districts in England, and 26 per cent of Muslims reporting they have no qualifications (MCB 2015). Pakistani and Bangladeshi Britons, the vast majority of whom identify as Muslim, report lower levels of satisfaction with their GPs (Nazroo and Williams 2006).

As British Muslims are predominantly a diasporic community, the wider impact that migration has had on their health cannot be overstated. Geronimus (1992) introduced a concept known as 'weathering' – an aggregate of disadvantage accumulated across generations due to poor socioeconomic conditions, which may be at play for Muslim communities in the West. Furthermore, the pressure of migration can result in 'acculturative stress' from adaptation to and identification with a new environment (Sam and Berry 2010). With rising Islamophobia and hostility to migrants, the complex and unsolved issues raised from the intersectionality of race and religion, and an increasingly polarised socioeconomic climate, public health interventions and issues affecting Muslim patients need to be addressed by engaging with commissioners, academics and policy makers.

What Health Inequalities Do Some Muslim Communities Face and What Are the Consequences?

National census data from the UK in 2011 (MCB 2015) indicates that elderly Muslims report a higher proportion of bad or very bad health (38 per cent for Muslim women, compared to 16 per cent for all women in England). These inequalities are confirmed by the 2018 GP Patient Survey which was analysed in the MCB report on End of Life (MCB 2019a). This data also indicates that diabetes and cardiovascular disease are more prevalent among Muslims compared to the rest of the population. Furthermore, the proportion of Muslims who feel their medical condition reduces their ability to carry out day-to-day duties, and the proportion of elderly people who are on more than five medications a day is 20 per cent higher than for the rest of the population.

The challenges found at the intersection of faith, race and gender are best highlighted by the inequalities that occur in maternal health and experiences for British Muslim mothers, where a lack of awareness of their needs and their inability to fully express their views leads to suboptimal care (Hasnain et al. 2011). Muslim women face a plethora of challenges during their childbearing journey – from difficulties in communication, lazy stereotyping and intolerant assumptions from those caring for them, to more overt instances of racism and Islamophobia (Ae and Gustafson 2008; Alshawish et al. 2013; Hassan et al. 2019). The situation is not helped by a general lack of research and understanding concerning the needs of women from such backgrounds, leading to a lethargic policy response (Ellis 2004; Hutchinson and Baqi-Aziz 1994; Walpole et al. 2013; Ali and Burchett 2004). The net effect of these issues has very serious implications: during childbirth Black and Asian women are, respectively, five times and twice more likely to die compared to White women (Knight et al. 2019). This is something we have known about and have been living with for a long time.

Mental health is another area where Muslim patients face unique challenges. Some Muslim patients' manifestations of mood disorders and other psychiatric conditions can have a religious basis (Walpole et al. 2013). This can range from their understanding of mental health itself to fatalistic beliefs and their confidence in their therapist. Notably this area has been identified as one where Islamic religious beliefs can be therapeutic, and there has been a demonstrative benefit in a religious approach for Muslim patients over conventional therapy (Meer and Mir 2014; Mir et al. 2015).

The list of inequalities for Muslims is extensive, with similar findings seen in diabetes care (Patel et al. 2015), cancer treatments and screening (Padela et al. 2016), and end-of-life care (MCB 2019a; Ahaddour 2018), to name but a few. Clearly there is an urgent need for solutions that can reach out to these communities.

Health Promotion through Faith Institutions

So, who is best placed to tackle these specific health challenges? No doubt these are complex, systematic issues that need urgent attention by public bodies and changes to government policy. In the absence of this, the third sector has provided invaluable faith-based organisations, especially those representing clinicians, that might provide effective health promotion to communities that have struggled to respond to conventional programmes. There is value in local healthcare professionals coming from within these very communities, educating their fellow congregants in their own language and addressing the specific barriers that they will be particularly well placed to understand and mitigate for.

There is some data that suggests faith institutions are effective at bridging this gap in populations which have strong traditional and cultural beliefs. Most of these studies come from the USA, where faith has a prominent and formative role in society. Several programmes have been published and evaluated, predominantly Christian church-based primary prevention or general health promotion programmes in African-American and Hispanic communities. A systematic review looked at 386 such interventions and whilst outcome data was poor or missing in many of these studies, those that did have it seemed to suggest there are benefits from interventions that involve both faith and health communities (DeHaven et al. 2004).

Good examples include the US Centers for Disease Control's faith organisations preparedness checklist for pandemic influenza and the UK Department of Health's work with the Muslim Council of Britain (MCB) to improve spiritual care for Muslim patients (CDC 2006; ONS 2016). More recently, there has been research into the feasibility of using a Muslim religious setting for childhood obesity prevention, with promising potential (Rai et al. 2019). Furthermore, studies suggest that health services should develop solutions to support Muslim patients both in treatment and in preventative measures (McFadden et al. 2013). Policy makers and commissioners are not able to address these issues without understanding the rich context of the diverse Muslim communities, which are varied in their faith traditions, language and cultural expressions (Sheikh 2007; McFadden et al. 2013).

Recent studies in the UK on the role of faith-based organisations have suggested that places of worship for BME communities may offer 'therapeutic landscapes' and synergise the formal public health delivery (Tomalin et al. 2019). Furthermore, religious leaders have been shown as influential change agents in their communities and gatekeepers, with an ability to leverage the relationship with the congregation to meet public health needs (Symonds et al. 2012). These roles can also be undertaken by social entrepreneurs, who can act as 'health brokers' to anchor the community to local policy makers and initiatives, and can link actors together as 'boundary spanners' (Harting et al. 2011; Steadman 1992). For the Muslim community specifically, some research has been undertaken already on the acceptability of health promotion through sermons (Padela et al. 2018a).

In summary, there is great potential for faith institutions and healthcare practitioners of faith to come together in partnership with health commissioners and third-sector organisations to address these health inequalities.

The British Islamic Medical Association

The British Islamic Medical Association (BIMA) is a non-profit organisation that represents Muslim healthcare professionals in the UK (BIMA n.d.). Its vision is to unite, inspire and serve its members and patients, and it has members in all parts of the country. The organisation is democratic, with an elected leadership, and all projects are organised, delivered and evaluated by a team of over 100 core volunteers. BIMA's membership, currently nearing 5,000 registered members, is open to all healthcare professionals licensed with UK regulators and to undergraduate students. The membership comprises many different health professional groups and there are special projects for international graduates and women, given the specific challenges these groups face.

BIMA has good connections with Muslim civic society and British Muslim leaders. As a national affiliate of the MCB, BIMA engages with various national bodies in the Muslim community and takes the lead on matters relating to health. On an international platform BIMA is also part of the Federation of International Islamic Medical Associations (FIMA n.d.) and is helping with the development of similar bodies for Muslim clinicians in neighbouring European countries in addition to collaborating closely with similar organisations in the Western world. BIMA also has active links with the wider health fraternity, sitting on several professional representative bodies and engaging regularly with NHS bodies, the UK government and with mainstream charities.

BIMA has six aims:

1. To promote better understanding and appreciation of the principles and values of Islam among all healthcare professionals
2. To protect and promote the health of patients and the public by adhering to the fundamentals of Islamic ethics and good clinical practice
3. To encourage professional and social interaction among Muslim medical healthcare professionals and with the wider medical community in the UK
4. To promote research and education in clinical disciplines, Islamic history and Islamic bioethics
5. To engage our professional skills in charitable activities locally and globally to help the needy, irrespective of colour, creed or faith
6. To advise and support Muslim healthcare professionals and students in career development, orientation and other work-related issues

BIMA's activities are centred on serving its membership through the above aims, and in serving the Muslim community through advocacy of Muslim health issues. To date, BIMA has organised several initiatives through mosques dealing with cancer screening (MCB 2019b), and diabetes and Ramadan (Bukhari 2017). Furthermore, BIMA organises events for newly qualified dentists, pharmacists and medics; professional development webinars; annual conferences; and networking events.

BIMA Lifesavers 2017

In 2014, BIMA started a project to teach basic life support (BLS) in mosques across the UK, which is now in its ninth consecutive year. This case study evaluates data from the 2017 event. Just as with the rest of BIMA, all the healthcare professionals and students who delivered BLS training were volunteers who organised and delivered the project in their spare time. Not only is the project benefiting communities in Britain, but it has expanded internationally in recent years to a number of Muslim-majority and Muslim-minority nations.

The Need for Community BLS

Approximately 60,000 out-of-hospital cardiac arrests (OHCA) occur each year in the UK (Resuscitation Council UK 2015). Survival rates vary between 2 and 12 per cent (Perkins and Cooke 2012), which is low compared with the European average, and far off the best OHCA rates seen in Norway (25 per cent), the USA (20 per cent), and the Netherlands (21 per cent) (OHCAO Registry 2018). Improving the UK average of 7 per cent to that of Norway could see an additional 4,500 lives being saved every year.

Around 70 per cent of cardiac arrests in London occur at home, and nearly half of these are witnessed by bystanders who have the potential to help in the situation if given the appropriate training (London Ambulance Service 2019). Bystander training equips people with the capability to buy time for the casualty until professional help arrives.

Cardiopulmonary resuscitation (CPR) given to a casualty immediately following a cardiac arrest can triple the chance of survival for shockable cardiac arrests (those that require a defibrillator to 'restart' the heart rhythm) that occur outside of the hospital setting.

The UK government announced in 2019 that schoolchildren would be taught CPR in schools (Department for Education 2019), which has gone a long way in improving bystander training and the likelihood of CPR being delivered. However, as is the case with healthcare professionals, these skills need continuous refreshing to boost confidence, especially when they are seldom used, and there are several generations of citizens who lack knowledge about CPR and how to deliver it.

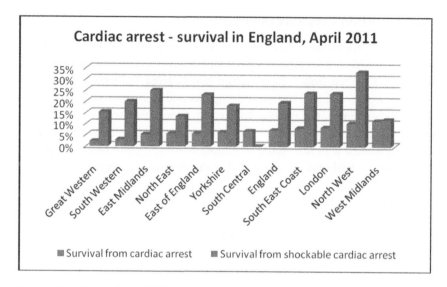

Figure 16.1 Rates of survival from a cardiac arrest as of 2011 in different regions of the UK. (Source: British Heart Foundation (2012).)

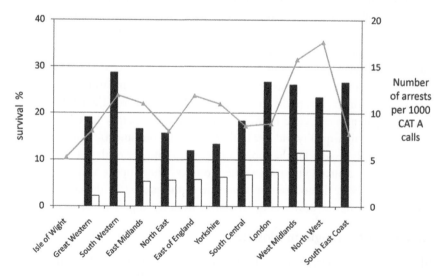

Figure 16.2 Cardiac arrest, return of spontaneous circulation (ROSC) and survival to discharge rates for UK Ambulance Services, April 2011. (Source: NHS England (2012) and figure from Perkins and Cooke (2012).)

The black bars show ROSC rates and the white bars survival to hospital discharge (left-hand axis). Survival to discharge rates were not available for South East Coast Ambulance. The line represents the number of cardiac arrest cases per 1,000 category A 999 calls (right-hand axis).

How Was BIMA Lifesavers Delivered?

Lifesavers 2017 was organised by initially recruiting a core team of fourteen people who worked with seventy mosque leads from March 2017 to start preparing for the event in September. Each mosque lead targeted and recruited a mosque that they frequented and had pre-existing ties and warm relations with. From March to September, the mosque leads enlisted local healthcare professional or student volunteers to teach BLS with the support of the national core team. They also worked with their respective mosques ensuring they had the appropriate equipment ready for the day and that the mosque was prepared to actively promote the event.

Training was offered to the volunteers in preparation for the day, covering how to teach BLS and the specifics of the day itself including a presentation to precede the actual BLS teaching. All local teachers had existing BLS certification from their place of work or study.

Quality assurance took the form of training days, with each region holding its own training day in mosques, hospitals and charity offices. In total, the mosque leads were able to recruit 625 volunteers to teach 3,652 individual members of the public in 70 mosques all over the UK on 30 September 2017.

The MCB, as a partner organisation, were able to facilitate conversations with their affiliates to help with recruitment of mosques to Lifesavers. They also published a Friday sermon (*khutbah*), which some imams in mosques delivered during Lifesavers week to draw further attention to the event (MCB 2017a). The national core team worked with the British Heart Foundation (BHF), and managed to gain their support in this project (MCB 2017b). The BHF have an active campaign to teach and train CPR in communities across the UK and have a number of high-quality videos, leaflets, presentations and training materials which are ready to use. Furthermore, a significant number of their resuscitation dummies were sourced and used at the mosques. The support of the BHF was important in both demonstrating the value of the project to the congregation and in illustrating the power of collaborative working to policy makers.

How Was BLS Taught in Mosques?

BIMA Lifesavers started after the participants had finished their afternoon (*dhuhr*) prayer in congregation, at around 1.30 p.m. People were welcome to join if they had not made the prayer, or if they were not Muslim and attending from the local community near the mosque. The training consisted of an initial presentation that highlighted the need to learn BLS. This included topics such as diet, smoking, alcohol and exercise. The presentations were tailored to their respective audiences and commentary on the various cultures was incorporated into many of them. This included delivering the event in a language other than English that was spoken by the congregation or making use of religious or cultural references to illustrate principles or reinforce messages.

The presentations were followed by a pre-event survey on the participants' confidence in performing CPR. Then a video was played, courtesy of the BHF, on how to deliver CPR. After this, Lifesaver volunteers performed a live demonstration on a dummy. Attendees were then divided into groups to practise on dummies with closer supervision from the Lifesavers volunteers.

The same sequence of video followed by a live demonstration followed by practice was repeated for teaching the recovery position and how to deal with choking. The day ended with feedback forms being given out to participants and certificates being awarded to volunteers.

What Was the Overall Response to Lifesavers 2017?

Feedback from the participants in Lifesavers 2017 (Figure 3) demonstrates a clear improvement in confidence in performing BLS. Volunteers who were teaching BLS comprised medical students, GPs, consultants, registrars and other doctors in training. Notably, 21 per cent of the volunteers consisted of other healthcare professionals demonstrating the importance of multi-professional community engagement. Instructors also received favourable ratings from participants.

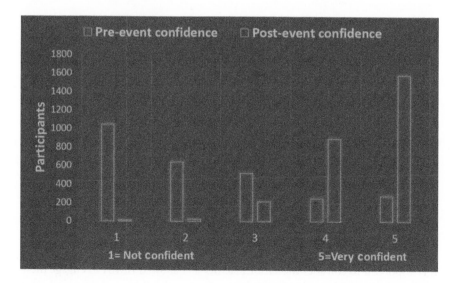

Figure 16.3 Aggregated survey responses pre- and post-event confidence in performing BLS following Lifesavers 2017.

What Demographics Were Engaged through BIMA Lifesavers?

Gender and age

There was an approximately even proportion of men and women being trained, at 47 per cent and 52 per cent respectively. In terms of age, there was a good spread of attendees across all age groups, with 39 per cent of attendees aged between 25 and 45.

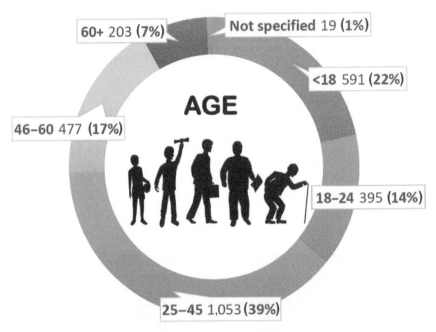

Figure 16.4 Age range of those who attended Lifesavers 2017.

Ethnicity

Most attendees (76 per cent) were from Asian ethnic backgrounds. This broadly mirrors the census data from 2011, where 68 per cent of British Muslims are Asian (MCB 2015). Most events were conducted in English, however 16 per cent of those who were taught BLS were taught in a language other than English.

Analysis of BIMA Lifesavers

It is important to consider the various factors that allowed BIMA to engage these communities, which are known to be hard to reach. These points are adapted from Memon et al. (2016) on the barriers to accessing mental health services for Black and minority ethnic communities.

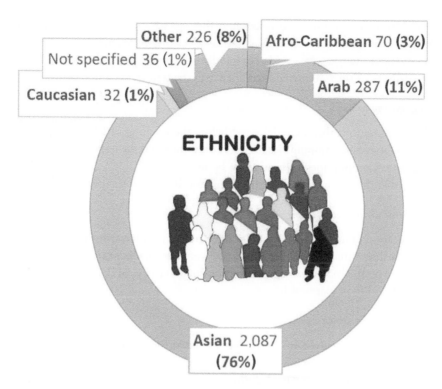

Figure 16.5 The different ethnic groups that attended Lifesavers 2017.

Social networks

The fact that mosques oversaw the publicising of the event to their congregation not only appealed to a large demographic but also allowed the project to become legitimised in the eyes of the congregation. The role of imams, social entrepreneurs and local clinicians was vital.

Power and authority

Volunteers teaching and interacting with members of the public automatically balances any power that laypeople might view as being vested in a professional's favour. Mosques also took ownership of the event and had agency to have their cultural nuances considered.

Cultural naivety and insensitivity

Many of the volunteers were already members of the congregation of their respective mosques, which mitigated any cultural misunderstandings, for example, the exclusion of music from the videos and the segregation of genders. Moreover, sectarian and intra-faith issues, such as those relating to religious motivation or behavioural change, were avoided or handled sensitively which further enhanced the delivery of the training and confidence in the trainer.

Responding to needs

The presentations that were delivered before the teaching of BLS incorporated the need for these communities to become healthier and the importance of learning BLS. Communities will naturally be more comfortable learning BLS in a locale that they frequent and so this automatically supports cultural preferences.

Discrimination and awareness of services

The location of the project goes a long way in showing inclusivity and so patients felt less discriminated against. Attendees were also made aware of the services provided by BIMA and were given an introduction to the BHF and their services around cardiovascular health.

Language and ethnic barriers

The volunteers involved in the project attended the mosques where the event took place and so in many cases belonged to the same ethnic group as many of the mosque goers; largely, therefore, many of them were confident in teaching BLS in a different language. Participants from ethnic minorities expressed a desire to see healthcare professionals from their own ethnic background as this is where they felt more comfortable and less intimidated.

* * *

There are some important aspects of the Lifesavers project that are worth noting:

1. The recruitment of healthcare professionals – this led to high-quality engagement and feedback from the communities, as they preferred providers who could understand and share their cultural characteristics (Terlizzi et al. 2019).
2. The venues that were chosen – mosques were deliberately chosen as venues as they were able to reach out many people, especially if the event took place after congregational prayers, and provided a culturally appropriate setting.
3. The importance given to volunteers and professionals being from within their own communities and localities – this further localised the delivery of the presentation, allowing for a highly tailored and nuanced approach, including language/dialect.

Overall, the BIMA Lifesavers project adopts a community-orientated grassroots method of delivering a national mainstream initiative. This is made possible because healthcare professionals from a diverse background went into the hubs of their own communities where they were able to successfully bridge the offer from BHF into their congregation.

What Can Be Learnt from BIMA Lifesavers?

Lifesavers demonstrates that faith institutions and health professionals can be effective partners in health promotion. Communities that are hard to reach (or those where we need to try harder to reach) are often those with higher risks of illness and carry a greater burden of poor health. Faith communities are often neglected in policy decisions and plans, and often bundled together with ethnicity and general cultural considerations. This lack of understanding and nuance can lead to further marginalisation as existing schemes may not have the projected impact.

This is an example of a project that is tailored to a wide demographic, directly related to known health inequalities amongst ethnic minorities. It makes use of the diverse workforce of the NHS, recognising the strength of their diversity and connections in a positive manner, and actively works with communities to create assets for healthcare systems among faith centres. It is a prime example of what a 'Health in All Policies' venture, as encouraged by Public Health England, could look like if external organisations like BIMA are harnessed and engaged with (Local Government Association 2016).

The Health Foundation (2011) established a Shared Leadership for Change Programme on how to improve care for BME groups. Many of BIMA Lifesavers' strengths are found in their concluding analysis of six initiatives that sought to improve BME health. These involved having a personal, innovative, and multidisciplinary approach that was designed with close coordination with the community and staff. Lifesavers is also unique in that it is independent of the NHS and local government, which helps with its credibility in BME communities where there may be a trust deficit from the mainstream providers.

The collaboration with a large third-sector health charity in the BHF is also key, as the logistical and material support that was provided to BIMA and the ability to reach out to a whole new segment of the population created a natural synergy. This is commendable on the part of BHF who correctly identified an important project and invested in it to become key stakeholders.

Harnessing the Islamic identity and narrative was also part of a novel approach which worked very well in practice. BIMA was able to recruit many volunteer healthcare professionals using religious and cultural motivation to inspire a call to action. Whilst the training material to the participants was largely based on BHF resources, they were adapted slightly with Islamic scriptural references. This needed to be done with tact and care, as faith communities can be sensitive to having their creed and beliefs co-opted for political purposes, no matter how benign the cause may be (Williams et al. 2012). Padela et al. (2018b) have mapped out a framework for delivering religiously tailored health messages which can help with interventions, using a process of reframing, reprioritising and reforming health behaviour.

Conclusions

Grassroots work is pivotal to ending health inequalities. It is only through working with BME communities that we gain valuable insight into how engage them. The NHS Confederation (2013) recognises the value these alliances bring, as when communities become invested in and empowered by the cause, it creates a foundation from which further steps can be taken to improve health and outcomes. Sadly, there remains a disconnect between BME communities and health system commissioners, researchers and policy makers. However, there are many health professionals, social entrepreneurs and third-sector organisations that have been working in partnership to bring real value to the communities they serve.

Lifesavers has demonstrated a method of dealing with faith communities in a way that champions their diversity and celebrates their contributions. This is done in a manner that invests in organisations that are already committed to and well known by the communities they serve. The potential of this model can be expanded further to other services.

BIMA Lifesavers has, to date, been funded by voluntary donations from the very healthcare professionals who deliver the CPR training to the community. If initiatives like these are to be scaled up to realise their benefits, they should be supported through funding and support from public health bodies and health system commissioners as part of their strategy to address disparities in outcomes, especially within BME communities and gender inequalities.

The role of faith organisations and communities is also key and must not be forgotten, nor aggregated in the discussion and context of ethnicity and race. Data is also sparse and conflated with ethnocultural confounders. There needs to be a greater emphasis on quality data collection of faith and belief so that impact, inequalities and progress can be tracked.

NHS England had announced an ambition to have a more localised approach to healthcare with the development of Primary Care Networks and called on them to work closely with communities to address health inequalities (Johnstone 2019; Fisher and Baird 2019). Initiatives like BIMA Lifesavers should therefore become regular features of public health promotion and community engagement by commissioners.

The BIMA Lifesavers project is a prime example of empowerment and is widely successful as it appeals to a demographic that had previously been classed as hard to reach. Its success hinges on the combined effect of having trusted individuals engaging mosques from within their own communities, partnerships with established national organisations and having culturally competent health professionals act as brokers. This project should be a template for others to consider and use. And in encouraging other grassroots movements spearheaded by communities we will continue the efforts of trying harder to reach those who have been left behind.

References

Ae, S. R. and Gustafson, D. L. (2008). '"They can't understand it": maternity health and care needs of immigrant Muslim women in St. John's, Newfoundland'. *Maternal and Child Health Journal*, 12, 101–11.

Ahaddour, C., van den Branden, S. and Broeckaert, B. (2018). 'Between quality of life and hope. Attitudes and beliefs of Muslim women toward withholding and withdrawing life-sustaining treatments'. *Medicine, Health Care and Philosophy*, 21, 347–61.

Akhter, M. W. (2019). 'Mosque Lifesavers – a public health revolution'. *Journal of the British Islamic Medical Association*, 2(1), 54.

Ali, N. and Burchett, H. (2004). 'Experiences of maternity services: Muslim women's perspectives'. The Maternity Alliance. Available at: www.maternityaction.org.uk/wp-content/uploads/2013/09/muslimwomensexperiencesofmaternityservices.pdf (last accessed 1 June 2022).

Alshawish, E., Marsden, J., Yeowell, G. and Wibberley, C. (2013). 'Investigating access to and use of maternity health-care services in the UK by Palestinian women'. *British Journal of Midwifery*, 21(8), 571–7.

British Heart Foundation (2012). 'Emergency Life Support'. Policy statement. Available at: www.bhf.org.uk/pdf/ELS_policy_statement_June2012.pdf (last accessed 5 Jul 2020).

British Islamic Medical Association (n.d.). Available at: www.britishima.org (last accessed 1 June 2022).

Bukhari, N. (2017). 'The Ramadan Initiative: addressing the healthcare profession's skills gap'. The Pharmaceutical Journal. Available at: https://pharmaceutical-journal.com/article/opinion/the-ramadan-initiative-addressing-the-healthcare-professions-skills-gap (last accessed 1 June 2022).

Centers for Disease Control (2006). 'Faith-based and community organizations pandemic influenza preparedness checklist'. Available at: www.cdc.gov/flu/pandemic-resources/pdf/faithbaseedcommunitychecklist.pdf (last accessed 13 July 2022).

DeHaven, M. J., Hunter, I. B., Wilder, L., Walton, J. W. and Berry, J. 'Health programs in faith-based organizations: are they effective?'. *American Journal of Public Health*, 94(6), 1030–6.

Department for Education (2019). 'Damian Hinds: Learning life-saving skills in school is crucial'. Available at: www.gov.uk/government/news/damian-hinds-learning-life-saving-skills-in-school-is-crucial (last accessed 1 June 2022).

Ellis, N. (2004). 'Birth experiences of South Asian Muslim women: marginalised choice within the maternity services', in M. Kirkham (ed.), *Informed Choice in Maternity Care*. Basingstoke: Palgrave Macmillan, pp. 237–55.

Federation of Islamic Medical Associations (2020). Available at: https://fimaweb.net/about-fima (last accessed 1 June 2022).

Fisher, R. and Baird, B. 'Primary care networks and the deprivation challenge: are we about to widen the gap?'. *The BMJ Opinion*. Available at: https://blogs.bmj.com/bmj/2019/05/08/primary-care-networks-and-the-deprivation-challenge-are-we-about-to-widen-the-gap (last accessed 2 June 2022).

Geronimus, A. T. (1992). 'The weathering hypothesis and the health of African-American women and infants: evidence and speculations'. *Ethnicity & Disease*, 2(3), 207–21.

Ghani, F. (2013). 'Most Muslims say they fast during Ramadan'. Pew Research Center. Available at: http://www.pewresearch.org/fact-tank/2013/07/09/global-median-of-93-of-muslims-say-they-fast-during-ramadan (last accessed 1 June 2022).

Harriss, K. (2007). 'Ethnicity and health' Available at: https://www.parliament.uk/globalassets/documents/post/postpn276.pdf (last accessed 1 June 2022).

Harting, J., Kunst, A. E., Kwan, A. and Stronks, E. (2011). 'A "health broker" role as a catalyst of change to promote health: an experiment in deprived Dutch neighbourhoods'. *Health Promotion International*, 26(1), 65–81.

Hasnain, M., Connell, K. J., Menon, U. and Tranmer, P. A. (2011). 'Patient-centered care for Muslim women: provider and patient perspectives'. *Journal of Women's Health*, 20(1), 73–83.

Hassan, S. M., Leavey, C. and Rooney, J. S. (2019). 'Exploring English speaking Muslim women's first-time maternity experiences: a qualitative longitudinal interview study'. *BMC Pregnancy and Childbirth*, 19, 156.

Hutchinson, M. K. and Baqi-Aziz, M. (1994). 'Nursing care of the childbearing Muslim family'. *Journal of Obstetric, Gynecologic, & Neonatal Nursing*, 23(9), 767–71.

Johnstone, P. W. (2019). 'A case study of new approaches to address health inequalities: Due North five years on'. *British Medical Bulletin*, 132(1), 17–31.

Karlsen, S. and Nazroo, J. Y. (2002). 'Relation between racial discrimination, social class, and health among ethnic minority groups'. *American Journal of Public Health*, 92(4), 624–31.

Knight, M., Bunch, K., Tuffnell, D., Shakespeare, J., Kotnis, R., Kenyon, S. and Kurinczuk, J. J. (2019). 'Saving lives, improving mothers' care: lessons learned to inform maternity care from the UK and Ireland confidential enquiries into maternal deaths and morbidity 2015–17'. MBRRACE-UK. Available at: www.

npeu.ox.ac.uk/downloads/files/mbrrace-uk/reports/MBRRACE-UK%20Maternal%20Report%202019%20-%20WEB%20VERSION.pdf (last accessed 13 July 2022).

Local Government Association (2016). *Health in All Policies: A Manual for Local Government.* London: Local Government Association.

London Ambulance Service NHS Trust (2019). 'Cardiac arrest annual report: 2018/19. Available at: www.londonambulance.nhs.uk/wp-content/uploads/2020/01/Cardiac-Arrest-Annual-Report-2018-2019.pdf (last accessed 1 June 2022).

Lynch, J. W., Smith, G. D., Kaplan, G. A. and House, J. S. 'Income inequality and mortality: importance to health of individual income, psychosocial environment, or material conditions'. *BMJ*, 320(7243), 1200–4.

Mcfadden, A., Renfrew, M. J. and Atkin, K. (2013). 'Does cultural context make a difference to women's experiences of maternity care? A qualitative study comparing the perspectives of breast-feeding women of Bangladeshi origin and health practitioners'. *Health Expectations*, 16(4), e124–e135.

Meer, S. and Mir, G. (2014). 'Muslims and depression: the role of religious beliefs in therapy'. *Journal of Integrative Psychology and Therapeutics*, 2(1):2.

Memon, A., Taylor, K., Mohebati, L. M., Sundin, J., Cooper, M., Scanlon, T. and de Visser, R. (2016). 'Perceived barriers to accessing mental health services among black and minority ethnic (BME) communities: A qualitative study in South-east England. *BMJ Open*, 6(11), e012337.

Mir, G. and Sheikh, A. (2010). '"Fasting and prayer don't concern the doctors . . . they don't even know what it is": communication, decision-making and perceived social relations of Pakistani Muslim patients with long-term illnesses'. *Ethnicity & Health*, 15(4), 327–42.

Mir, G., Meer, S., Cottrell, D. and McMillan, D, House, A. and Kanter, J. W. (2015). 'Adapted behavioural activation for the treatment of depression in Muslims'. *Journal of Affective Disorders*, 180, 190–9.

Muslim Council of Britain (2015). 'British Muslims in numbers: a demographic, socio-economic and health profile of Muslims in Britain drawing on the 2011 census'. Available at: https://www.mcb.org.uk/wp-content/uploads/2015/02/MCBCensusReport_2015.pdf (last accessed 1 June 2022).

Muslim Council of Britain (2017a). 'Sample Friday prayer speech (Khutbah). Saving lives'. Available at: https://mcb.org.uk/wp-content/uploads/2017/09/Lifesavers2017-SampleFridaySermon.pdf (last accessed 2 June 2022).

Muslim Council of Britain (2017b). 'Learn basic life support for free at over 70 mosques'. Available at: https://mcb.org.uk/press-releases/learn-basic-life-support-for-free-at-over-70-mosques (last accessed 2 June 2022).

Muslim Council of Britain (2019a). 'Elderly and end of life care for Muslims in the UK'. Available at: www.hospicefoundation.org/endoflife (last accessed 1 June 2022).

Muslim Council of Britain (2019b). 'Tackling cancer in Muslim communities, screening campaign aims to raise awareness'. Press release, 1 February. Available at: https://mcb.org.uk/press-releases/cancer-screening-campaign-launches-to-raise-awareness-in-muslim-communities (last accessed 1 June 2022).

Nazroo, J. Y. and Williams, D. R. (2006). The Social Determination of Ethnic/Racial Inequalities in Health, in M. Marmot and R. G. Wilkinson (eds), *Social Determinants of Health*. 2nd edn. Oxford: Oxford University Press, pp. 238–66.

NHS Confederation (2013). 'Engaging with BME communities: insights for impact. Personal views from NHS leaders'. Available at: www.networks.nhs.uk/news/engaging-with-bme-communities-insights-for-impact (last accessed 13 July 2022).

NHS England (2012). 'Ambulance Quality Indicators Data 2011–12'. Available at: www.england.nhs.uk/statistics/statistical-work-areas/ambulance-quality-indicators/ambqi-data-2011-12 (last accessed 13 July 2022).

Office for National Statistics (2016). 'Case study: Muslim Council of Britain and Muslim spiritual care provision in the NHS'. Available at: www.ons.gov.uk/census/2011census/2011censusbenefits/howothersusecensusdata/thirdsectorandcommunitygroups/casestudymuslimcouncilofbritainandmuslimspiritualcare-provisioninthenhs (last accessed 1 June 2022).

OHCAO (2018). 'Out of Hospital Cardiac Arrest Outcomes (OHCAO) Registry'. Available at: https://warwick.ac.uk/fac/sci/med/research/ctu/trials/ohcao/publications/showcase/57904_ctu_report-final.pdf (last accessed 1 June 2022).

Padela, A. I., Malik, S. and Ahmed, N. (2018a). 'Acceptability of Friday sermons as a modality for health promotion and education'. *Journal of Immigrant and Minority Health*, 20(5), 1075–84.

Padela, A. I., Malik, S., Vu, M., Quinn, M. and Peek, M. (2018b). 'Developing religiously-tailored health messages for behavioral change: introducing the reframe, reprioritize, and reform ("3R") model'. *Social Science and Medicine*, 204, 92–9.

Padela, A. I., Vu, M., Muhammad, H., Marfani, F., Mallick, S., Peek, M. and Quinn, M. T. (2016). 'Religious beliefs and mammography intention: findings from a qualitative study of a diverse group of American Muslim women'. *Psycho-Oncology*, 25(10), 1175–82.

Patel, N. R., Kennedy, A., Blickem, C., Rogers, A, Reeves, D. and Chew-Graham, C. (2015). 'Having diabetes and having to fast: a qualitative study of British Muslims with diabetes'. *Health Expectations*, 18(5), 1698–708.

Perkins, G. D. and Cooke, M. W. (2012). 'Variability in cardiac arrest survival: the NHS Ambulance Service Quality Indicators'. *Emergency Medicine Journal*, 29(1), 3–5.

Rai, K. K., Dogra, S. A., Barber, S., Adab, P. and Summerbell, C. (2019). 'A scoping review and systematic mapping of health promotion interventions associated with obesity in Islamic religious settings in the UK'. *Obesity Reviews*, 20(9), 1231–61.

Rassool, G. (2014). *Cultural Competence in Caring for Muslim Patients.* Basingstoke: Palgrave Macmillan.

Resuscitation Council UK (2015). Consensus Paper on out-of-hospital cardiac arrest in England. Available at: www.resus.org.uk/library/publications/publication-consensus-paper-out-hospital-cardiac-arrest (last accessed 1 June 2022).

Sam, D. L. and Berry, J. W. (2010). 'Acculturation: when individuals and groups of different cultural backgrounds meet'. *Perspectives on Psychological Science,* 5(4), 472–81.

Sheikh, A. (2007). 'Should Muslims have faith based health services?' *BMJ,* 334(7584), 74.

Steadman, H. J. (1992). 'Boundary spanners: a key component for the effective interactions of the justice and mental health systems'. *Law and Human Behavior,* 16(1), 75–87.

Symonds, R. P., Lord, K., Mitchell, A. J. and Raghavan, D. (2012). 'Recruitment of ethnic minorities into cancer clinical trials: experience from the front lines'. *British Journal of Cancer,* 107, 1017–21.

Terlizzi, E. P., Connor, E. M., Zelaya, C. E., Ji, A. M. and Bakos, A. D. (2019). 'Reported Importance and Access to Health Care Providers Who Understand or Share Characteristics with their patients among adults, by race and ethnicity'. National Health Statistics Reports 130. Available at: www.cdc.gov/nchs/products/index.htm (last accessed 2 June 2022).

The Health Foundation (2011). 'Shared Leadership for Change (BME) . Available at: www.health.org.uk/publications/shared-leadership-for-change-bme (last accessed 2 June 2022).

Tomalin, E., Sadgrove, J. and Summers, R. (2019). 'Health, faith and therapeutic landscapes: places of worship as Black, Asian and Minority Ethnic (BAME) public health settings in the United Kingdom'. *Social Science & Medicine,* 230, 57–65.

Walpole, S, McMillan D, House A, Cottrell, D. and Mir, G. (2013). 'Interventions for treating depression in Muslim patients: a systematic review'. *Journal of Affective Disorders,* 145(1), 11–20.

Williams, A., Cloke, P. and Thomas, S. (2012). 'Co-constituting neoliberalism: faith-based organisations, co-option, and resistance in the UK'. *Environment and Planning A: Economy and Space,* 44(6), 1479–501.

17

BRITISH MUSLIMS, COMMUNITY ENGAGEMENT AND PARTNERSHIP FOR HEALTH PROMOTION: CASE STUDIES FROM BRADFORD

Sufyan Abid Dogra and Ishtiaq Ahmed

Mosques and madrassas continue to retain their influence and relevance as places of worship, education and social connectivity, and hold the fabric of Muslim communities together in Bradford and elsewhere in the UK (Dogra 2019). Throughout Islamic history, wherever Muslims travelled to distant places or migrated from one place to another, instinctively their first step for community organisation has been to establish a mosque. They do this to follow the tradition of Prophet Muhammad (PBUH), who established a mosque after his migration to the city of Medina from Makkah in the seventh century. Building a mosque in Medina was the first collective social action taken by Prophet Muhammad and His followers to demonstrate a community in the making. The mosque provided a physical space to build meaningful social relations with diverse religious, political and kinship-based groups living in that part of the Arabian peninsula.

The story of assembling social life around mosques has been repeated by forthcoming generations of Muslims for centuries whenever they have migrated from one place to another and for whatever reason. In recent decades, there has been a growing body of literature on how mosques have been instrumental in building the Muslim community and its identity (McLoughlin 2005; Gilliat-Ray 2010; Mughal 2015; Rai et al. 2019; Dogra et al. 2021). British Muslims' daily life, social organisation, identity preservation and continuity are centred around mosques.

The emergence of mosques in Bradford, in northern England, is no exception to the Islamic tradition. Bradford has a sizeable Muslim population and Bradford

Muslims take pride in pioneering the idea of mosques and madrassas collaborating with mainstream local and national health promotion programmes. In this chapter, we present three case studies from Bradford on the role of mosques in health promotion and explain how research, evidence, partnership, community engagement and activism through mosques and madrassas work side by side with health professionals for the delivery of health promotion initiatives. These three case studies will inform readers about the contributions that British Muslims are making in saving millions for the NHS by volunteering for health promotion and using religious spaces to educate and inform mostly disadvantaged populations who attend these religious settings as captive audience.

Case Study 1: Trailblazer Childhood Obesity Prevention Programme in Mosques/Madrassas (2019–22)

The Trailblazer Childhood Obesity Prevention Progamme is funded by the Local Government Association and is a government initiative to tackle childhood obesity in Bradford. This is a three-year programme led by local councils to deliver on innovative actions in their local communities to tackle childhood obesity. In 2019, around 102 local councils from across England submitted an expression of interest by presenting innovative ideas to tackle childhood obesity. Thirteen councils were shortlisted and were awarded funding for a three-month discovery phase to further develop their innovative idea. In the final round, five local councils including Bradford were awarded three years' funding in June 2019 to implement their innovative Trailblazer Childhood Obesity Prevention Progamme. Born in Bradford (a longitudinal health study for the city's multi-ethnic population) is the Trailblazer Programme's partner and implementing organisation in collaboration with Bradford Council. The programme is built upon the research and evidence generated by the Born in Bradford longitudinal study on how mosques and madrassas can deliver health promotion initiatives (Rai et al. 2019; Dogra et al. 2021).

Trailblazing the Potential of Mosques/Madrassas for Health Promotion

Bradford Council, Born in Bradford and Faith in Communities (a Bradford community group promoting health by using faith settings) have formed a unique partnership to explore the opportunities for working with Islamic settings, in particular madrassas, to tackle childhood obesity by supporting healthier behaviours and influencing positive social and structural change for better health in the local environment. This targeted action seeks to address the higher rates of excess weight in South Asian children in Bradford, of which a large majority identify as Muslim. Ninety-one per cent of South Asian Muslim children attend the madrassa after school for around two hours a day from the age of 4 to 15 (Dogra et al. 2021). This innovative project is being implemented by Islamic settings like madrassas to co-produce evidence-based madrassa curriculum materials and training for Islamic leaders aligned to the Islamic narrative. Ten place-based groups affiliated with madrassas are established within participating faith settings to explore how to mobilise and connect existing community assets to further joined-up local approaches to promote health and identify enablers for systems change with wider partners. The project is coproducing a dynamic model of best practice and guidance to support and facilitate change that can be tailored to a range of Islamic settings both within the district and further afield.

The Trailblazer Childhood Obesity Prevention was launched in June 2019 and has set up governance structure for the implementation team and local participating madrassas. Born in Bradford is leading and implementing the programme and is coproducing a toolkit for the delivery of obesity prevention programme in madrassas with place-based groups. This toolkit has three major components: physical activity, healthy diet and places to achieve organisational behaviour change needed for religious settings. The programme facilitates partnerships between madrassas and other wider health promotion programmes.

Involvement and Engagement

The discovery phase (January to April 2019), before the funding was awarded, explored the potential of mosques and madrassas to coalesce community assets (people, networks and places) together with business, local authorities and health partners to tackle the cultural and environmental drivers of obesity. Through community engagement, the programme convened a multi-disciplinary steering group which identified a pioneering madrassa in Girlington (a deprived neighbourhood of Bradford). The steering group included the commissioners (Bradford Council Public Health, Bradford Clinical Commissioning Group), researchers (Born in Bradford), religious leaders (Council of Mosques), voluntary community organisations and two madrassas (Islam Bradford and the Al Mustafa Centre). We conducted several focus group discussions with children in the madrassa, and multiple community consultation meetings for the same. The purpose of these was to identify the cultural, organisational and structural drivers of obesity and how community in partnership with health partners would like to approach, understand and address the barrier in prevention of childhood obesity by harnessing the potential of community assets using a madrassa. The findings of data collected from all sources identified cultural and community drivers for obesity as diet (traditionally South Asian community members favouring food high in fats and sugar, and consumption of takeaways), physical activity (financial/time barriers and parents' busy lifestyles). Structural and environmental barriers were unsafe neighbourhoods for children to play, unhealthy food provision systems and an environment conducive to planning permissions for takeaway premises being granted. Children, community members, Islamic leaders, and steering groups and researchers identified solutions as child/parent education after Friday prayer, madrassas providing healthy food for children, low-cost or free physical activity and access to green spaces. Participants recommended that madrassas receive support and noted that any action taken should consider cultural sensitivity and appropriateness.

Evidence and Research for Using Mosques/Madrassas for Health Promotion

The Trailblazer Programme in Bradford is a pioneering case study for using mosques/madrassas for health promotion in a systematic way. This approach is embedded in longitudinal research like Born in Bradford, substantiated with academic evidence, and is facilitated by community activism. Islamic leaders influence British Muslims' life choices in relation to everyday practices (Dogra 2019). The pioneering research on the role of mosques and madrassas in the UK for health promotion was conducted in a scoping review and systematic mapping (Rai et al. 2019) with the purpose of exploring whether mosques and madrassas are being used for the delivery of health promotion interventions for British Muslims. This review was part of the Born in Bradford programme on how to capitalise on and collaborate with an effective network of more than 120 mosques and madrassas in Bradford to improve the growing-up experience of South

Asian children, the majority of whom are of the Islamic faith. The study found that religious settings are not only places of worship for British Muslims but also locations of trust and social support for Muslim communities living in deprivation and are willing to deliver health promotion initiatives. This study highlighted the enablers of and barriers to the delivery of health promotion with an emphasis on the delivery of childhood obesity prevention intervention.

Dogra et al. (2021) conducted a pioneering ethnography and qualitative research in Bradford to build upon the previously conducted scoping review and systematic mapping to find out how diverse stakeholders in mosques and madrassas such as parents of children attending madrassa, Islamic leaders, madrassa staff, volunteers and community activists would like to deliver a health promotion intervention using religious settings. Dogra et al. (2021) maintained that because of the reach and influence, mosques and madrassas may be appropriate places for the delivery of obesity prevention initiatives. The research asserts that obesity prevention intervention in South Asian/British Muslims can be delivered using the example of Prophet Muhammad (PBUH) as a role model on healthy living, tackling cultural influences on healthy diet and physical activity, and making organisational behavioural changes within mosques and madrassas. The research also found that the majority of parents, Islamic leaders and volunteers emphasised the need to invest in physical activities for South Asian girls, rejected South Asian cultural stereotypes around girls being active during puberty, and invoked the Islamic narrative on females living active lives and on healthy eating. The findings suggested that an intervention delivered through mosques and madrassas should be co-developed, both religiously and culturally sensitive, and coupled with the evidence-based guidelines on a healthy lifestyle with the Islamic narrative on the importance of healthy diet and physical activity.

This research laid the foundation for Bradford Council to forge a partnership with the Born in Bradford study and pursue funding for the Trailblazer Childhood Obesity Prevention Progamme from the Local Government Association. This resulted in Bradford Council, the Bradford Council for Mosques and Born in Bradford building a unique partnership to investigate the opportunities for working with Islamic settings like madrassas in order to tackle childhood obesity.

Case Study 2: The Journey of Bradford Council for Mosques for Health Promotion

The very first collective action by the novice Muslim community in Bradford was the establishment of the mosque in 1958 in a terraced house. The subsequent years saw a steady increase in these religious establishments as the Muslim population grew in the district. Currently, the combined figure for mosques and madrassas stands at around 130 in the Bradford District. This is a reflection of how much importance the city's growing Muslim population attaches to their social organisation revolving around their faith institutions, predominantly mosques and madrassas. In Bradford, mosques and madrassas are diverse in terms of size and capacity – from a purpose-built structure catering for thousands of worshippers to a small terraced house set-up with a limited shared space for five daily prayers and very basic faith-based education for around fifty to sixty children. Therefore, the community reach of each mosque or madrassa varies according to its size and resources available for the establishment. Each mosque and associated or independent madrassa are individual entities, managed by local people often from the same neighbourhood. A smaller number of mosques are loosely connected in terms of organisation and coordination with each other by virtue of their denominational affiliations to various streams of practising Islam in daily life.

The word mosque (*masjid* in Arabic) is a derivative of the Arabic root word *sajda* (prostration before Allah). It is a place of worship, dedicated to the formal individual and collective five daily prayers, weekly *Jumma* (Friday) prayer and other congregational prayers in the Islamic calendar such as Eid al-Fitr and Eid al-Adha. In many smaller mosques, the prayer space also doubles up as a locale for basic religious instruction.

The Arabic word *madrassa* means school. A madrassa can provide instruction on a full-time or part-time basis, with Muslim children learning about Islam and how to read the Qur'an at evenings and weekends. A madrassa can be part of a mosque or a standalone building. Standalone madrassas (faith schools) usually have a dedicated space for formal prayers. Almost all mosques have a religious provision but not all madrassas are mosques. This is a useful way of explaining the difference when informing and defining the engagement approach for external partners or those working on health promotion. Historically in Bradford, when the Muslim community set about establishing mosques, they ensured mosques included a madrassa provision. Madrassas were set up in the buildings converted for the purpose of educating Muslim children and young people, usually in terraced houses, warehouses, cinemas, former churches and church halls. As the Muslim community began to lay down its roots and grow in confidence, it established new grand mosques which now dominate the Bradford skyline. For forthcoming generations of British Muslims, Bradford is truly recognised as their only home. In recent years, along with mosques and madrassas, there has been a significant growth in the numbers of full-time Muslim faith schools and academies providing mainstream education along similar lines to those of Jewish and Catholic faith schools. Currently there are twelve academic institutions for formal education offering a full curriculum to children.

Historically, mosques developed as places of worship and then gradually became social hubs that provided various services like Islamic education for young people and a space for community gatherings. In addition, they offered a locale for making friends and connecting with people from the same place of origin before migration and with those who spoke the same language. These linguistic, cultural and social similarities are evident among the majority of regular attendees of any particular mosque and madrassa in Bradford. The familiarisation with and understanding of the diversity of people attending mosques is paramount in any successful engagement with these institutions. Mosques and madrassas play a dominant role in the life of the Muslim community. They serve as important religious and social hubs for local communities for worship, religious gatherings, and educational and social activities. In this sense, these are institutions of influence that are accessed by their local communities five times a day with an average attendance ranging from 80 to 500. On Fridays, attendance at some of the purpose-built mosques with a large infrastructure could be anything from 500 to 1,500, including children, young people and women. It is also estimated that around 10,000–15,000 children from age 4 to 18 attend mosques and faith schools for religious instruction on a daily basis. Therefore, mosques and madrassas offer a unique and elaborate network for engaging and cascading any preventative or educational work through the Muslim community. The Islamic settings in Bradford have the potential to be strong allies for external partners on health promotion with regard to reaching out to the Muslim community. In our observation, this opportunity that Islamic settings provide is often not capitalised on by those who want to engage the Muslim community for their programmes.

Using a case study of the delivery of a health promotion project through mosques in Bradford, we can demonstrate how engagement and partnership with mosques and madrassas can result in effective delivery of such a programme. Although the case study is based around the health promotion project delivered in Bradford, the principal learnings could apply anywhere in the UK.

Healthier Lives Project by Council for Mosques, Bradford

In 2013, NHS Bradford City and NHS Bradford Districts Clinical Commissioning Groups (CCGs) awarded non-recurrent funding to projects that would deliver benefits to patients and communities in Bradford and support the delivery of the CCGs' strategic goals. One of the areas the CCGs wanted to focus on was social innovation, an approach deployed by the CCGs to work with local people and organisations differently. For this, Khidmat Centre's Healthier Lives project was chosen as one of the innovative schemes to be taken forward. Khidmat Centres are local community organisations embedded in deprived neighbourhoods of Bradford and provide various social needs like elderly care, disability care, loneliness support, sports, organisation of community events and so on, and additionally are delivery arms of the Bradford Council of Mosques for various programmes with external partners. The project focused on delivering health messages to tackle four key health challenges in Bradford that South Asian communities in particular and disadvantaged communities in general live with:

- diabetes
- mental health
- obesity
- cardiovascular disease

The network of mosques offered a unique way to share important health messages with the communities living with these chronic and non-communicable health issues. The project was delivered over eighteen months. Working with five mosques, 2,400 beneficiaries from diverse backgrounds, gender and age profiles were engaged in the programme of healthier lives activities rolled out in the five hubs in the first instance. However, we know from feedback that the actual number of people impacted by the project was much higher as the learnings and awareness created by the project filtered through families and the community. The project also served to change the outlook and outreach of the mosques that participated in the design and the delivery of the projected, expanding their mindsets and horizons through positive experiences.

The Healthier Lives programme through mosques was funded by CCGs for the period of September 2013 to March 2015. The evaluation draws on feedback from the five mosques organised into 'health hubs', the imams and faith teachers who participated in the training and the feedback from the beneficiaries and the stakeholders on how informed the messages delivered were.

Project Rationale

Twenty-four per cent of the Bradford population are of South Asian origin, according to the 2011 census (MCB 2015). Within the South Asian population, the largest community are Muslim, mainly Pakistani with a smaller but significant presence from Bangladesh and India. The CCGs' strategic plans cited obesity, diabetes, mental health, premature deaths, respiratory diseases and infant mortality as being disproportionally prevalent in the Muslim community. Hence, it was rightly felt that prevention work would be better targeted and channelled through networks of mosques. It was hoped that this would provide the best opportunity to reach out to a large number of people, engage and enable mosque-based faith leadership to champion the preventative education work by leading from the front, and to identify possible models of engagements that could be cascaded elsewhere.

The mosques hierarchy presented some major delivery challenges. First, each mosque functions as an independent entity with a unique and standalone modus of administrative operation. This meant that arrangements for developing this unique piece of work had to be negotiated with each mosque separately. Second, not all mosques had capacity in terms of space, finances or personnel to accommodate a health hub. Hence, these issues and challenges had to be given due consideration in our selection of the five mosques to be health hubs. Mosques are essentially centres for worship and religious education or instruction. Anything outside these parameters is perceived as extracurricular and optional activities, only accommodated and encouraged if these do not impinge on the core activities and if there are sufficient resources in terms of finance and space. Mosques are entirely community-funded by way of individual donations; these donations are made for the performance of core activities, meaning that it is often impossible for resources to be used for anything else.

Mosques as Health Promotion Hubs

The aims of the mosque-based health hubs were

1. to deliver a preventative programme of education through the network of mosques in Bradford via three strands
2. to engage, train and empower imams and mosque-based faith teachers, giving them knowledge and awareness on key health issues prevalent in the Muslim community
3. to offer a range of health-based activities
4. to communicate the importance of regular health checks as a means of preventing chronic diseases

The project managers for mosques as health promotion hubs set certain communication objectives for the people attending the mosques. They decided that all mosques would be informed in writing about the project. The project was launched at a meeting of mosque representatives. Leaflets and posters about the project were widely distributed through the network of mosques. Information sessions for mosque representatives were organised throughout the project along with project briefing meetings for imams and teachers. The health hub mosques organised one-to-one sessions with individuals attending mosques. The criteria for the selection of the five mosques to be health hubs were:

- commitment to the objectives of the project
- capacity for delivery of the main strands
- commitment to partnership work
- geographical spread to widen the impact of the project

From the start, it was anticipated that not all the selected mosques would be able to achieve all the expected outcomes, as some were better placed to perform better in some areas than others. A service agreement was signed with each of the five mosques. This outlined clearly what was expected of the mosques. The service agreement helped to clarify and define the arrangement for the partnership work between mosques and the Khidmat Centres as the delivery arm of the Council for Mosques for the project. For all partners, this was a new area of work and presented new arrangements for working with external partners like CCGs and the NHS. Volunteers and imams in the health hubs actively delivered health information messages to people attending the mosques. It allowed mosques to adjust their delivery to maximise participation alongside their existing activities.

Partnership for the Project Delivery

In order to maximise the benefits of the project, other providers had to get involved, including local doctors and other healthcare staff who happened to be attending mosque for their routine prayers. Volunteers from within mosques greatly enhanced the delivery of a number of key project strands, for example the health information open days at health hub mosques and the training elements of the project. Feedback following the open days indicated that providers and public alike found the events extremely useful. The contact between professional healthcare staff, imams and volunteers made the partnership work extremely effective in delivering health information days.

The project required thinking out of the traditional and accepted norms on how a mosque should be functioning on a daily basis for ritual worshipping. There was also the issue of capacity for many mosques in terms of space and human resources. It is worth stating that contrary to the general perception, many mosques are financially constrained and there is little scope to try out new ideas, particularly if these do not fit with the perceived main objectives. These considerations and challenges had to be sensitively negotiated and overcome. This meant that at least two of our originally selected mosques had to be dropped from the programme and replaced.

The tangible delivered outcomes were as follows:

1. Sixty imams and ustads (faith teachers), male and female, took part in a training session held at a number of mosques, such as Al-Hira, Minhaj ul Quran and Islami Markaz. Each participant received six hours of training in the four priority areas: diabetes, mental health, obesity and heart-related illnesses. Each session was carefully planned within an agreed framework and delivered by a highly reputable trainer with input from a number of providers. The input from the providers on the related areas added realism and interest to the training sessions. The feedback received suggests that participants found the training useful, relevant, challenging and interesting.
2. Five mosque health hubs were established. The participating mosques from Bradford were Islami Markaz, Madni (Thornbury), Jamiyiat Tabligh ul Islam (Hilton Road), Al-Hira and Minhaj ul Quran.

3. Each of the hubs offered a range of activities based on expressed interest of their congregational members. In each of the hubs activities were offered for both male and female attendees as well as a range of activities for different age groups. The experimental nature of the programme meant that Health Hubs were able to try different activities out and be more flexible in their approach in order to maximise engagement and participation. The project received significant numbers of women participating in the activities and these mosques as health hubs were gender inclusive.

4. Health open days: all five mosque health hubs were required to organise a Health Awareness Open Day. Each open day had the support and participation of a number of other providers and was attended by both male and female members of the community.

5. To give added value to the project, a Healthier Lives website was set up to cascade information about health-related activities for the duration of the project. The website proved to be a useful tool for mosques to share their health-related activities with members of the public and for various providers to promote their facilities and services.

6. The project has contributed significantly to widen the understanding of health risks in the four priority areas, has generated interest among the mosque community and has demonstrated that mosques can be very useful tools for encouraging and promoting healthy lifestyles, certainly within the Muslim community. The project has also helped to bring about a cultural change and a different mindset within the Mosque hierarchy, pushing the traditional parameters around the perceived role of a mosque.

All five hubs offered a varied programme of activities reflecting the expressed preferences of their congregations, for example Madni delivered a sports-based programme involving young people and adults, Jamiyiat Tabligh ul Islam targeted hard-to-reach women, Al-Markaz Islami offered a varied programme with mental health as a key focus and the Minhaj ul Quran integrated physical education into its teaching curriculum. This approach of assigning one speciality in health promotion to each mosque health hub was effective as mosques chose an area where they felt they had better capacity and resources.

The following physical activities were delivered by the health hubs to children and adults:

- weight management sessions
- healthier eating sessions

- relaxation sessions (silent meditation)
- reflection sessions
- regular sports activities for students attending mosques and madrassas
- physical exercise sessions as part of the madrassa curriculum
- moraqba and yoga sessions
- keep-fit classes
- health circles
- massage sessions
- group walking
- archery and ju-jitsu
- information days
- health clinics
- health and wellbeing weekend activities
- recruitment and training of community health champions

Project Impact

The project had a major impact on the five mosques that signed up as health hubs. Before the delivery of the project, these mosques and their management committees had an anecdotal understanding of disseminating health information but had no overall appreciation of the scale and severity of the health issues among the city's Muslim population. Signing up to the Healthier Lives project required the mosques to commit to health-related work as a major priority. The project therefore embedded health promotion in the daily lives and activities of those attending mosques. This shifted the approach and culture of the mosques' priorities towards health promotion and made it part of the role of mosques within Bradford's Muslim community. Islamic leaders, imams and volunteers participated in activities, training and delivery which enhanced the capacity of staff for health promotion. More service users became aware of the various health support networks available to them and an increasing number of people attended the health hub mosques regularly. The impact of mosques providing accurate health information and delivering activities related to health issues and ill-health prevention strategies was well noted. Some mosques did not have a system for keeping, recording and presenting health information. The Healthier Lives project provided a platform of knowledge, awareness, training and support for those who needed it.

Recent research has suggested that involving faith-based settings always improves engagement and reach for health promotion within Muslim communities (Grace et al. 2008; Shirazi et al. 2015; Dogra et al. 2021). The majority of health experts and health promotion programmes targeted at ethnic minorities tend to collaborate with and rely upon the so-called 'community leaders' for delivery. This has proved to be less effective than using Islamic settings like mosques and madrassas, which can ensure sustainability of health promotion initiatives that individual community leaders cannot. Involving mosques and madrassas can help national organisations and programmes gain community trust and dispel the perceptions among Bradfordian Muslims that these organisations and programmes always bring 'outsiders' as experts instead of showing confidence in local partners by using Islamic settings. In our experience, policy makers, experts and service providers who have no understanding of the dynamics of mosques and madrassas harbour misconceptions and fears that prevent them from reaching out to wider audiences effectively. Equally, it is to be noted that some Islamic institutions are still evolving and are at different stages of development, and so may have capacity issues around resource management.

Case Study 3: Bradford Muslims and their COVID-19 Response

The experience of delivering a community-driven project such as 2015's Healthier Lives by turning mosques into health hubs an evidence-/research-driven programme such as the Trailblazer Childhood Obesity Prevention Progamme became a significant community learning asset to build upon when the Bradford Muslim community faced COVID-19. The learning from the Trailblazer programme and Healthier Lives project was capitalised upon by mosques in Bradford as they acted as health hubs to protect Muslims and the general population from COVID-19.

COVID-19 first surfaced in China towards the end of 2019 and was reported to the World Health Organization on 31 December that year (WHO 2020). The virus then travelled to other parts of the world, making its way to Europe. By February 2020, all the indicators clearly pointed to COVID-19 taking a firm hold in the UK with predicted devastating consequences. It was becoming inevitable that the UK authorities could no longer delay the necessary action required to protect its citizens. The early instructions from the UK government, Public Health England and other health authorities were that people should practise social distancing, wash their hands at regular intervals, use hand sanitiser, wear masks and stay at home when possible.

The government's key message was 'Stay at Home, Protect the NHS, Save Lives'. The Council for Mosques, Bradford was made aware of the risks to the health and wellbeing of the Muslim population of the district with an indication that Muslims could be at greater risk because of a number of prevalent adverse health conditions among the Muslim community. Based on this advice and information, Council for Mosques, Bradford made the safety and wellbeing of the Muslim community its topmost priority. The Muslim community's lives, particularly those of the first generation who are at most risk from the deadly virus, revolves around daily congregational prayers, religious gatherings and activities, and events taking place at mosques. Equally, Muslim children attend mosques or independent faith schools in the evenings and at weekends. Social distancing in these settings can be very difficult. Council for Mosques, Bradford as a responsible faith body, had to act fast and show decisive leadership to help mitigate the potential risks to Muslim lives in the district. It started taking advice from key stakeholders, Muslim scholars and Muslim medical experts regarding concerns around the COVID-19 pandemic and what could or should be done to safeguard the lives of Muslim people in the district. All this started in earnest in February 2020. Council for Mosques, Bradford's team took extensive soundings from NHS, Public Health England and Bradford Council to ensure that their own thinking and plans were in sync with those of the district-wide thinking. There also followed a series of consultative and action planning meetings at the organisation's central office, by now set up to support and coordinate its strategic plans and actions. Council for Mosques, Bradford established a COVID-19 Advisory Group comprising Islamic scholars of different Islamic denominations in the district, Muslim medical experts, mosque representatives and a number of other Muslim professionals from various fields.

Following a series of deliberations, Council for Mosques, Bradford agreed to focus its attention on the following areas:

1. congregational prayers, religious gatherings, events and activities in mosques and madrassas
2. management of Muslim cemeteries to allow safe and dignified Muslim burials throughout the pandemic
3. partnership and joined-up work with key stakeholders to ensure a reciprocal approach
4. a multi-strand communication strategy to consistently push home and reinforce 'staying safe' messages that joined up with other stakeholders to ensure consistency

At the general membership meeting on 18 March 2020, in the presence of senior Muslim religious scholars, Muslim doctors and Muslim professionals, Council for Mosques, Bradford took the unprecedented and momentous decision to recommend to mosques and madrassas that they suspend all congregational daily and *Jumma* prayers, religious gatherings, events and activities. This was a painful decision to arrive at but given the exceptional risks to Muslim lives, it was deemed essential and appropriate action. In hindsight, this proved to be a judicious decision which significantly contributed to limiting the rate of infection and hence the COVID-19 related Muslim deaths in the district. It should be noted that Council for Mosques, Bradford started its local lockdown in Islamic religious settings in Bradford a week before the UK government announced the first national lockdown.

Mosque Support Fund

Council for Mosques, Bradford was made acutely aware of the likely financial impact on mosques and madrassas of the decision to suspend congregational prayers and other activities. These settings rely hugely on donations from members of their congregations for their survival. Lockdown meant no congregations and other collective activities and hence no collections or contributions. In order to ease the financial difficulties, particularly of smaller settings who rely entirely on their weekly collections, Council for Mosques, Bradford set aside £100,000 for the 'Mosque Support Fund'. Mosques could apply for a payment of up to £1,000 from this fund. This initiative was greatly welcomed by mosques and acted as a lifeline.

In line with government advice and guidelines, and working in partnership with Bradford Council and Muslim Funeral Directors, Council for Mosques, Bradford moved promptly to implement appropriate arrangements to allow Muslim burials to take place with dignity and in accordance with religious requirements, whether or not the person had died of COVID-19. This meant putting the following arrangements in place:

- All *Janazah* (Islamic funerals) were to take place at the Scholemoor Cemetery, Bradford.
- *Janazah* congregations should not exceed ten people, all of whom should observe social distancing rules.
- Restricted visits to the cemetery would be facilitated and managed in partnership with Bradford Council.
- Those attending *Janazah* should wear face masks and gloves and apply hand sanitiser, provided by the funeral directors.

Apart from a few isolated incidents, the above arrangements worked extremely efficiently. This would not have been possible without the cooperation and goodwill of the partner organisations and the families of the deceased.

Council for Mosques, Bradford was in close liaison with Bradford Council, the NHS and CCGs and West Yorkshire Police and is represented on the Council's Gold, Silver and Bronze groups. These groups were set up to have an overview of the impact of COVID-19 and brought together various key partners to coordinate an effective and efficient response in the district to the pandemic. Various aspects of the joined-up approach are reflected in the management of burials, the communication strategy, Muslim chaplaincy support in hospitals and so on. Council for Mosques, Bradford implemented a high-profile multi-faceted communication strategy to ensure that the Muslim community was kept abreast of what needed to be done individually and collectively to stay safe. Among other things, this included:

- extensive use of social media messaging, using platforms such as Facebook, Twitter, Instagram, YouTube and WhatsApp, as well as SMS messaging and the Council for Mosques website
- short videos on social media based around key messages
- regular slots on Radio Fast and Muslim Community Radio: two weekly 90-minute slots on Fast FM and a weekly one-hour slot on Muslim community radio
- regular appropriate radio jingles to reinforce key safety messages
- double-page spreads in the *Asian Express* and *Asia Sunday*.
- proactive media stories featuring positive activities of the Muslim community during the crisis

Challenges in COVID-19 Response

The main challenges included:

- managing Bradford Muslims' fears and anxieties around their personal and family safety
- suspension of congregational prayers, religious gatherings, events and other collective activities at the mosques and madrassas, which was unprecedented, painful and challenging. Having taken this action, Council for Mosques, Bradford had to work diligently and sensitively to ensure compliance, which was not an easy thing to do when trying to mitigate people's natural emotional instincts and religious sensitivities

- identifying and managing misinformation, competing 'conspiracy theories' and ambiguities in a highly charged climate
- managing Muslim burials safely, with dignity and in compliance with religious and government stipulations. This meant striking a workable balance between competing elements
- managing the particular requirements of and sensitivities around Ramadan and Eid, knowing that the advice being given was against the traditions and customs of the faith
- developing, resourcing and implementing an all-embracing and multifaceted communication strategy

Conclusion

The Trailblazer Childhood Obesity Prevention Programme in Bradford conducted a systematic and scientific research on how religious settings can be used for the delivery of health promotion initiatives. This has opened up new pathways of collaboration, partnership and involvement between mainstream health providers and religious settings across the country where there are pockets of British Muslim populations.

Council for Mosques, Bradford started as an organisation to attend to the religious needs of the novice Muslim community. Over time, it has developed capacity, trained people and improved its resources to become an effective body to deliver on health promotion programmes in Bradford. The first of these was a CCG-funded programme in 2013–15 which helped significantly with its robust and effective COVID-19 response. We believe that delivering health promotion initiatives through mosques and madrassas can be a win-win situation for service providers, mainstream health promotion programmes and, most importantly, British Muslims, the majority of whom live in deprived neighbourhoods and are a high-risk group for chronic and non-communicable diseases.

References

Dogra, S. A. (2019). 'Living a piety-led life beyond Muharram: becoming or being a South Asian Shia Muslim in the UK'. *Contemporary Islam*, 13(3), 307–24.

Dogra, S. A., Rai, K., Barber, S., McEachan, R. R., Adab, P. and Sheard, L. (2021). 'Delivering a childhood obesity prevention intervention using Islamic religious settings in the UK: What is most important to the stakeholders?' *Preventive Medicine Reports*, 22, 101387.

Gilliat-Ray, S. (2010). *Muslims in Britain*. Cambridge: Cambridge University Press.

Grace, C., Begum, R., Subhani, S., Kopelman, P. and Greenhalgh, T. (2008). 'Prevention of type 2 diabetes in British Bangladeshis: qualitative study of community, religious, and professional perspectives'. *BMJ*, 337, a1931.

McLoughlin, S. (2005). 'Mosques and the public space: conflict and cooperation in Bradford'. *Journal of Ethnic and Migration Studies*, 31(6), 1045–66.

Mughal, M. A. Z. (2015). 'An anthropological perspective on the mosque in Pakistan'. *Asian Anthropology*, 14(2), 166–81.

Muslim Council of Britain (2015). 'British Muslims in numbers: a demographic, socio-economic and health profile of Muslims in Britain drawing on the 2011 census'. Available at: https://www.mcb.org.uk/wp-content/uploads/2015/02/MCBCensusReport_2015.pdf (last accessed 29 April 2022).

Rai, K. K., Dogra, S. A., Barber, S., Adab, P., Summerbell, C., on behalf of the Childhood Obesity Prevention in Islamic Religious Settings' Programme Management Group (2019). 'A scoping review and systematic mapping of health promotion interventions associated with obesity in Islamic religious settings in the UK'. *Obesity Reviews*, 20(9), 1231–61.

Shirazi, M., Shirazi, A. and Bloom, J. (2015). 'Developing a culturally competent faith-based framework to promote breast cancer screening among Afghan immigrant women'. *Journal of Religion and Health*, 54(1), 153–9.

World Health Organization (2020). 'Listings of WHO's response to COVID-19'. Available at: www.who.int/news/item/29-06-2020-covidtimeline (last accessed 13 July 2022).

18

THE WAY FORWARD TO REDUCE HEALTH INEQUALITIES AMONG BRITISH MUSLIMS

Sufyan Abid Dogra

This book has discussed why British Muslims live with ill-health indicators and how they experience health inequalities in their daily lives. It has argued that the sociopolitical experience of being British Muslim and British Muslims' religious identity can be wider determinants of health along with class, ethnicity, racism and deprivation. The book advocates a revision in the policy of delivering health promotion interventions and initiatives targeting high-risk groups. British Muslims live with multiple and multi-layered factors negatively affecting their health. We present the following recommendations to improve the health and wellbeing of British Muslims, ethnic minorities and people living with disadvantages in deprived neighbourhoods across the country.

1. A new perspective on involving people in the design and delivery of health promotion initiatives and interventions meaningfully is required. This renewed thinking among health practitioners, researchers and policy makers should involve an intersectional approach by acknowledging religion as a wider determinant of health for British Muslims along with ethnicity and social class, and consider factors like structural violence, discrimination, racism and Islamophobia, all of which affect ill-health experiences.

2. Applied health researchers, when developing and delivering health promotion interventions for marginalised groups and British Muslims, need to avoid a neo-eugenics inspired mindset, stereotypes regarding the health practices of ethnic minorities and the use of research methodologies that ignore nuances. When designing theoretical frameworks and logic models of health interventions, and collecting/analysing data, applied health researchers and academics should avoid reinforcing or buttressing racist and neo-eugenics driven assumptions about

high-risk groups, disadvantaged populations and ethnic minorities. A careful dissemination of applied health research findings is needed when academics and practitioners engage with mainstream media to showcase and/or promote their research.

3. In the broader systems of management and administration within the NHS, public health organisations and other health bodies, there needs to be an acknowledgement of how Islamophobia and racism are part of the service delivery and how the systems of profiling patients and service delivery can be improved for healthcare staff and patients or service users.

4. There is a need for modern and culturally sensitive ways of providing information and services on genetic health for ethnic minorities and British Muslims.

5. Health promotion and delivery programmes on preventive health initiatives should target men from ethnic minorities and British Muslims for involvement in mental, emotional and parental services. Healthcare staff should be able to deliver health information sensitively to third- and fourth-generation British Muslims and avoid cultural stereotypes during the delivery of health services.

6. Mental health is a very serious issue for BME and British Muslims. The methodologies and therapies provided in mainstream mental health services need to be updated through incorporating religious and cultural narratives on living healthily. Equally, researchers and academics designing guidelines and toolkits for supporting mental health services should learn how instrumental the cultural and religious narratives can be in the overall wellbeing of people from ethnic minority backgrounds. Further, people from deprived parts of the country should be prioritised for the provision of mental health services.

7. When a patient is in the care of health professionals, the personal aspects of their identity should be acknowledged when they are provided with pain relief, elderly care, end-of-life care and dementia care. For these health conditions, staff should be trained, and need-based treatments should be provided that are compatible with patients' values and priorities.

8. Women and children's health needs should be met with a broader understanding of their personal and family circumstances. Healthcare staff and social services need to have an empathetic approach for issues like domestic violence and abuse and learn how the existing standard procedures of addressing the issue might be harmful for the victims or families.

9. Applied health research methodologies need to have their conceptual frameworks revised to collect meaningful data from groups living with trauma. The research methodologies need to translate lived experiences of research participants and should be more reflective. The transnational links of migrant communities and how these links shape their health practices and priorities should be incorporated in research methodologies and analytical categories of knowledge production on health and wellbeing.

10. Islamic faith settings like mosques, madrassas, Muslim organisations working on health promotion, and Muslim women's circles are effective mechanisms and sites for involving high-risk groups in health promotion. We strongly recommend that Islamic faith settings and Islamic narratives on living healthily be incorporated into health promotion interventions targeting British Muslims. Public involvement in the development and delivery of targeted and complex health interventions is crucial. Co-production, partnership, collaboration and utilisation of Islamic settings can reduce the cost of health promotion and ensure effective delivery for high-risk groups.

11. We recommend public health practitioners, policy makers and health promotion bodies involve young leaders affiliated with Islamic faith settings in Britain. This will ensure higher uptake of service delivery and will help avoid the tunnel vision of some elderly members on mosque management committees who might consider that the sole purpose of Islamic faith settings is to conduct ritual worship for the congregation.

12. We believe that mere 'talking to imams' to disseminate health promotion messages does not work effectively or sustainably, although it can be helpful for one-off messages. Imams are generally very busy and can work more effectively if a small group of dedicated volunteers is there to help them. We recommend organising and establishing small health groups comprising individuals affiliated with faith settings who might be willing to volunteer and actively participate in the delivery of health promotion initiatives on a long-term basis. The involvement of women and young people in these health groups can ensure families' wider participation and uptake. Local authorities and other wider health promotion programmes should provide capacity-building funding and relevant training to these groups.

13. Co-production and the involvement of service users should be the guiding principles of the design and delivery of health promotion initiatives. We recommend that patients and the public should contribute to the design and development of research questions and implementation strategies for community-based health initiatives.

14. Senior leadership in local authorities and health funding bodies need to work on developing new models of awarding major funding by ensuring that neighbourhood- based small groups, women and young people, and marginalised voices contribute to the drafting of funding applications and the development of programme proposals for health promotion.

INDEX

Note: f indicates figure; t indicates table